Urticaria

Editor

MALCOLM W. GREAVES

IMMUNOLOGY AND ALLERGY CLINICS OF NORTH AMERICA

www.immunology.theclinics.com

Consulting Editor
RAFEUL ALAM

February 2014 • Volume 34 • Number 1

ELSEVIER

1600 John F. Kennedy Boulevard • Suite 1800 • Philadelphia, Pennsylvania, 19103-2899
http://www.theclinics.com

IMMUNOLOGY AND ALLERGY CLINICS OF NORTH AMERICA Volume 34, Number 1
February 2014 ISSN 0889–8561, ISBN-13: 978-0-323-26662-8

Editor: Jessica McCool
Developmental Editor: Stephanie Carter

Immunology and Allergy Clinics of North America (ISSN 0889–8561) is published quarterly by Elsevier Inc., 360 Park Avenue South, New York, NY 10010-1710. Months of issue are February, May, August, and November. Periodicals postage paid at New York, NY and additional mailing offices. Subscription prices are $320.00 per year for US individuals, $454.00 per year for US institutions, $150.00 per year for US students and residents, $395.00 per year for Canadian individuals, $220.00 per year for Canadian students, $577.00 per year for Canadian institutions, $445.00 per year for international individuals, $577.00 per year for international institutions, $220.00 per year for international students. To receive student/resident rate, orders must be accompanied by name of affiliated institution, date of term, and the *signature* of program/residency coordinator on institution letterhead. Orders will be billed at individual rate until proof of status is received. Foreign air speed delivery is included in all *Clinics* subscription prices. All prices are subject to change without notice. **POSTMASTER**: Send address changes to *Immunology and Allergy Clinics of North America,* Elsevier Health Sciences Division, Subscription Customer Service, 3251 Riverport Lane, Maryland Heights, MO 63043. **Customer Service: 1-800-654-2452 (U.S. and Canada); 314-447-8871 (outside U.S. and Canada). Fax: 314-447-8029. E-mail: journalscustomerservice-usa@elsevier.com (for print support); journalsonlinesupport-usa@elsevier.com (for online support).**

Reprints. For copies of 100 or more, of articles in this publication, please contact the Commercial Reprints Department, Elsevier Inc., 360 Park Avenue South, New York, New York 10010-1710. Tel. 212-633-3874, Fax: 212-633-3820, E-mail: reprints@elsevier.com.

Immunology and Allergy Clinics of North America is covered in MEDLINE/PubMed (Index Medicus), Current Contents/Life Sciences, Science Citation Index, ISI/BIOMED, Chemical Abstracts, and EMBASE/Excerpta Medica.

Printed and bound by CPI Group (UK) Ltd, Croydon, CR0 4YY

Transferred to digital print 2012

Contributors

CONSULTING EDITOR

RAFEUL ALAM, MD, PhD
Professor and Chief, Division of Allergy and Immunology, National Jewish Health, University of Colorado Denver School of Medicine, Denver, Colorado

EDITOR

MALCOLM W. GREAVES, MD, PhD, FRCP
Emeritus Professor of Dermatology, Consultant Specialist in Dermatology and Allergy, Cutaneous Allergy Clinic, St Johns Institute of Dermatology, St Thomas' Hospital; The London Allergy Clinic, London, United Kingdom

AUTHORS

MARINA ABAJIAN
Resident Physician, Department of Dermatology and Allergy, Allergie – Centrum Charité/ECARF, Charité – Universitätsmedizin Berlin, Berlin, Germany

SABINE ALTRICHTER, MD
Resident Physician, Department of Dermatology and Allergy, Allergie – Centrum Charité/ECARF, Charité – Universitätsmedizin Berlin, Berlin, Germany

RICCARDO ASERO, MD
Ambulatorio di Allergologia, Clinica San Carlo, Paderno Dugnano, Milano, Italy

KONRAD BORK, MD
Department of Dermatology, Johannes Gutenberg University, Mainz, Germany

MELODY C. CARTER, MD
Laboratory of Allergic Diseases, National Institute of Allergy and Infectious Diseases, National Institutes of Health, Bethesda, Maryland

MASSIMO CUGNO, MD
Medicina Interna, Dipartimento di Fisiopatologia Medico-Chirurgica e dei Trapianti, Università degli Studi di Milano, IRCCS Fondazione Ca' Granda, Ospedale Maggiore Policlinico, Milano, Italy

GEORGE DU TOIT, FRCPCH
Department of Children's Allergies, Guy's and St Thomas' Hospital NHS Foundation Trust, King's College London, London, United Kingdom

CARSTEN FLOHR, BM, BCh, MA, MSc, MRCPCH, PhD
Departments of Paediatric Dermatology and Children's Allergies, St John's Institute of Dermatology, Guy's and St Thomas' Hospitals NHS Foundation Trust, King's College London, London, United Kingdom

MALCOLM W. GREAVES, MD, PhD, FRCP
Emeritus Professor of Dermatology, Consultant Specialist in Dermatology and Allergy, Cutaneous Allergy Clinic, St John's Institute of Dermatology, St Thomas' Hospital; The London Allergy Clinic, London, United Kingdom

MICHIHIRO HIDE, MD, PhD
Department of Dermatology, Integrated Health Sciences, Institute of Biomedical and Health Sciences, Hiroshima University, Hiroshima, Japan

MAKIKO HIRAGUN, MD
Department of Dermatology, Integrated Health Sciences, Institute of Biomedical and Health Sciences, Hiroshima University, Hiroshima, Japan

TAKAAKI HIRAGUN, MD, PhD
Department of Dermatology, Integrated Health Sciences, Institute of Biomedical and Health Sciences, Hiroshima University, Hiroshima, Japan

NOBUO KANAZAWA, MD, PhD
Assistant Professor, Department of Dermatology, Wakayama Medical University, Wakayama, Japan

HIRSH D. KOMAROW, MD
Laboratory of Allergic Diseases, National Institute of Allergy and Infectious Diseases, National Institutes of Health, Bethesda, Maryland

FRANCES LAWLOR, MB.BCh.BAO, DCh, DObst RCOG, MD, FRCP(Irel), FRCP(Lond)
Department of Cutaneous Allergy, St Thomas' Hospital; The London Clinic, London, United Kingdom

MARCUS MAURER, MD
Professor of Dermatology and Allergy, Director of Research, Department of Dermatology and Allergy, Allergie – Centrum Charité/ECARF, Charité – Universitätsmedizin Berlin, Berlin, Germany

JOHN MCFADDEN, DM, FRCP
Consultant Dermatologist, Department of Cutaneous Allergy, St John's Institute of Dermatology, King's College, St Thomas' Hospital, London, United Kingdom

DEAN D. METCALFE, MD
Chief, Laboratory of Allergic Diseases, National Institute of Allergy and Infectious Diseases, National Institutes of Health, Bethesda, Maryland

BRIGID F. O'DONNELL, MD, MRCPI, DCH
Consultant Dermatologist, Department of Dermatology, Children's University Hospital; Mater Misericordiae Hospital, Dublin, Ireland

RUTH A. SABROE, FRCP, MD
Consultant Dermatologist and Honorary Senior Lecturer, Royal Hallamshire Hospital, Sheffield Teaching Hospitals NHS Foundation Trust, Sheffield, United Kingdom

SARBJIT S. SAINI, MD
Associate Professor of Medicine, Division of Allergy and Clinical Immunology, Johns Hopkins Asthma and Allergy Center, Johns Hopkins University School of Medicine, Baltimore, Maryland

NICOLE SCHOEPKE, MD
Resident Physician, Department of Dermatology and Allergy, Allergie – Centrum Charité/ECARF, Charité – Universitätsmedizin Berlin, Berlin, Germany

ALBERTO TEDESCHI, MD
U.O. Allergologia e Immunologia Clinica, Fondazione IRCCS Ca' Granda, Ospedale Maggiore Policlinico, Milano, Italy

TERESA TSAKOK, BM, BCh, MA, MRCP
Academic Clinical Fellow/Core Medical Trainee, Guy's and St Thomas' Hospital NHS Foundation Trust, King's College London, London, United Kingdom

H.C. TORSTEN ZUBERBIER, MD
Professor of Dermatology and Allergy, Director of Clinic, Department of Dermatology and Allergy, Allergie – Centrum Charité/ECARF, Charité – Universitätsmedizin Berlin, Berlin, Germany

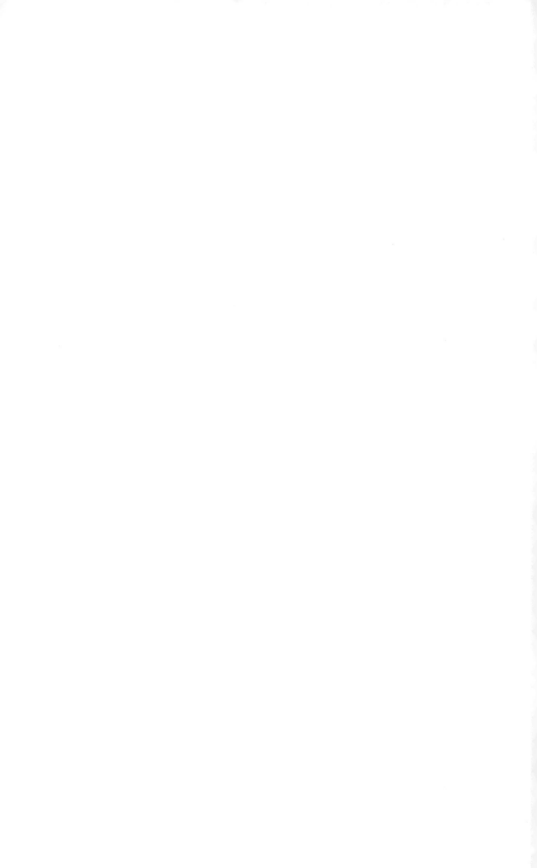

Contents

> Chronic urticaria is defined as daily or almost daily urticaria for more than 6 weeks. Chronic urticaria is normally subdivided into physical urticaria (wheals evoked by a physical stimulus such as pressure friction or cold contact) and spontaneous urticaria. A patient with a history of less than 6 weeks is traditionally designated as having acute urticaria. Patients with chronic spontaneous urticaria have an increased frequency of HLA-DR and HLA-DQ alleles characteristically associated with autoimmune disease. Some of these patients have functional anti-FceR1 and/or anti-IgE autoantibodies which are considered to be the cause of the urticaria.

> Acute urticaria is a common condition, which presents in all age groups and to multiple specialties. It may be a presenting symptom of anaphylaxis. The following article describes the epidemiology, etiology, clinical features, differential diagnosis, investigations, management, and prognosis of acute urticaria. Contact urticaria and angioedema without urticarial weals are not covered, as these are described elsewhere in this issue.

> Urticarial wheals and angioedema are two different clinical symptoms. Both belong to various disease entities, and may occur in combination or be isolated. Increased vasodilation and vasopermeability is a common feature. Histamine and bradykinin are well-known mediators. For clinical purposes, three groups of diseases can be differentiated: diseases with urticaria and angioedema, diseases with angioedema alone, and diseases with urticarial lesions without angioedema. This article presents an overview of these groups and the role of the main mediators, and the clinical features of urticaria and angioedema.

> Urticaria affects individuals of all ages and is commonplace. Nearly 1 in 5 individuals will experience an episode of urticaria in their lifetime, while the

chronic form of disease has an estimated annual prevalence of approximately 1% of the population. Given the similarity of chronic urticaria symptoms to those seen in patients suffering an allergic reaction, the condition often leads to a search for an external cause. In most cases, no external trigger factor is identified. At present several theories of pathogenesis exist, none of which is firmly established.

most antihistamine-resistant patients who require long-term corticosteroid treatments to control their disease. Omalizumab is effective in most subsets of chronic urticaria sufferers who do not respond to other treatments but its high cost represents a limitation to its widespread use.

Although urticaria is not a life-threatening disease, its impact on quality of life in children should not be overlooked. A systematic search of online databases, including Medline, was performed to inform a review aiming to equip clinicians with an evidence-based approach to all aspects of pediatric urticaria. This review hinges on an illustrative case and includes a summary table of studies pertaining to disease management in children. The multiple issues faced by patients, their families, and treating clinicians are highlighted, and the current literature on the presentation, natural history, investigation, and management of this poorly understood condition is assessed.

Both urticarial vasculitis and Schnitzler syndrome are serious diseases but an improved understanding of their underlying pathomechanism allows better treatment options than what was available only a decade ago.

Urticaria is part of the management of pregnancy, labor, delivery, and the puerperium in some women. The urticaria can be acute, chronic, or physical, presenting with whealing, angioedema, or both. Contact urticaria can occur. Acquired angioedema, usually with urticaria, must be differentiated from hereditary angioedema. An approach to management of these conditions in pregnancy is proposed.

The wheal and flare reaction from direct contact with a chemical or protein agent is known as *contact urticaria*. Contact urticaria can be either nonimmunologic (no sensitization required) or immunologic (sensitization required). Immunologic contact urticaria often gives a more aggravated response and has the potential to spread from the local vicinity. Skin testing in immunologic contact urticaria gives a quicker response compared with skin testing in nonimmunologic contact urticaria. There are a wide variety of agents that can cause immunologic contact urticaria, and they can be either low-molecular-weight chemicals (haptens) or proteins.

The latest clinical guideline includes three major hereditary disorders presenting with urticaria: urticaria pigmentosa (mastocytosis), hereditary angioedema, and cryopyrin-associated periodic syndromes. Understanding

IMMUNOLOGY AND ALLERGY CLINICS OF NORTH AMERICA

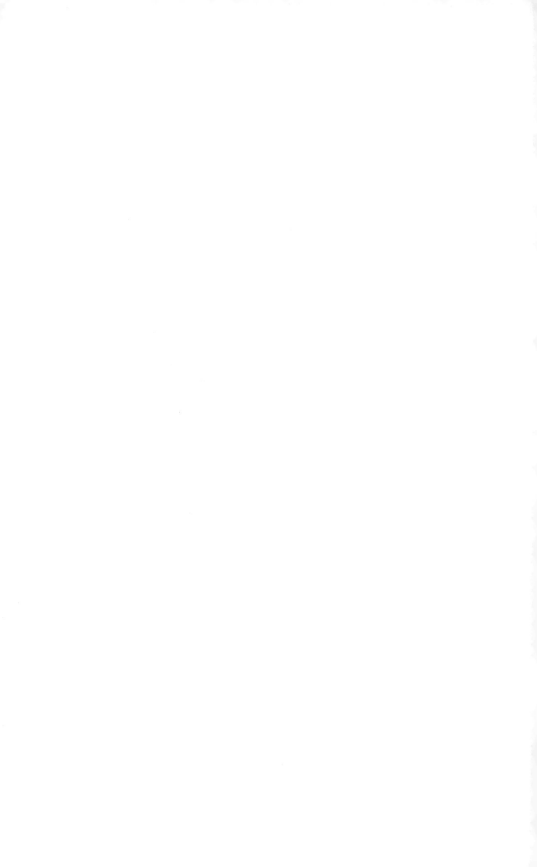

Foreword

Urticaria: An Evolving Story

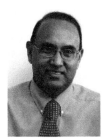

Rafeul Alam, MD, PhD
Consulting Editor

Chronic spontaneous urticaria affects nearly 20% of the population. Although it is commonly considered a mast cell-mediated disease, the mechanism of mast cell activation remains a medical mystery. A number of new developments in this field got us quite excited. The demonstration of the presence of an anti-IgE receptor autoantibody and sometimes an anti-IgE autoantibody in serum from urticaria patients suggested an autoimmune mechanism. Although some studies have shown that these autoantibodies are more prevalent in patients with severe urticaria, the clinical correlation is not very strong. This is similar to autoantibodies found in rheumatologic disorders. It is possible that the anti-IgE autoantibody primes the mast cells, which require a second trigger for full activation and manifestation of the disease. We need to further understand the specific role of these autoantibodies in pathogenesis. There are a number of tests that detect this autoantibody. We need a standardized approach for optimal detection of the autoantibodies.

Another important development in the field is the impressive efficacy of omalizumab in antihistamine-resistant urticaria. The clinical implication of this finding is huge. However, the result raises questions about how omalizumab exerts its beneficial effect in urticaria. Omalizumab reduces the level of unbound IgE in the serum. This is associated with reduced FcεRI on mast cells and basophils. If reduced FcεRI is key to clinical improvement, it would imply a fundamental role for this receptor in the pathogenesis of urticaria.

Finally, there is a subgroup of urticaria patients whose basophils are unresponsive to activating stimulation, such as an anti-IgE antibody. This subgroup is called the nonresponder. Some preliminary observations suggest an increased expression of certain cytosolic phosphatases (SHIP1 and 2) in this subgroup. These phosphatases downregulate FcεRI signaling by inhibiting the activating kinases. It would be important to

Supported by NIH Grants RO1 AI091614 and N01 HHSN272200700048C.

immunology.theclinics.com

demonstrate that the tissue mast cells also manifest a similar increase. If this is confirmed in larger populations, it would suggest that this subgroup utilizes a mechanism of mast cell activation that is different from FcεRI. These are exciting findings, indeed. To update us on these evolving stories, I have invited Dr Malcolm Greaves as guest editor. Dr Greaves is an internationally recognized leader in the field. He has brought together an outstanding group of authors and topics for this issue.

Rafeul Alam, MD, PhD
Division of Allergy and Immunology
National Jewish Health
University of Colorado Denver School of Medicine
1400 Jackson Street
Denver, CO 80206, USA

E-mail address:
alamr@njc.org

Preface

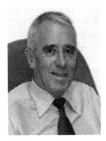

Malcolm W. Greaves, MD, PhD, FRCP
Editor

Urticaria, particularly in its chronic forms, and especially when complicated by angioedema, can have a devastating effect on quality of life, but its etiology remains controversial. Evidence in the 1990s that autoimmunity plays a role in some patients has generally held up, but it is puzzling that other clinically indistinguishable patients have no evidence of an autoimmune basis. Surprisingly, immunotherapy also seems to be equally effective in autoimmune and apparently nonautoimmune patients. More recently additional pathomechanisms have been proposed, including primary defects of signal transduction in basophil leucocytes and mast cells and abnormalities of the coagulation pathway. Up to now these approaches have not led to significant advances in investigation or treatment. Despite slow progress in these areas, encouraging advances in treatment are imminent. Omalizumab, a monoclonal antibody directed against IgE and currently licensed in several countries for the indication of allergic asthma, is proving effective in the majority of patients with severe, treatment-resistant chronic urticaria. Because of its apparent freedom from serious adverse effects, it offers an attractive alternative to systemic steroids and immunosuppressants such as cyclosporine or methotrexate. Up to now (2013), omalizumab is not licensed for the indication of urticaria in Europe or North America.

It is hoped that this collection of contributions from acknowledged experts in this field will help the clinician to understand what we do know and, equally importantly, what remains enigmatic about the causation of this sometimes confusing group of diseases. It is also hoped that these accounts will provide an up-to-date platform for the clinician to formulate a rational management plan for individual patients.

Interestingly, recent impressive progress has been made in unraveling the molecular mechanisms and genetic basis of hereditary angioedema, mastocytosis, and the cryopyrin-associated autoinflammatory syndromes. These entities, although comparatively rare, do present with angioedema and/or urticaria and the opportunity has therefore been seized to include contributions from recognised authorities on these topics including striking advances in treatment.

Immunol Allergy Clin N Am 34 (2014) xv–xvi
http://dx.doi.org/10.1016/j.iac.2013.10.001
0889-8561/14/$ – see front matter **immunology.theclinics.com**

Overall it is hoped that a reasonable balance has been achieved that will meet the needs of the practicing clinician and the investigator who seeks a sound clinical context for research in this exciting group of disorders.

Malcolm W. Greaves, MD, PhD, FRCP
Cutaneous Allergy Clinic
St Johns Institute of Dermatology
St Thomas' Hospital
Lambeth Palace Rd
London SE1 7EH UK

E-mail address:
mwatsong@hotmail.com

Pathology and Classification of Urticaria

Malcolm W. Greaves, MD, PhD, FRCP[a,b,*]

KEYWORDS

- Chronic urticaria • Physical urticaria • Autoimmune urticaria • Acute urticaria

KEY POINTS

- Chronic urticaria is normally defined as daily or almost daily urticaria for more than 6 weeks. Chronic urticaria has been traditionally subdivided into physical urticaria (wheals evoked by a physical stimulus, such as pressure, friction, cold contact, or sun exposure) and spontaneous urticaria.
- A patient with a length of history less than 6 weeks is designated as having acute urticaria, although most patients with acute urticaria have a much shorter duration.
- Depletion of the peripheral blood basophil leukocyte count occurs in some patients with chronic spontaneous urticaria.
- Patients with chronic urticaria have an increased frequency of HLA-DR and HLA-DQ alleles that are characteristically associated with autoimmune diseases. Some of these patients have functional anti-FceR1 and/or anti-IgE autoantibodies which are considered to be the cause of the urticaria.

WHAT IS URTICARIA?

In 1480, King Richard III of England, whose mortal remains have recently been discovered under a public car park in Leicester, developed an itchy red rash after consuming strawberries procured by a courtier. Accused by the king of witchcraft, the courtier was put to death.[1] Fortunately, even when accompanied by angioedema, urticaria is rarely fatal. The term, urticaria, was first used by Johann P Frank in 1792 in his classic *De curandis hominum morbus epitome praelectionibus dicata*. Aided by Thomas Bateman, Robert Willan, in his *A Practical Synopsis of Cutaneous Diseases* (1813), attempted classification of subtypes of urticaria.[2] He recognized *urticaria febrilis* (urticaria associated with fever), *urticaria evanida* (corresponding with spontaneous chronic urticaria), and *urticaria perstans*, in which individual wheals last several days, consistent with urticarial vasculitis or possibly delayed pressure urticaria.

[a] Cutaneous Allergy Clinic, St John's Institute of Dermatology, St Thomas' Hospital, Lambeth Palace Road, London SE1 7EH, UK; [b] The London Allergy Clinic, 66 New Cavendish Street, London W1G 8TD, UK
* Cutaneous Allergy Clinic, St John's Institute of Dermatology, St Thomas' Hospital, Lambeth Palace Road, London SE1 7EH, United Kindom.
E-mail address: mwatsong@hotmail.com

Immunol Allergy Clin N Am 34 (2014) 1–9
http://dx.doi.org/10.1016/j.iac.2013.07.009
0889-8561/14/$ – see front matter © 2014 Elsevier Inc. All rights reserved.

The role of mast cells and histamine in the pathogenesis of urticaria was not revealed for many decades. In 1879, Paul Ehrlich,[3] a medical student, using recently discovered basic dyes as histochemical stains, proposed the name, *mastzellen* (well-fed cells), for these cells whose granules exhibited metachromatic properties and water solubility. More than 30 years later, Dale[4] identified histamine as an important pharmacologic mediator of vasodilation and vascular permeability, and in the 1920s, Lewis,[5] in his description of the actions of histamine in the skin, drew attention to its potential role as a mediator of urticaria.

Urticarial wheals are clinically characterized by central swelling due to local increased permeability of cutaneous capillaries and postcapillary venules. The redness of the urticarial wheal is due to vasodilation, the more central component of which is caused by a direct action of histamine on postcapillary venules, but the surrounding bright red, often patchily distributed, flare is a result of an axon reflex, these (wheal, central redness, axon flare) being components of Lewis' famous triple response.[5] Increased blood flow causes the affected skin to be warm and also often causes a visible halo of pallor surrounding the wheal, which is due to a steal effect. Curiously, in his otherwise comprehensive treatise on actions of histamine in human skin, Lewis omits mention of itch. It was not until the 1950s that Riley and West[6] firmly confirmed the localization of histamine in tissue mast cells of the skin and other organs, thereby establishing the dermal mast cell as the target cell in urticaria.

Angioedema is frequently associated with most subtypes of urticaria, although it occurs alone without urticaria in hereditary forms, and angioedema evoked as an adverse reaction to ACE inhibitors. Credit for clear descriptions of the clinical features of angioedema should be shared jointly by John Milton of Edinburgh[7] and Heinrich Quincke,[8] although the latter frankly acknowledges that he was essentially describing the work entitled, "Uber akutes Odem," of one of his graduate students, Eugen Dinkellacker. Unlike urticaria, angioedema affects mucous membranes as well as skin, with a predilection for mucocutaneous junctions, including eyelids and lips. Increased vascular permeability is abrupt and massive and located deep in the dermis, subcutaneous tissue, and submucosa. Vasodilation is variable and often angiedema swellings are the color of normal skin and painful rather than itchy.

The histopathology and immunopathology of urticaria have been insufficiently studied and vary depending on the subtype of urticaria studied. The histopathologic findings in a physical urticaria, such as symptomatic dermographism, in which the wheal lasts only a few minutes before fading without leaving a trace, are different from the findings in chronic spontaneous urticaria, in which the duration of each individual wheal is usually 12 to 18 hours. There are certain common features, however. Dermal edema, vasodilation, and a perivascular cellular infiltrate are microscopically evident with variations in all subtpypes of urticaria. Although prominent in urticarial vasculitis, endothelial cell damage is not seen in any form of nonvasculitic urticaria. Available data on the histopathology of the wheal in urticaria are mainly derived from studies in chronic spontaneous urticaria.

THE DERMAL MAST CELL IN URTICARIA

Despite their central role in the pathogenesis of urticaria, histologic studies have not convincingly demonstrated quantitative or qualitative abnormalities in dermal mast cells in any subtype of urticaria. Using a double-labeling immunohistochemical technique, no significant difference in mast cell numbers in lesional, nonlesional, or control (healthy) skin were observed.[9] Human mast cells are of 2 types, based on the protease content of the granules. Mast cells of the Tc type (MC Tc) contain tryptase and chymase); the granules of the MC T type contain tryptase only. MC Tcs predominate in human skin, whereas pulmonary mast cells are predominantly the MC T type.[10,11] Expression of the C5a receptor (CD88) on MC Tc dermal mast cells but not on pulmonary MC T mast cells explains the absence of pulmonary involvement in autoimmune (IgG anti-FcεR1) chronic spontaneous urticaria. Dermal mast cell activation in this condition is known to be complement dependent.[12]

THE BASOPHIL LEUKOCYTE IN URTICARIA

It has long been recognized that depletion of the peripheral blood basophil leukocyte count occurs in some patients with chronic spontaneous urticaria.[13,14] This abnormality is strongly associated with the presence of functional IgG anti-FcεR1 autoantibodies (autoimmune chronic urticaria), suggesting active recruitment of blood basophils into lesional skin.[15–17] Circulating basophils in patients with chronic urticaria show reduced reactivity to activation via the high-affinity IgE receptor,[18] and this has recently been associated with abnormalities in the FcεR1 signaling pathway.[19] The late-phase reaction, which is IgE dependent and shows histologic appearances resembling those seen in some forms of chronic urticaria, manifests basophil infiltration.[20] Caution should be exercised, however, in interpretation of these findings. The importance of the basophil leukocyte relative to the dermal mast cell in the pathogenesis of chronic urticaria is unclear, although its accessibility compared with dermal mast cells has prompted its use in urticaria research as a convenient mast cell surrogate.

THE INFLAMMATORY INFILTRATE IN CHRONIC URTICARIA

That the inflammatory infiltrate plays a major role in the pathogenesis of chronic spontaneous urticaria (CSU) is evidenced by the almost invariably positive response to systemic corticosteroids, which have little or no direct effect on dermal mast cells. Conversely, physical urticarias, such as symptomatic dermographism, in which there is little or no perivascular infiltrate, respond poorly if at all to systemic corticoids.

The dermal perivascular infiltrate of lesional skin in CSU contains mainly $CD3^+$, $CD4^+$, $CD8^+$, and $CD25^+$ T lymphocytes with a mainly T_H0 cytokine profile predominantly expressing mRNA for interleukin (IL)-4, IL-5, and interferon γ.[20] An intense perivascular neutrophilic infiltrate without vasculitis is seen in a minority (approximately 15%) in involved skin of patients with chronic urticaria.[21,22] The significance of this neutrophilic urticaria is unclear, but it may be a nonspecific acute-phase reaction. A neutrophilic histology is often seen in involved skin in the rare Schnitzler syndrome (urticaria, arthralgia, fever, bone pain, and an IgM kappa paraproteinemia). Although not a dominant feature of the infiltrate in CSU, neutrophil as well as eosinophil infiltration is found predominantly in early (<4 h duration) wheals.[23]

PHARMACOLOGIC MEDIATORS OF CHRONIC URTICARIA

The wheals of physical urticarias, including symptomatic dermographism and cold contact urticaria, are short-lived and closely resemble the triple response of skin to intradermal injection of histamine (central wheal, erythema, and an axon flare)[5] together with itching. This, and the effective suppression of symptoms and signs by H_1 antihistamines encourages the view that histamine, derived from dermal mast cells, is the main, if not the only, mediator of these physical urticarias. As indicated previously, the wheal of CSU is of a different character, lasting individually for 12 h to 18 h, usually responding only partially to H_1 antihistamines. Tissue histamine levels in lesional skin of patients with CSU are elevated.[24] Although H_1 antihistamines provide symptomatic relief in CSU, they are usually more effective in relieving the itching than the whealing. Furthermore, no convincing evidence has emerged that H_2 or H_3 histamine receptors[25,26] play a clinically significant part in the response of human skin to histamine. Although histamine mediates the pruritus, it is not the exclusive mediator of the whealing in CSU.

The role of mediators other than histamine in the generation of wheals in CSU has received little attention. There is some indirect evidence suggesting that the arachidonic acid transformation products, leukotrienes C_4, D_4, and E_4, may play a role. Human mast cells secrete leukotrienes and leukotrienes C_4, D_4, and E_4 are vasoactive in the skin of healthy human subjects and patients with chronic urticaria.[27] The leukotriene antagonist, montelukast, and the 5-lipoxygenase inhibitor, zafirlukast, have shown some evidence of efficacy in patients with chronic urticaria in small studies.[28] Abnormalities of the coagulation pathway have been demonstrated in some patients with chronic urticaria.[29,30] Whether these abnormalities are of pathogenetic significance or are secondary epiphenomena, consequent on extensive urticaria, is unclear. Therapeutic efficacy of the coumarin oral anticoagulant warfarin, however, has been claimed.[31]

Chronic urticaria is generally recognized as exacerbated by anxiety and stress, raising the possibility of a neurogenic component in its pathophysiology.[32] Several neuropeptides are known to activate mast cells, including substance P, calcitonin gene-related peptide, vasoactive intestinal peptide, and nerve growth factor. Attempts to measure tissue and plasma levels of these neuropeptides in relation to disease activity in chronic urticaria have yielded conflicting results.[33,34]

PATHOPHYSIOLOGY OF ITCH IN URTICARIA

Itch is the dominant symptom of urticaria. Most patients with urticaria rub rather than scratch their itchy wheals. In the urticaria clinic, prominent excoriation is a rarity, which, if present, calls into question the diagnosis. Itch is usefully classified as pruritogenic (generated in the skin), neurogenic (generated in the central nervous system in response to circulating pruritogens), neuropathic (due to anatomic lesions in the peripheral or central nervous sytem), and psychogenic (stress related or, rarely, delusional parasitosis).[35–37] In urticaria, itching originates in the skin and is, therefore, pruritogenic. It is due to release from mast cells of pruritogenic mediators, of which histamine is prominent. Itching evoked by histamine is due to ligation of G protein–coupled H_1 receptors on dorsal root ganglion (DRG) unmyelinated C neurons, which are distinct from pain-transmitting neurons. This leads to increased intracellular calcium and causes depolarization of the nerve terminal via membrane ion channels. Recent evidence in different murine models suggests that H_4 receptors may also be involved in itching[26,38,39] and in experimental models H_4 receptor antagonists show some promise in alleviating histamine-evoked itch. DRG C neurons also express receptors selective for the mast cell–derived protease tryptase. These receptors are termed, proteinase-activated receptor 2, and may contribute to the intense pruritus experienced by many patients with mastocytosis, in which serum tryptase levels are elevated, as well as in urticaria in which cutaneous DRG neurone terminals and dermal mast cells exist in close proximity.[40]

A small rise in skin temperature causes a lowering of the threshold for itch[41] and this may be a factor in the observation by most patients with urticaria that their pruritus is worse in the evening and night-time. More importantly, inhibitory neuronal circuits located in the substantia gelatinosa of the posterior horns of the gray matter of the spinal cord form a gated mechanism whereby afferent itch traffic is modulated.[42,43]

Increased tone in the descending pathways has been shown by functional positron emission tomography (PET) scan studies to originate in the reticular formation of the periacqueductal gray and is the result of visual auditory and other sensory stimuli. Outside working hours, these stimuli are diminished, resulting in reduced inhibitory tone, opening, in turn, the regulatory gated mechanism and increased itching. Cold ameliorates itch. The transient receptor potential (TRP) ion channels expressed on afferent itch transmitting nociceptor cutaneous nerve terminals are temperature sensitive.[44] One subset of these receptors, TRPV1, may account for the cooling sensation conferred by topical menthol products that are widely used in the symptomatic relief of itching in urticaria.[45] Immediate, but temporary, relief of itching in urticaria is normally achieved by rubbing, although occasional patients obtain a better response by slapping the affected skin with the palm of the hand. These physical stimuli cause surround inhibition due to activation of fast-conducting myelinated low-threshold Aβ neurons, which are inhibitory on itch traffic in the C neurons[46] and on spinothalamic tract neurons that transmit itch.[47] Recent functional PET scan imaging of the cerebral cortex has also demonstrated deactivation of brain areas that are involved in processing unpleasant itch sensation, such as the anterior cingulate cortex by scratching.[48] Thus, itch in urticaria can, in a sense, be relieved by rubbing the brain.

AUTOIMMUNITY IN CHRONIC URTICARIA

A close association between chronic urticaria and autoimmune disease has long been recognized. In the 1980s, Leznoff drew attention to the frequent occurrence of autoimmune thyroid disease and chronic urticaria. Of 182 patients with chronic urticaria, 22 (12%) had antithyroid microsomal autoantibodies. Leznoff went as far as to propose a syndrome of autoimmune thyroid disease and chronic urticaria.[49–51] In a recent large Israeli study, chronic urticaria was associated with an increased odds ratio for hypothyroidism and hyperthyroidism and thyroid autoimmunity and there was also a significantly higher incidence of lupus erythematosus, type 1 diabetes mellitus, and several other autoimmune diseases in patients with chronic urticaria.[52] The basis of this linkage is unclear; 30% to 60% of patients with CSU have functional IgG autoantibodies directed against the high-affinity IgE receptor (FcεR1) expressed on dermal mast cells and basophil leulocytes and these autoantibodies are believed the cause of the wheals in the patients who have them. The extensive evidence for this has recently been reviewed[53,54] and is not detailed here. The high prevalence of anti-FcεR1 and thyroid antimicrosomal autoantibodies in CSU is not explained by a shared epitope recognized by these 2 autoantibodies[55] and is likely due to genetic predisposition to development of autoimmune disease shared by patients with these 2 diseases. In favor of this interpretation, patients with chronic urticaria have an increased frequency of HLA-DR and HLA-DQ alleles that are characteristically associated with autoimmune diseases.[56–58]

CLASSIFICATION OF URTICARIA

To describe a patient as having urticaria and/or angioedema is not to make a diagnosis but rather to characterize in a general way the signs and symptoms that the patient has. The subtypes of urticaria are different in etiology, pathogenesis, prognosis, and treatment. Classification of urticaria is only of value if it aids clinicians in formulation of an investigational and therapeutic strategy for individual patients. An internationally recognized classification should also be useful to investigators involved in research in the urticarial disorders. Too often, research publications on urticaria leave readers unsure of the particular subtypes studied. Traditionally, urticaria (with or without angioedema) has been classified as acute or chronic. Chronic urticaria is normally defined as daily or almost daily urticaria for more than 6 weeks. It follows that a patient with a length of history less than 6 weeks is designated as having acute urticaria, although most patients with acute urticaria have a much shorter duration. Chronic urticaria has been traditionally subdivided into physical urticaria (wheals evoked by a physical stimulus, such as pressure, friction, cold contact, or sun exposure) and idiopathic urticaria. The latter term reflects that up to the 1990s, the cause for the vast majority of these patients was elusive.

The first attempt at an international consensus–based classification was published in 2006.[59] Three main subtypes were proposed. The subtype, CSU, distinguished those patients with chronic urticaria in whom the wheals appeared spontaneously, without a triggering physical stimulus, from those in whom a local physical eliciting stimulus, such as friction, heat, cold, or sun exposure, evokes whealing (subtype, physical urticaria). The third subtype consisted of a miscellaneous urticaria group, including cholinergic urticaria and contact urticaria.

This classification was modified in 2009[60] to further subdivide CSU into CSU due to known causes and CSU due to unknown causes (the latter corresponding with the traditional term, idiopathic). This modification can be criticized on the grounds that some of the cited known causes (chronic infection, dietary pseudoallergens, and stress) are, to say the least, controversial. A further minor modification was to substitute the subtype, physical urticaria, with chronic inducible urticaria. This subtype includes both physical urticarias and miscellaneous urticarias, such as cholinergic urticaria and contact urticaria.

In a further recent communication, the same group[60] reasonably advised that the term, idiopathic, as applied to chronic urticaria, should be dropped on the grounds that it is often indiscriminately applied to all subtypes of chronic urticaria and that not all CSU is of unknown causation.[61] Their claim that "chronic idiopathic urticaria is no longer idiopathic"[61] is misleading, however; in reality, thorough investigation of at least 50% of patients with CSU leads to the conclusion that their urticaria is idiopathic—no cause can be substantiated.

A classification that is of use to clinicians and that incorporates the substance of the previously discussed versions but that seeks to avoid their drawbacks is set out in **Table 1**.

Table 1 Chronic urticaria: classification	
Chronic Spontaneous Urticaria	**Chronic Inducible Urticaria**
Autoimmune etiology	Physical urticarias
Unknown etiology (idiopathic)	Symptomatic dermographism
	Simple dermographism
	Cold urticaria
	Delayed pressure urticaria
	Solar urticaria
	Heat urticaria
	Vibratory angioedema
	Aquagenic urticaria
	Cholinergic urticaria
	Contact urticaria

Data from Zuberbier T, Asero R, Bindslev-Jensen C, et al. Guideline: definition, classification and diagnosis of urticaria. Allergy 2009;64:1417–26; and Maurer M, Bindslev-Jensen C, Gimenez-Arnaud A, et al. Chronic idiopathic urticaria (CIU) is no longer idiopathic: time for an update. Br J Dermatol 2013;168:426–60.

REFERENCES

1. Shakespeare W. (1591) The life and death of King Richard 111. Act 3, scene 4.
2. Bateman T. A practical synopsis of cutaneous diseases. London: Longman, Hurst, Rees, Orme and Brown; 1813.
3. Ehrlich P. Bertrage zur Kenntis der Granulierten Bindegewebszellen und der eosinopholen leucocyten. Arch Anat Physiol (Lpz) 1879;3:166–9.
4. Dale HH. Some chemical factors in the control of the circulation. Lecture 2, local vasodilator reactions – histamine. Lancet 1929;1:1233–7.
5. Lewis T. The blood vessels of the human skin and their responses. London: Shaw and Sons; 1927. p. 47.
6. Riley JF, West GB. Presence of histamine in tissue mast cells. J Physiol 1953; 120:528–37.
7. Milton JL. On giant urticaria. Edinb Med J 1876;22:513–26.
8. Quincke H. Concerning the acute localised oedema of the skin. Prakt Dermatol 1882;1:129–31.
9. Smith CH, Kepley C, Schwartz LB, et al. Mast cell number and phenotype in chronic idiopathic urticaria. J Allergy Clin Immunol 1995;96:360–4.
10. Irani AA, Schecter NM, Craig SS, et al. Two types of human mast cells that have distinct neutral protease compositions. Proc Natl Acad Sci U S A 1986;83: 4464–8.
11. Fureder W, Agis H, Willheim M, et al. Differential expression of complement receptors on human basophils and mast cells. J Immunol 1995;155:3152–60.
12. Ferrer M, Nakazawa K, Kaplan AP. Complement dependence of histamine release in chronic urticaria. J Allergy Clin Immunol 1999;104:169–72.
13. Greaves MW, Plummer VM, McLaughlan P, et al. Serum and cell bound IgE in chronic urticaria. Clin Allergy 1974;4:265–71.
14. Sabroe RA, Francis DM, Barr RM, et al. Anti-Fc(epsilon)R1 autoantibodies and basophil histamine releasability in chronic idiopathic urticaria. J Allergy Clin Immunol 1998;102:651–68.
15. Grattan CE, Walpole D, Francis DM, et al. Flow cytometric analysis of basophil numbers in chronic urticaria: basopenia is related to serum histamine releasing activity. Clin Exp Allergy 1997;27:1417–24.
16. Grattan CE, Dawn G, Gibbs S, et al. Blood basophil numbers in chronic ordinary urticaria and healthy controls: diurnal variation, influence of loratidine and prednisolone and relationship to disease activity. Clin Exp Allergy 2003;33:337–41.
17. Hoskin SL, Wilson SJ, Sabroe RA, et al. Basophil infiltration of wheals in chronic idiopathic urticaria. J Allergy Clin Immunol 2002;109:A229.
18. Vonakis BM, Vasagar K, Gibbons SP, et al. Basophil FcεR1 histamine release parallels expression of Src-homology 2-containing inositol phosphatises in chronic idiopathic urticaria. J Allergy Clin Immunol 2007;119:441–8.
19. Irani AM, Huang C, Xia HZ, et al. Immunohistochemical detection of human basophils in late phase skin reactions. J Allergy Clin Immunol 1998;101:354–62.
20. Ying S, Kikuchi Y, Meng Q, et al. Th1/Th2 cytokines and inflammatory cells in skin biopsy specimens from patients with chronic idiopathic urticaria: comparison with allergen induced late phase cutaneous reaction. J Allergy Clin Immunol 2002;109:694–700.
21. Peters MS, Winkelmann RK. Neutrophilic urticaria. Br J Dermatol 1985;113: 25–30.
22. Toppe E, Haas N, Henz BM. Neutrophilic urticaria: clinical features, histological changes and possible mechanisms. Br J Dermatol 1998;138:248–53.

23. Sabroe RA, Poon E, Orchard G, et al. Cutaneous inflammatory cell infiltrate in chronic idiopathic urticaria: comparison of patients with and without anti-FcεR1 or anti- IgE autoantibodies. J Allergy Clin Immunol 1999;103(3 Pt 1): 484–93.
24. Kaplan AP, Horakova Z, Katz SI. Assessment of tissue fluid histamine levels in patients with urticaria. J Allergy Clin Immunol 1978;61:350–4.
25. Lovenberg TW, Roland BL, Wilson SJ, et al. Cloning and functional expression of the human histamine H3 receptor. Mol Pharmacol 1999;55:1101–7.
26. Dunford PJ, Williams KN, Desai PJ, et al. Histamine H4 receptor antagonists are superior to traditional antihistamines in the attenuation of experimental pruritus. J Allergy Clin Immunol 2007;119:176–83.
27. Maxwell DL, Atkinson BA, Spur BW, et al. Skin responses to intradermal histamine and leukotrienes C4, D4, E4 in patients with chronic idiopathic urticaria and in normal subjects. J Allergy Clin Immunol 1990;86:759–65.
28. Erbagei Z. The leukotriene receptor antagonist montelukast in the treatment of chronic idiopathic urticaria: single blind placebo-controlled cross over clinical study. J Allergy Clin Immunol 2002;110:484–8.
29. Asero R, Tedeschi A, Coppola S, et al. Activation of the tissue pathway of blood coagulation in patients with chronic urticaria. J Allergy Clin Immunol 2007;119: 705–10.
30. Wang F, Tang H, Xu J, et al. Activation of the blood coagulation cascade is involved in patients with chronic urticaria. J Allergy Clin Immunol 2009;123: 972–3.
31. Vedanthan PK, Mahesh PA, Holla AD, et al. Warfarin sodium as a steroid sparing agent in severe chronic idiopathic urticaria. J Allergy Clin Immunol 2008;121: S103.
32. Dimitrijevic M, Stanojevic S, Kustrimovic N, et al. End-point effector stress mediators in neuroimmune interactions: their role in immune system homeostasis and autoimmune pathology. Immunol Res 2012;52:64–80.
33. Wallengren J, Moller H, Ekman R. Occurrence of substance P, vasoactive intestinal peptide and calcitonin gene-related peptide in dermographism and cold urticaria. Arch Dermatol Res 1987;279:512–5.
34. Tedeschi A, Lorini M, Asero R. No evidence of increased serum substance P levels in chronic urticaria patients with and without demonstrable circulating vasoactive factors. Clin Exp Dermatol 2005;30:171–5.
35. Twycross R, Greaves MW, Handwerker H, et al. Itch: scratching more than the surface. QJM 2003;96:7–26.
36. Yosipovitch G, Greaves MW, Schmeltz M. Itch. Lancet 2003;361:690–4.
37. Greaves MW. Pathogenesis and treatment of pruritus. Curr Allergy Asthma Rep 2010;10:236–42.
38. Bell JK, McQueen DS, Rees JL, et al. Involvement of histamine H4 and H1 receptors in scratching induced by histamine receptor agonists in Balb C mice. Br J Pharmacol 2004;142:374–80.
39. Yamaura K, Oda M, Suwa E, et al. Expression of histamine H4 receptor in human epidermal tissues and attenuation of epidermal pruritus using H4 receptor antagonist. J Toxicol Sci 2009;34:427–31.
40. Steinhoff M, Neisius U, Ikoma A, et al. Proteinase-activated receptor -2 mediates itch: a novel pathway for pruritus in human skin. J Neurosci 2003;23:6176–80.
41. Fruhstorfer H, Hermanns M, Latzke L. The effects of thermal stimulation on clinical and experimental itch. Pain 1986;24:259–69.
42. Greaves MW, Wall PD. Pathophysiology of itching. Lancet 1996;348:938–40.

43. Wall PD, Melzack R. Textbook of pain. 3rd edition. Edinburgh (United Kingdom): Churchill Livingstone; 1995.
44. McKemy DD, Neuhasser WM, Julius D. Identification of a cold receptor reveals a general role for TRP channels in thermosensation. Nature 2002;416:52–8.
45. Stander S, Moormann C, Schumacher M, et al. Expression of vanilloid receptor subtypes in cutaneous sensory fibres, mast cells, and epithelial cells of appendage structures. Exp Dermatol 2004;13:129–34.
46. Wall PD, Sweet WH. Temporary abolition of pain in man. Science 1967;155:108–9.
47. Davidson S, Zhang X, Khasabov SG, et al. Relief of itch by scratching: state-dependent inhibition of primate spinothalamic neurons. Nat Neurosci 2009;12:544–6.
48. Vierow V, Fukuoka M, Ikoma A, et al. Cerebral representation of the relief of itch by scratching. J Neurophysiol 2009;102:3216–24.
49. Leznoff A, Josse RG, Denburg J, et al. Association of chronic urticaria and angioedema with thyroid autoimmunity. Arch Dermatol 1983;119:636–40.
50. Leznoff A, Sussman GL. Syndrome of idiopathic urticaria and angioedema with thyroid autoimmunity: a study of 90 patients. J Allergy Clin Immunol 1989;84:66–71.
51. O'Donnell BF, Francis DM, Swana GT, et al. Thyroid autoimmunity in chronic urticaria. Br J Dermatol 2005;153:331–5.
52. Confino-Cohen R, Chodick G, Shalev V, et al. Chronic urticaria and autoimmunity: associations found in a large population study. J Allergy Clin Immunol 2012;129:1307–13.
53. Kaplan AP. Chronic urticaria: pathogenesis and treatment. J Allergy Clin Immunol 2004;114:465–74.
54. Greaves MW, Tan KT. Chronic urticaria: recent advances. Clin Rev Allergy Immunol 2007;33:134–43.
55. Mozena JD, Tinana A, Negri J, et al. Lack of a role for cross reacting anti-thyroid antibodies in chronic idiopathic urticaria. J Invest Dermatol 2010;130:1860–5.
56. O'Donnell BF, O'Neill CM, Francis DM, et al. Human leucocyte antigen type 11 associations in chronic idiopathic urticaria. Br J Dermatol 1999;140:853–8.
57. Aydogan K, Karadogan SK, Akdag I, et al. HLA class I and class II antigens in Turkish patients with chronic ordinary urticaria. Clin Exp Dermatol 2006;31:424–9.
58. Calamita Z, Calamita AB. HLA in patients with chronic spontaneous urticaria who are positive for anti-thyroid antibodies. J Eur Acad Dermatol Venereol 2013;27:661–2.
59. Zouberbier T, Bindslev-Jensen T, Canonica W, et al. EAACI/GA[2] LEN/EDF guideline: definition, classification and diagnosis of urticaria. Allergy 2006;61:316–20.
60. Zuberbier T, Asero R, Bindslev-Jensen C, et al. Guideline: definition, classification and diagnosis of urticaria. Allergy 2009;64:1417–26.
61. Maurer M, Bindslev-Jensen C, Gimenez-Arnaud A, et al. Chronic idiopathic urticaria (CIU) is no longer idiopathic: time for an update. Br J Dermatol 2013;168:426–60.

Acute Urticaria

Ruth A. Sabroe, FRCP, MD

KEYWORDS

• Acute urticaria • Anaphylaxis • Antihistamines

KEY POINTS

- Acute urticaria is common in adults and children.
- Acute urticaria is most often idiopathic, but it may follow infection, exposure to drugs, or less commonly food ingestion.
- Acute urticaria may be a presenting symptom of anaphylaxis.
- Acute urticaria by definition resolves within 6 weeks, but it often settles within 2 to 3 weeks. It may recur in a small proportion of patients.
- Acute urticaria may be treated with antihistamines or oral steroids if needed.

INTRODUCTION

Urticaria consists of transient red itchy swellings, or weals. Swellings are variable in size and usually last for less than 24 hours. Acute urticaria is defined as the occurrence of weals for less than 6 weeks, after which the disease instead becomes chronic urticaria.[1]

Acute urticaria is common, and presents in all age groups.[2–4] Its transient and usually benign nature means that it may not come to the attention of doctors. Thus, the incidence may be underestimated, typical disease severity may be overestimated, the proportion with causative factors is difficult to ascertain, and the response to treatment is difficult to quantify. Such problems are compounded because patients also present to various different specialties, including generalists, emergency departments, pediatricians, immunologists or allergists, and dermatologists. This situation may explain why there are few publications including large cohorts of patients specifically with acute urticaria. However, the following article summarizes current knowledge on the condition.

EPIDEMIOLOGY

Acute urticaria is common in both adults and children. Indeed, it is one of the most common dermatologic conditions presenting to many emergency departments.[3,5,6]

Disclosures/Conflict of Interest: None.
Department of Dermatology, Royal Hallamshire Hospital, Sheffield Teaching Hospitals NHS Foundation Trust, Glossop Road, Sheffield S10 2JF, UK
E-mail address: rsabroe@doctors.org.uk

Immunol Allergy Clin N Am 34 (2014) 11–21
http://dx.doi.org/10.1016/j.iac.2013.07.010   immunology.theclinics.com

Overall, 12% to 22% of the general population will suffer from at least one subtype of urticaria at some time in their lives,[7–9] with a prevalence of 0.11% to 0.6%.[10,11] Of all patients with urticaria, only a low proportion of 7.6% to 16% have acute urticaria,[12–14] although in one study the percentage was much higher at 56%.[15] The variation may be related to the population studied and the interests of the department or doctor to whom patients are referred.

The age group studied may be particularly important, because acute urticaria seems to be more common than chronic disease in very young children. Indeed, in one report, all children presenting at less than age 6 months had acute urticaria, and 85% of children less than age 2 years had this subtype.[16] In older children, the ratio of chronic to acute urticaria seems to be similar to that in adults.[17–19]

The overall age range for presentation with acute urticaria is wide, in one study 3 months to 88 years,[2] with an average in the early twenties.[2–4]

Most,[2–4] but not all,[15] reports find a female preponderance of about 60%. However, in young children the male to female ratio may be roughly equal.[20–22]

ETIOLOGY

Attacks of acute urticaria are thought to be idiopathic in 30% to 50% of cases.[2,15,23,24] Otherwise attacks may be triggered by infections, drugs, or foodstuffs (**Table 1**). The relative proportion of patients with each precipitant varies from study to study.

In children, many studies find respiratory tract and other infections to be the most common trigger for urticaria.[22,24,25] The association with respiratory tract infections may be related to a seasonal variation in incidence.[25] Infections, of many types

Table 1
Some of the reported causes of acute urticaria

Cause		Reference
Idiopathic		2,15,23,24
Infection		
Viral	Adenovirus	26,56
	"Common cold"	4
	Cytomegalovirus	57
	Enterovirus	26,56,57
	Epstein-Barr	26,57
	Hepatitis A, B, C	56,58
	Herpes simplex	57,59
	Influenza A	57
	Parvovirus B19	57
	Respiratory syncytial virus	26
	Rotavirus	26
	Varicella/Zoster	26
Bacterial	Group A beta-hemolytic streptococcus	60,61
	Haemophilus influenzae	62
	Staphylococcus aureus	62
Other	*Anisakis simplex*	33
	Blastocystis hominis	63,64
	Malaria	65
	Mycoplasma	57,66
	Scabies	15

(continued on next page)

Table 1 (continued)		
Cause		**Reference**
Drugs	ACE inhibitors	67
	Antibiotics/anti-infective drugs, especially cephalosporins and penicillins	3,4,15,23,24,26,29,30,32
	Antihistamines	68
	Anti-TNF alpha drugs	69
	Aspirin and other nonsteroidal antiinflammatory drugs	3,4,15,24,26,30,53
	Blood products	70,71
	Candesartan	23
	Epidural hyaluronidase	72
	Gadolinium-containing radiocontrast media	73
	Intravenous immunoglobulins	74
	Iodine-based contrast agents, eg, iopromide	3,75
	Isotretinoin	76
	Methylprednisolone (oral)	77
	Opiates and tramadol	53,78
	Paracetamol	29,49,53
	Proton pump inhibitors	79
	Vaccination	2,80,81
Food	Cow's milk	16,17,24,26,82
	Egg	24,26
	Fish and seafood	3,17
	Fruit, eg, peach and kiwi	12,24,26
	Nuts	12,24,26
	Tomato and other vegetables	12,17
	Wheat	19
	Yeast	23
Other	"Gomutra" (cow's urine) gargle	83
	Hedgehog spines	84
	Insect bites or stings	2–4,15,23,24
	Latex	12,26
	Systemic lupus erythematosus	34
	Thyroid papillary carcinoma or other thyroid disease	23,85

(see **Table 1**), may also be associated with urticaria in adults.[2,4] However, it may be difficult to know if the urticaria was due to the infection itself or the drug used to treat it.[2,4,16,24,26]

Urticaria/angioedema is one of the most common types of drug-induced rash, and has been reported to account for 11.3% and 16.6% of drug eruptions in hospitalized patients aged 13 to 88 years and children, respectively.[27,28] It may be more common for a drug eruption to be of an urticarial nature in younger patients.[29] Urticaria may be more commonly drug induced in the elderly, especially due to nonsteroidal antiinflammatory drugs (NSAIDs).[3] Overall, drugs are reported as being the cause of acute urticaria in 9.2% to 27% of cases.[3,4] Multiple drugs have been implicated in acute urticarial reactions (see **Table 1**). In a recent study, 147 drugs were presumed to have caused attacks.[30] However, the most common are antibiotics and NSAIDs.[29,30] Reactions to one cephalosporin or one NSAID may or may not indicate cross-reactivity with other drugs in the same group.[31,32]

Various foodstuffs have been reported as causing urticaria (see **Table 1**). In children younger than 6 months, cow's milk allergy may be important.[16] However, generally food is implicated less often in more recent reports, with estimates of causality ranging from 0% to 18% of cases.[2–4,24]

Some other causes of acute urticaria are listed in **Table 1**, and include contact with latex,[12] insect bites or stings,[2,3,15,23] ingestion of the fish nematode *Anisakis simplex*,[33] and rarely acute urticaria may occur as part of a systemic disease such as systemic lupus erythematosus.[34] Acute contact urticaria is not covered in this article.

DISEASE MECHANISMS

The mechanism for mast cell degranulation in acute urticaria is not always understood.

In some cases, acute urticaria is due to a type I hypersensitivity reaction, in which case the urticaria may occur alone or as part of an anaphylactic reaction. A broad range of allergens may trigger urticaria in this way, including some antibiotics, latex, foodstuffs such as peanuts or tomatoes, and insect stings.[12] However, type I hypersensitivity reactions are now thought to be less common than before as an etiologic factor in acute urticaria.[4,24]

Other mechanisms are thought to be involved in mast cell degranulation in urticaria induced by opiates, angiotensin-converting enzyme (ACE) inhibitor, and NSAIDs. Opiates trigger mast cell degranulation independent of IgE receptor activation.[35] ACE inhibitor-induced urticaria may be due to elevated levels of bradykinin.[36]

In NSAID-induced urticaria, the arachidonic acid pathway is implicated, possibly with an inhibition of prostaglandin synthesis and an increase in leukotrienes.[37] There may be a genetic tendency for patients to develop aspirin sensitivity. Indeed, several promoter polymorphisms have been identified, such as in *TBXA2R* (the thromboxane A2 receptor) gene,[38] in the genes of aspirin-metabolizing enzymes,[39] and in other genes encoding enzymes and receptors of the arachidonic acid pathway.[40] In aspirin sensitivity, promoter polymorphisms have also been identified in some cytokine genes, including *IL-18*,[41] *IL-10*,[42] and *TNFα*.[43]

CLINICAL FEATURES

During an attack of acute urticaria, weals are variable in number and size. More than 50% of the body surface area may be involved, and in one study the rash was described as generalized in 48% patients.[3,4]

Urticarial weals may occur alone or with angioedema. Coexistent angioedema has been reported in 16% to 31% of patients[3,23] but may be more common in children younger than 3 years (60%) who may also get hemorrhagic weals.[16,26]

Systemic symptoms occur in up to a quarter of patients.[23] Wheezing, breathlessness, cough, rhinorrhea, dizziness, flushing, gastrointestinal upset (nausea, vomiting, diarrhea, or abdominal pain), headache, fever, tachycardia, joint pain, or conjunctivitis can occur with an attack of acute urticaria.[3,4] Such symptoms may indicate anaphylaxis if of rapid onset.

DIFFERENTIAL DIAGNOSIS

The key feature distinguishing urticaria from other rashes is the transient nature of the weals, and this usually makes it easy to diagnose within 24 to 36 hours. In addition, weals usually do not blister or form scales and disappear without residual changes. A detailed review of the differential diagnoses was published in 2010.[44]

The differential diagnosis includes the following:

- Erythema multiforme. Urticarial weals can sometimes clear centrally and spread out, giving an annular appearance. However, true target lesions do not occur in urticaria, and the lesions of erythema multiforme persist for several days in the same place, sometimes with central blisters and sometimes with associated mucous membrane erosions.

- Toxic erythema. The lesions of a toxic erythema may be urticated and so initially confused with urticaria, but the lesions are usually symmetric, and remain fixed in the same place for several days.
- Acute eczema or acute contact dermatitis. Eczema may be red and swollen, but unlike urticaria it is associated with epidermal changes (weeping or vesicle formation followed by scaling) and takes a few days to settle.
- Autoimmune bullous diseases. Prodromal lesions may be urticarial or urticated.
- Polymorphic eruption of pregnancy. This condition may present with urticated lesions, but the distribution on stretch marks on the abdomen and duration of the lesions, which again are more prolonged than in urticaria, should distinguish the two.
- Cellulitis or erysipelas. These can be confused with large urticarial weals, but involved areas are unilateral, persistent and painful and the patient may be pyrexial and unwell. Similarly, in Well's syndrome or eosinophilic cellulitis, the areas of redness persist, and here a skin biopsy may aid diagnosis.
- Progesterone-induced dermatosis. Here, weals recur premenstrually.
- Urticarial vasculitis. Prolonged urticarial weals followed by bruising may suggest urticarial vasculitis, especially if associated with systemic symptoms. A skin biopsy should then be taken to look for features suggestive of urticarial vasculitis, such as red cell extravasation, endothelial cell swelling, leukocytoclasia, and rarely fibrinoid necrosis.[45]
- Systemic lupus erythematosus. Urticaria or urticarial vasculitis may occur as a presenting feature of systemic lupus erythematosus, and so if other suspicious features are present, an autoimmune screen should be performed.
- Scrombroid fish poisoning. Acute urticaria may be a presenting symptom.[46]

INVESTIGATIONS

In many cases no investigations, other than a thorough history, are required (**Box 1**).[47] Overinvestigation should be avoided.

Sometimes a full blood count may be helpful, as alterations in the differential white cell count may indicate infection.

An elevated C-reactive protein (CRP) level and/or erythrocyte sedimentation rate may point toward an infective or inflammatory cause, and the CRP level may also be elevated in NSAID-induced urticaria.[48]

Box 1
Investigations to consider

Thorough history

? Nothing else

Full blood count, with differential white cell count

CRP level and/or erythrocyte sedimentation rate

Culture relevant specimens

Serum allergen-specific IgE tests

Prick tests

Oral drug challenge tests

Relevant samples should be sent for culture if infection is suspected.

If indicated, serum allergen-specific immunoglobulin E tests and/or prick tests may be used to investigate suspected type 1 hypersensitivity reactions.[47] To minimize risks of misinterpretation of false-positive and false-negative test results, careful correlation of exposure history and relevant ancillary allergic history is required.

It may be difficult to work out which drug if any was causative, particularly if several were given, or if drugs were given after an infection that might itself have caused the urticaria. On occasion, progression to skin prick or intradermal tests or structured oral drug challenge tests in a qualified immunology unit or expert center may be needed to correctly identify any culprit drugs and make relevant plans for possible future exposures.[31] Oral drug challenge tests may also be helpful in defining cross-reactivity between similar drugs.[31,32,49]

MANAGEMENT

In mild cases, treatment may not be required (**Box 2**). However, if an infection is present, this should be treated appropriately. Causative drugs should be withdrawn and known allergens avoided.

Topically, 1% to 2% menthol in aqueous cream may be helpful to reduce itching.[50]

If further treatment is needed, H1 receptor antagonists are usually introduced first.[47,51] Low sedating drugs are preferable, but if the patient is still unable to sleep, then sedating drugs, particularly hydroxyzine, may be beneficial for a short period.[2,4,52] The patient should be warned that such drugs may slow reactions when driving, even if they are not feeling sedated. Some patients known to develop urticaria after taking NSAIDs may be able to tolerate them if an antihistamine, or an antihistamine and a leukotriene receptor antagonist such as montelukast, is given beforehand.[53,54]

For severe urticaria, particularly if associated with angioedema or marked systemic symptoms, and provided infection is ruled out or treated, oral corticosteroids may be given for a few (3–5) days. Fairly high doses, up to 20 to 50 mg daily of prednisolone, are sometimes needed. Oral corticosteroids may shorten the duration of an attack and reduce symptom severity.[4,52]

If the urticaria is part of an anaphylactic reaction, then national guidelines and local protocols for anaphylaxis should be followed.[55] Intramuscular adrenaline, intravenous antihistamines, intravenous corticosteroids, oxygen, salbutamol, fluid replacement, and other supportive treatment may be needed.

Box 2
Management options to consider

? No treatment

Stop causative drugs

Avoid relevant allergens

Treat infection

Menthol, 1% to 2%, in aqueous cream

H1 antihistamines

Oral corticosteroids

Treatment of anaphylaxis according to guidelines

Medic alert bracelet

Self-injectable adrenaline

Medic Alert bracelets may be recommended if there is a confirmed type 1 hypersensitivity reaction, particularly if the urticaria has occurred as part of an anaphylactic reaction. In the latter case, self-injectable adrenaline may be carried provided the patient has been shown how to use it and is capable and willing to do so.[55]

PROGNOSIS

Most attacks of acute urticaria settle within 2 to 3 weeks.[2,4,22] In a study of 1075 children with urticaria, disease duration was shortest for infants and adolescents, but more prolonged attacks were associated with having an atopic background, an infective cause, or the presence of systemic symptoms.[22] This study also reported an association between short attack duration and the presence of angioedema. However, this finding was probably explained by the fact that children with angioedema were treated more aggressively, because the authors also found that aggressive management decreased episode length.[22]

Attacks may recur, particularly if the patient is inadvertently exposed to the same allergen or culprit drug. The percentage of children developing a second episode or chronic disease has been variously reported as 20% to 30% in 2 years[26] or 3.5% to 5% in 8 years.[21] In one study, 12% of 109 patients aged 5 to 86 years reported an attack of acute urticaria in the 10 years preceding the presenting episode, again indicating the possibility of recurrent episodes.[4] None of the patients in this study went on to develop chronic disease, but the follow-up period was only 8 weeks. In another study of 50 patients aged 3 months to 88 years, 5 patients went into remission at 3 months and 2 patients had disease for more than 1 year.[2] Overall, there are few reports documenting the proportion of patients progressing from acute to chronic disease.

SUMMARY

Acute urticaria is common in adults and children. It is a self-limiting condition, defined by its resolution within 6 weeks, although it usually disappears within 2 to 3 weeks. However, it may be recurrent and can progress to chronic disease. It is most often idiopathic but can be triggered by infection, drugs, and less frequently by foodstuffs. Although acute urticaria can occur as part of a type I hypersensitivity reaction, and sometimes as part of anaphylaxis, the mechanism leading to mast cell release is often unknown. The diagnosis is usually straightforward because of the transient nature of the urticarial weals, but it can be confused with several other conditions, especially in the first 24 hours. Investigations may be unnecessary. Management is aimed at removing or treating any cause, and symptom control, usually with H1 antihistamines. Anaphylaxis should be treated according to current guidelines.

REFERENCES

1. Zuberbier T, Asero R, Bindslev-Jensen C, et al. EAACI/GA(2)LEN/EDF/WAO guideline: definition, classification and diagnosis of urticaria. Allergy 2009;64: 1417–26.
2. Aoki T, Kojima M, Horiko T. Acute urticaria: history and natural course of 50 cases. J Dermatol 1994;21:73–7.
3. Simonart T, Askenasi R, Lheureux P. Particularities of urticaria seen in the emergency department. Eur J Emerg Med 1994;1:80–2.
4. Zuberbier T, Ifflander J, Semmler C, et al. Acute urticaria: clinical aspects and therapeutic responsiveness. Acta Derm Venereol 1996;76:295–7.

5. Wang E, Lim BL, Than KY. Dermatological conditions presenting at an emergency department in Singapore. Singapore Med J 2009;50:881–4.
6. Grillo E, Vano-Galvan S, Jimenez-Gomez N, et al. Dermatologic emergencies: descriptive analysis of 861 patients in a tertiary care teaching hospital. Actas Dermosifiliogr 2013;104:316–24.
7. McKee WD. The incidence and familial occurrence of allergy. J Allergy 1966;38: 226–35.
8. Sheldon JM, Mathews KP, Lovell RG. The vexing urticaria problem: present concepts of etiology and management. J Allergy 1954;25:525–60.
9. Swinny B. The atopic factor in urticaria. South Med J 1941;34:855–87.
10. Gaig P, Olona M, Munoz Lejarazu D, et al. Epidemiology of urticaria in Spain. J Investig Allergol Clin Immunol 2004;14:214–20.
11. Hellgren L. The prevalence of urticaria in the total population. Acta Allergol 1972;27:236–40.
12. Nettis E, Pannofino A, D'Aprile C, et al. Clinical and aetiological aspects in urticaria an angio-oedema. Br J Dermatol 2003;148:501–6.
13. Humphreys F, Hunter JA. The characteristics of urticaria in 390 patients. Br J Dermatol 1998;138:635–8.
14. Nizami RM, Baboo MT. Office management of patients with urticaria: an analysis of 215 patients. Ann Allergy 1974;33:78–85.
15. Sehgal VN, Rege VL. An interrogative study of 158 urticaria patients. Ann Allergy 1973;31:279–83.
16. Legrain V, Taieb A, Sage T, et al. Urticaria in infants: a study of forty patients. Pediatr Dermatol 1990;7:101–7.
17. Kauppinen K, Juntunen K, Lanki H. Urticaria in children. Retrospective evaluation and follow-up. Allergy 1984;39:469–72.
18. Ghosh S, Kanwar AJ, Kaur S. Urticaria in children. Pediatr Dermatol 1993;10: 107–10.
19. Sackesen C, Sekerel BE, Orhan F, et al. The etiology of different forms of urticaria in childhood. Pediatr Dermatol 2004;21:102–8.
20. Liu TH, Lin YR, Yang KC, et al. First attack of acute urticaria in pediatric emergency department. Pediatr Neonatol 2008;49:58–64.
21. Haas N, Birkle-Berlinger W, Henz BM. Prognosis of acute urticaria in children. Acta Derm Venereol 2005;85:74–5.
22. Lin YR, Liu TH, Wu TK, et al. Predictive factors of the duration of a first-attack acute urticaria in children. Am J Emerg Med 2011;29:883–9.
23. Kulthanan K, Chiawsirikajorn Y, Jiamton S. Acute urticaria: etiologies, clinical course and quality of life. Asian Pac J Allergy Immunol 2008;26:1–9.
24. Ricci G, Giannetti A, Belotti T, et al. Allergy is not the main trigger of urticaria in children referred to the emergency room. J Eur Acad Dermatol Venereol 2010; 24:1347–8.
25. Konstantinou GN, Papadopoulos NG, Tavladaki T, et al. Childhood acute urticaria in northern and southern Europe shows a similar epidemiological pattern and significant meteorological influences. Pediatr Allergy Immunol 2011;22: 36–42.
26. Mortureux P, Leaute-Labreze C, Legrain-Lifermann V, et al. Acute urticaria in infancy and early childhood: a prospective study. Arch Dermatol 1998;134:319–23.
27. Lee HY, Tay LK, Thirumoorthy T, et al. Cutaneous adverse drug reactions in hospitalised patients. Singapore Med J 2010;51:767–74.
28. Khaled A, Kharfi M, Ben Hamida M, et al. Cutaneous adverse drug reactions in children. A series of 90 cases. Tunis Med 2012;90:45–50.

29. Zhong H, Zhou Z, Wang H, et al. Prevalence of cutaneous adverse drug reactions in Southwest China: an 11-year retrospective survey on in-patients of a dermatology ward. Dermatitis 2012;23:81–5.
30. Rutnin NO, Kulthanan K, Tuchinda P, et al. Drug-induced urticaria: causes and clinical courses. J Drugs Dermatol 2011;10:1019–24.
31. Chaudhry T, Hissaria P, Wiese M, et al. Oral drug challenges in non-steroidal anti-inflammatory drug-induced urticaria, angioedema and anaphylaxis. Intern Med J 2012;42:665–71.
32. Pipet A, Veyrac G, Wessel F, et al. A statement on cefazolin immediate hypersensitivity: data from a large database, and focus on the cross-reactivities. Clin Exp Allergy 2011;41:1602–8.
33. Falcao H, Lunet N, Neves E, et al. Anisakis simplex as a risk factor for relapsing acute urticaria: a case-control study. J Epidemiol Community Health 2008;62: 634–7.
34. Cooper KD. Urticaria and angioedema: diagnosis and evaluation. J Am Acad Dermatol 1991;25:166–76.
35. Barke KE, Hough LB. Opiates, mast cells and histamine release. Life Sci 1993; 53:1391–9.
36. Caballero T, Baeza ML, Cabanas R, et al. Consensus statement on the diagnosis, management, and treatment of angioedema mediated by bradykinin. Part I. Classification, epidemiology, pathophysiology, genetics, clinical symptoms, and diagnosis. J Investig Allergol Clin Immunol 2011;21:333–47 [quiz follow: 347].
37. Nettis E, Dambra P. Comparison of montelukast and fexofenadine for chronic idiopathic urticaria. Arch Dermatol 2001;137:99–100.
38. Palikhe NS, Kim SH, Lee HY, et al. Association of thromboxane A2 receptor (TBXA2R) gene polymorphism in patients with aspirin-intolerant acute urticaria. Clin Exp Allergy 2011;41:179–85.
39. Palikhe NS, Kim SH, Nam YH, et al. Polymorphisms of aspirin-metabolizing enzymes CYP2C9, NAT2 and UGT1A6 in aspirin-intolerant urticaria. Allergy Asthma Immunol Res 2011;3:273–6.
40. Cornejo-Garcia JA, Jagemann LR, Blanca-Lopez N, et al. Genetic variants of the arachidonic acid pathway in non-steroidal anti-inflammatory drug-induced acute urticaria. Clin Exp Allergy 2012;42:1772–81.
41. Kim SH, Son JK, Yang EM, et al. A functional promoter polymorphism of the human IL18 gene is associated with aspirin-induced urticaria. Br J Dermatol 2011;165:976–84.
42. Palikhe NS, Kim SH, Jin HJ, et al. Association of interleukin 10 promoter polymorphism at -819 T>C with aspirin-induced urticaria in a Korean population. Ann Allergy Asthma Immunol 2011;107:544–6.
43. Choi JH, Kim SH, Cho BY, et al. Association of TNF-alpha promoter polymorphisms with aspirin-induced urticaria. J Clin Pharm Ther 2009;34:231–8.
44. Peroni A, Colato C, Schena D, et al. Urticarial lesions: if not urticaria, what else? The differential diagnosis of urticaria: part I. Cutaneous diseases. J Am Acad Dermatol 2010;62:541–55 [quiz: 555–6].
45. Mehregan DR, Hall MJ, Gibson LE. Urticarial vasculitis: a histopathologic and clinical review of 72 cases. J Am Acad Dermatol 1992;26:441–8.
46. Ward DI. 'Mass allergy': acute scombroid poisoning in a deployed Australian Defence Force health facility. Emerg Med Australas 2011;23:98–102.
47. Grattan CE, Humphreys F. Guidelines for evaluation and management of urticaria in adults and children. Br J Dermatol 2007;157:1116–23.

48. Kasperska-Zajac A, Grzanka A, Czecior E, et al. Acute phase inflammatory markers in patients with non-steroidal anti-inflammatory drugs (NSAIDs)-induced acute urticaria/angioedema and after aspirin challenge. J Eur Acad Dermatol Venereol 2013;27(8):1048–52.
49. Rutkowski K, Nasser SM, Ewan PW. Paracetamol hypersensitivity: clinical features, mechanism and role of specific IgE. Int Arch Allergy Immunol 2012;159:60–4.
50. Bromm B, Scharein E, Darsow U, et al. Effects of menthol and cold on histamine-induced itch and skin reactions in man. Neurosci Lett 1995;187:157–60.
51. Zuberbier T, Greaves MW, Juhlin L, et al. Management of urticaria: a consensus report. J Investig Dermatol Symp Proc 2001;6:128–31.
52. Pollack CV Jr, Romano TJ. Outpatient management of acute urticaria: the role of prednisone. Ann Emerg Med 1995;26:547–51.
53. Asero R. Cetirizine premedication prevents acute urticaria induced by weak COX-1 inhibitors in multiple NSAID reactors. Eur Ann Allergy Clin Immunol 2010;42:174–7.
54. Nosbaum A, Braire-Bourrel M, Dubost R, et al. Prevention of nonsteroidal inflammatory drug-induced urticaria and/or angioedema. Ann Allergy Asthma Immunol 2013;110:263–6.
55. Simons FE, Ardusso LR, Bilo MB, et al. World Allergy Organization anaphylaxis guidelines: summary. J Allergy Clin Immunol 2011;127:587–93.e1–22.
56. Weston WL, Badgett JT. Urticaria. Pediatr Rev 1998;19:240–4.
57. Bilbao A, Garcia JM, Pocheville I, et al. Round table: urticaria in relation to infections. Allergol Immunopathol (Madr) 1999;27:73–85 [in Spanish].
58. van Aalsburg R, de Pagter AP, van Genderen PJ. Urticaria and periorbital edema as prodromal presenting signs of acute hepatitis B infection. J Travel Med 2011;18:224–5.
59. Zawar V, Godse K. Recurrent facial urticaria following herpes simplex labialis. Indian J Dermatol 2012;57:144–5.
60. Schuller DE, Elvey SM. Acute urticaria associated with streptococcal infection. Pediatrics 1980;65:592–6.
61. Calado G, Loureiro G, Machado D, et al. Streptococcal tonsillitis as a cause of urticaria: tonsillitis and urticaria. Allergol Immunopathol (Madr) 2012;40:341–5.
62. Sakurai M, Oba M, Matsumoto K, et al. Acute infectious urticaria: clinical and laboratory analysis in nineteen patients. J Dermatol 2000;27:87–93.
63. Hameed DM, Hassanin OM, Zuel-Fakkar NM. Association of Blastocystis hominis genetic subtypes with urticaria. Parasitol Res 2011;108:553–60.
64. Zuel-Fakkar NM, Abdel Hameed DM, Hassanin OM. Study of Blastocystis hominis isolates in urticaria: a case-control study. Clin Exp Dermatol 2011;36:908–10.
65. Godse KV, Zawar V. Malaria presenting as urticaria. Indian J Dermatol 2012;57:237–8.
66. Kano Y, Mitsuyama Y, Hirahara K, et al. Mycoplasma pneumoniae infection-induced erythema nodosum, anaphylactoid purpura, and acute urticaria in 3 people in a single family. J Am Acad Dermatol 2007;57:S33–5.
67. Inman WH, Rawson NS, Wilton LV, et al. Postmarketing surveillance of enalapril. I: results of prescription-event monitering. Br Med J 1988;297:826–9.
68. Bobadilla-Gonzalez P, Perez-Rangel I, Camara-Hijon C, et al. Positive basophil activation test result in a patient with acute urticaria induced by cetirizine and desloratadine. Ann Allergy Asthma Immunol 2011;106:258–9.
69. de Moraes JC, Aikawa NE, Ribeiro AC, et al. Immediate complications of 3,555 injections of anti-TNFalpha. Rev Bras Reumatol 2010;50:165–75.

70. Henderson RA, Pinder L. Acute transfusion reactions. N Z Med J 1990;103: 509–11.
71. Shemin D, Briggs D, Greenan M. Complications of therapeutic plasma exchange: a prospective study of 1,727 procedures. J Clin Apher 2007;22:270–6.
72. Kim JH, Choi GS, Ye YM, et al. Acute urticaria caused by the injection of goat-derived hyaluronidase. Allergy Asthma Immunol Res 2009;1:48–50.
73. Dillman JR, Ellis JH, Cohan RH, et al. Frequency and severity of acute allergic-like reactions to gadolinium-containing i.v. contrast media in children and adults. AJR Am J Roentgenol 2007;189:1533–8.
74. Hamrock DJ. Adverse events associated with intravenous immunoglobulin therapy. Int Immunopharmacol 2006;6:535–42.
75. Palkowitsch P, Lengsfeld P, Stauch K, et al. Safety and diagnostic image quality of iopromide: results of a large non-interventional observational study of European and Asian patients (IMAGE). Acta Radiol 2012;53:179–86.
76. Saray Y, Seckin D. Angioedema and urticaria due to isotretinoin therapy. J Eur Acad Dermatol Venereol 2006;20:118–20.
77. Jang EJ, Jin HJ, Nam YH, et al. Acute urticaria induced by oral methylprednisolone. Allergy Asthma Immunol Res 2011;3:277–9.
78. Nasser SM, Ewan PW. Opiate-sensitivity: clinical characteristics and the role of skin prick testing. Clin Exp Allergy 2001;31:1014–20.
79. Chang YS. Hypersensitivity reactions to proton pump inhibitors. Curr Opin Allergy Clin Immunol 2012;12:348–53.
80. Humphreys F. Acute urticaria and angio-oedema following *Haemophilus influenzae* b vaccination. Br J Dermatol 1994;131:582–3.
81. Barbaud A, Trechot P, Reichert-Penetrat S, et al. Allergic mechanisms and urticaria/angioedema after hepatitis B immunization. Br J Dermatol 1998;139: 925–6.
82. Caffarelli C, Baldi F, Bendandi B, et al. Cow's milk protein allergy in children: a practical guide. Ital J Pediatr 2010;36:5.
83. Bhalla M, Thami GP. Acute urticaria following 'gomutra' (cow's urine) gargles. Clin Exp Dermatol 2005;30:722–3.
84. Fairley JA, Suchniak J, Paller AS. Hedgehog hives. Arch Dermatol 1999;135: 561–3.
85. Kartal O, Abdullah B, Ramazan E, et al. Acute urticaria associated with thyroid papillary carcinoma: a case report. Ann Dermatol 2012;24:453–4.

Angioedema

Konrad Bork, MD

KEYWORDS

- Urticaria • Angioedema • Histamine • Bradykinin • Hereditary angioedema
- Acquired angioedema • C1 esterase inhibitor • Factor XII gene mutations

KEY POINTS

- Wheals of urticaria and angioedema are due to short-lived edema in different layers of the skin, and differ in clinical and pathogenetic respects.
- The factors involved in the opening and closure of endothelial cell-cell adherens junctions, which are largely composed of vascular endothelial cadherin, are still unknown in urticaria and angioedema.
- In the spectrum urticaria/angioedema, 3 groups of diseases can be differentiated: diseases with urticaria and angioedema, diseases with angioedema alone, and diseases with urticarial lesions without angioedema.

INTRODUCTION

Urticaria and angioedema have several features in common, some of which are clinical. Both are based on a relatively short-lived edema in the skin and may be associated with edema episodes of other organs. Urticarial wheals and angioedema may be single or multiple. The individual lesion of either may persist for from a few hours to some days. Both belong to various disease entities (**Table 1**), and may occur in combination or in isolation. Local vasodilation and increased vascular permeability are the main changes in urticaria and angioedema.

PATHOPHYSIOLOGY
Common Pathophysiologic Features

Single urticaria and angioedema lesions have a localized fluid extravasation in common. The plasma passes through the vessel wall and, when extravascular, becomes interstitial fluid. The passage through the interstitial gaps of the endothelial cells has attracted more attention in recent years. Endothelial cells control the passage of plasma constituents from blood to underlying tissues. Endothelial permeability is mediated by transcellular and paracellular pathways (**Fig. 1**), which means that blood

The author has received consultancy fees from CSL Behring, Shire, and ViroPharma.
Department of Dermatology, Johannes Gutenberg University, Langenbeckstr. 1, 55131 Mainz, Germany
E-mail address: bork@hautklinik.klinik.uni-mainz.de

Table 1
Diseases with urticaria and/or angioedema

Diseases with Urticaria Combined with Angioedema	Diseases with Angioedema and Without Urticaria	Diseases with Urticaria and Without Angioedema
Acute urticaria	Hereditary angioedema due to C1-INH deficiency (HAE-C1-INH); types I and II	Cholinergic urticaria
Chronic spontaneous urticaria	Hereditary angioedema with normal C1-INH (HAE-nCl; HAE type III), subtypes HAE-FXII and HAE-unknown	Factitial urticaria
Cold urticaria	Acquired angioedema with C1-INH deficiency (AAE-C1-INH)	Delayed-pressure urticaria
Urticarial vasculitis	Angioedema due to ACE inhibitors (AE-ACEI)	Heat contact urticaria
Exercise-induced anaphylaxis/urticaria	Angioedema with unknown cause (AE-UC) responsive to antihistamines (AE-UC-h) or unresponsive to antihistamines (AE-UC-nh)	Solar urticaria
Episodic angioedema with eosinophilia		Aquagenic urticaria
Vibration-induced urticaria/angioedema		Contact urticaria

Abbreviations: ACE, angiotensin-converting enzyme; C1-INH, C1-inhibitor.

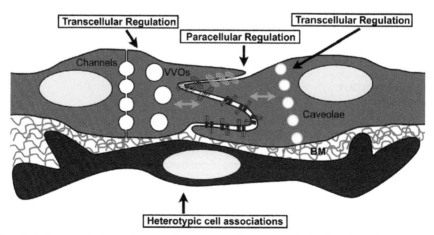

Fig. 1. Pathways that regulate barrier function in endothelial cells. The scheme shows 2 endothelial cells and the subendothelial space. Vascular permeability is regulated and maintained through 3 compartments: paracellular junctions (adherent and junctional complexes), transcellular pathways, and heterotopic cell interactions (usually pericytes). The details of this cross-talk remain largely unclear. BM, basement membrane; VVOs, vesiculovacuolar organelles. (*From* Goddard LM, Iruela-Arispe ML. Cellular and molecular regulation of vascular permeability. Thromb Haemost 2013;109:408; with permission.)

constituents may pass through or between endothelial cells. The paracellular pathway is mediated by the coordinated opening and closure of endothelial cell-cell adherens junctions. These junctions are largely composed of vascular endothelial cadherin (VE-cadherin), an endothelium-specific member of the cadherin family of adhesion protein that may bind to several protein partners.[1] The barrier between the bloodstream and tissues may be influenced not only by endothelial cells but also by other mural cells. These endothelial-associated cells, pericytes, smooth muscle cells, and macrophages, might not form a permanent sheath, but instead are dynamically associated with capillaries and functional participants of the "vascular unit."[2]

The exact mechanism of edema formation at the vascular level in urticaria and angioedema is still unknown, and this also holds true for the mechanism of reabsorption of the fluid after hours to days.

Different Pathophysiologic Features

Urticaria and angioedema belong to various disease entities. Both are complex reactions and occur through various pathogenetic pathways. Some types of angioedema may be hereditary and others not; this is also true for urticaria. Wheals and angioedema are clinically different lesions. The underlying process concerns superficial vessels in urticaria and deep vessels in angioedema. The structural or functional differences of the vessels leading to the different clinical signs are not known. Some of the diseases forms are described here.

Urticaria

A wheal is a single lesion of an urticaria, and is a short-living edema of the upper and mid-dermal layer of the skin, with dilation of the postcapillary venules and lymphatic vessels of the upper dermis. Urticaria is a mast-cell–driven disease, the pathogenesis of which is complex. The release of histamine from dermal mast cells plays a major role. After activation, the cutaneous mast cells release preformed mediators such as histamine, heparin, proteases, newly formed mediators such as prostaglandins and leukotrienes, and cytokines such as tumor necrosis factor α and interleukin-8. The mediators released from activated mast cells result in sensory nerve activation, vasodilation, and plasma extravasation, as well as cell recruitment to urticarial lesions. The mast-cell–activating signals in urticaria are ill defined and are likely to be heterogeneous and diverse.

Angioedema

Angioedema is a short-lived edema in the deep dermal layer of the skin and the subcutaneous tissue. Similar edema episodes may occur in the submucosal tissue of various organs. Little is known about the pathogenesis of angioedema associated with the clinical subtypes of urticaria. Histamine might play a major role. Many patients with angioedema associated with chronic spontaneous urticaria (CSU) respond to antihistamines, partially or completely. This finding confirms that histamine is involved at least in part in angioedema in patients with CSU. To date it remains unknown as to which other mediators are involved in angioedema of CSU. Bradykinin does not seem to play a major role in the pathogenesis of angioedema associated with urticaria.

In recurrent angioedema alone (ie, without urticaria), the vasoactive mediator bradykinin is clearly involved, at least in most of the diseases. Bradykinin is a vasoactive nonapeptide. High bradykinin levels in plasma may result from an overproduction of bradykinin caused by activation of the kallikrein-kinin system, or may result from an inhibited degradation of bradykinin. The role of the involvement of bradykinin and other mediators in the various angioedema diseases is discussed later in this article.

CLINICAL FEATURES
Urticaria

A wheal is a single lesion of an urticaria. The clinical manifestation of this circumscribed lesion depends, among other factors, on properties of the tissue. Swellings of thin skin with a thin dermis and a loose subcutaneous tissue may appear as larger and not well-circumscribed lesions, as seen in the regions of the eyelids and the genitals, similarly to angioedema.

Angioedema

Angioedema is a diffuse swelling of deeper skin layers. Under the heading of angioedema in a broader sense, swellings of other organs are subsumed, including self-limiting edema attacks of the gastrointestinal tract and laryngeal edema.

DISEASES WITH URTICARIA AND/OR ANGIOEDEMA
Diseases with Urticaria Combined with Angioedema

Acute spontaneous urticaria or acute urticaria

An acute urticaria is a frequent reaction, persisting for less than 6 weeks by definition, in most patients lasting only 1 day or a few days.

Usually it is a "one-off" occurrence, with recurrences only occurring on repeated exposure. The usual triggers are infections, foods, drugs including acetylsalicylic acid and other nonsteroidal anti-inflammatories, and insect stings and bites. In less than 50% the trigger remains unknown.

In this common type of urticaria, angioedema is a frequent symptom. However, the exact incidence is unknown and is difficult to determine. Probably less than 50% of cases are associated with an angioedema. Angioedema usually occurs in the form of facial swelling, which usually responds to corticosteroids and antihistamines.

Chronic spontaneous urticaria

Angioedema is a frequent symptom of CSU. Because CSU is a frequent disease (about 1%–5% of the population are affected), angioedema associated with CSU is a considerable clinical problem.

Angioedema in CSU may occur as an angioedema of the skin or as a gastrointestinal edema (rare), a tongue edema, or an edema of the upper airways. In more than 50% of patients with CSU, recurrent angioedema of the skin or other organs occurs in addition to urticarial lesions. An urticaria without angioedema occurs in about 30% to 40% of patients with CSU. About 10% of patients have recurrent angioedema without or nearly without an urticaria. However, the precise percentages of patients with urticaria alone or with angioedema with concurrent urticaria or with angioedema alone vary within different studies.[3–7]

Angioedema associated with CSU is most frequently localized in the eye region, lips, and tongue. Less frequently hands, feet, and genitals are affected. Associated symptoms such as fever, headache, arthralgia, gastrointestinal symptoms, and dyspnea may occur. Angioedema may occur when hives are present or at times when hives are not present.

Thus there are 2 different lesions in CSU, urticarial lesions and angioedema. Both may respond to antihistamines, which is true for a large proportion of patients. However, in other patients with CSU antihistamines do not work for either the urticaria or angioedema component.

Accordingly, the mediator for angioedema in CSU is histamine in many patients. Obviously, however, further mediators are involved (see earlier discussion), although their exact role in the development of the cutaneous edema of hives and angioedema is unknown at present. Antihistamines may not work at low doses, but may be effective at higher doses. Omalizumab is a chimeric monoclonal antibody that works by reducing circulating free immunoglobulin (Ig)E, thereby reducing expression and function of FceR1 on mast cells and basophils. It has shown to be effective in patients with CSU (urticarial lesions and angioedema) who exhibited IgE against thyroperoxidase.[8]

Cold urticaria
In cold urticaria, urticarial lesions and angioedema occur after exposure to cold. In more than 70% of patients the urticarial lesions are combined with angioedema.

Urticarial vasculitis
Urticarial vasculitis is a rare disease, characterized histopathologically by vessel-wall necrosis, which is a hallmark of this disease. Urticaria-like skin lesions with a faint residual pigmentation, and systemic symptoms including arthralgia and renal and lung involvement are frequent. Angioedema often occurs concurrently with urticarial vasculitis.

Exercise-induced anaphylaxis/urticaria
Exercise-induced urticaria/anaphylaxis (EIA) is a special entity. Urticarial lesions with or without angioedema may occur; more rarely, recurrent angioedema alone may also occur.

Episodic angioedema with eosinophilia (Gleich syndrome)
Episodic angioedema with eosinophilia is defined by bouts of angioedema, urticaria, fever, weight gain, eosinophilia, and an increase in IgM.[9]

Vibration-induced urticaria/angioedema
In rare cases, vibratory forces lead to urticaria or angioedema. This condition has been observed in patients after working with a pneumatic hammer, bicycling on cobbles, using massage devices, and playing musical instruments.

Diseases with Angioedema and Without Urticaria

Hereditary angioedema due to C1-inhibitor deficiency
Hereditary angioedema (HAE) due to C1-INH deficiency (HAE-C1-INH) is a rare disease with an autosomal dominant pattern of inheritance.

C1-INH controls the spontaneous autoactivation of the first complement component (C1) and activated C1. A deficiency in functional C1-INH leads to activation of the initial phase of the complement system, resulting in a permanent reduction of plasma levels of C4. It is now known, however, that it is the inhibitory effect of C1-INH not on the complement system, but on the kallikrein-kinin system, that has the essential pathogenetic role in HAE-C1-INH. C1-INH is responsible for the inhibition of the greater part of plasma kallikrein and factor XIIa, and is thus the most important regulator of activation of the kallikrein-kinin system. During acute attacks of HAE, kallikrein is insufficiently inhibited because of the deficiency in C1-INH, the kallikrein-kinin system (contact system) becomes activated, and at the end of the cascade there is an increased amount of bradykinin, the main mediator of increased vascular permeability, and hence of the edema seen in HAE-C1-INH.

Clinically, HAE-C1-INH is characterized by recurring swelling of the skin (extremities, face, genitals), gastrointestinal attacks (painful abdominal cramps, mostly accompanied by circulatory symptoms caused by hypotension, sometimes vomiting, and diarrhea), and by edema of the larynx and other organs. Urticaria does not belong to the clinical signs of HAE-C1-INH. Among the 420 patients with HAE-C1-INH surveyed at the Angioedema Outpatient Service in Mainz, only 2 patients have additional urticaria.

HAE-C1-INH manifests most often early in the second decade of life, also frequently in the first, and in a few patients in the third decade or even later. Recurring attacks of edema follow, the frequency of which varies greatly from patient to patient. In one study series, about 70% of patients had 12 attacks or fewer per year, and 30% more than 12 attacks.[10]

Attacks are triggered by trauma, pressure, situations of psychological stress, menstruation, ovulation, or infectious diseases. The tendency to edema attacks can be greatly increased by ingestion of angiotensin-converting enzyme (ACE) inhibitors; these are contraindicated in patients with HAE. Angiotensin convertase II (ATII) receptor blockers can also increase a tendency to edema attacks, albeit more rarely. In the same way, attacks may become more frequent in women receiving estrogen in contraceptives or as hormone replacement therapy.[11]

Hereditary angioedema with normal C1-INH

In 2000, a novel type of HAE was described that was not associated with C1-INH deficiency and occurred mainly in women.[12] All patients had normal C1-INH concentration and activity with respect to C1 esterase inhibition and normal C4, ruling out both types of HAE-C1-INH (HAE-C1-INH types I and II). This hitherto unknown disease was proposed to be termed "hereditary angioedema with normal C1 inhibitor" (HAEnCI) or "hereditary angioedema type III." HAEnCI is autosomally inherited with incomplete phenotypical penetrance.[12]

In 2006, 2 different missense mutations in a nonconservative gene region were identified in German patients, located in exon 9 of the gene coding for the coagulation factor XII (Hageman factor).[13] In 2011 a further HAE mutation was identified, a large deletion of 72 base pairs (c.971_1018+24del72).[14] To date, numerous families have been reported that include members having HAEnCI, with affected women bearing these mutations (HAE-FXII). The clinical symptoms of HAEnCI include recurrent skin swellings, abdominal pain attacks, tongue swellings, and laryngeal edema. Urticarial lesions do not belong to the clinical symptoms of HAEnCI. Oral contraceptives, pregnancy, and hormone replacement therapy often play a particular role as triggering or aggravating factors. HAEnCI has been observed predominantly in women, but male patients have been reported. Antihistamines and corticosteroids are not effective. Icatibant, a bradykinin-B2 receptor antagonist, and C1-inhibitor concentrate, as well as tranexamic acid and danazol, are effective, at least in some patients.[15]

Acquired angioedema with C1-INH deficiency

This form of angioedema is seen in patients whose C1-INH deficiency is due to increased C1-INH catabolism. Accordingly, C1q is usually decreased. The symptoms are the same as those of HAE-C1-INH.[16] In a significant proportion of these patients there is an underlying B-cell disorder (eg, monoclonal gammopathy of unknown significance or malignant lymphoma), and it can often happen that angioedema is the presenting feature of lymphoreticular disease. In some patients autoantibodies against C1-INH are found.[17]

Angioedema due to ACE inhibitors

Approximately 0.1% to 2.2% of patients treated with ACE inhibitors develop recurrent angioedema, often facial or lip swelling or edema of the tongue (angioedema induced by ACE inhibitors, AE-ACEI).[18,19] Several cases of death by asphyxiation following closure of the upper airways have been reported.[20] The interval between the start of treatment with and the appearance of the first angioedema can be months or several years, so that the causal connection between the angioedema and the triggering ACE inhibitors is sometimes unrecognized or recognized late. Because of the enormously high use of ACE inhibitors, cases of AE-ACEI are not rare. ATII receptor blockers can also trigger the same forms of angioedema, though more rarely. Occasionally chronic urticaria is associated with AE-ACEI.

Angioedema with unknown cause (idiopathic angioedema)
Angioedema of unknown cause (AE-UC), or idiopathic angioedema, is the name given to cases of angioedema that cannot be identified as any of the recognized forms of angioedema. In these cases, none of the patient's relatives are affected, C1-INH deficiency is not present, and the angioedema cannot be determined to be caused by drugs or any other triggers. Knowledge about the pathogenesis and treatment of this form of angioedema is still very limited.[21] It is one of the most frequent forms of angioedema and is therefore important in daily practice.

Some of these cases respond to antihistamines and corticosteroids, either at normal or higher doses. The name "idiopathic histaminergic angioedema" has been proposed for this type of angioedema.[22] The author prefers the name "angioedema of unknown cause responding to antihistamines" (AE-UC-h). This type of recurrent angioedema obviously is mast-cell driven. Most probably these cases correspond to antihistamine-sensitive CSU.

The problem may arise that angioedema does not respond to antihistamines, even at high doses. The author prefers the name "angioedema of unknown cause not responding to antihistamines" (AE-UC-nh) for this condition. The response to antihistamine is a clinical feature pointing toward the pathomechanism. If patients with AE-UC do not respond to antihistamines, other pathomechanisms can be taken into consideration. It is possible that subtypes exist according to the following pathomechanisms. First, recurrent angioedema could develop from mast-cell mediators other than histamine. This type of angioedema might correspond to those patients with CSU who do not respond to antihistamines. Second, the main mediator could be bradykinin. In bradykinin-induced angioedema, such as HAE-C1-INH, AAE-C1-INH, and HAE-nCl (HAE type III), histamine plays a minor role, if any. Accordingly, urticarial lesions are usually not observed in these diseases. If bradykinin was the main mediator in AE-UC-nh, a response to icatibant would be expected. Information about this proposal is still sparse. Third, other and hitherto unknown pathways might play a role that differs from that of from mast-cell mediators and bradykinin.

Diseases with Urticaria Without Angioedema
Several forms of urticaria are not associated with angioedema.

Cholinergic urticaria
Cholinergic urticaria is a frequent form of urticaria, clinically characterized by tiny urticarial lesions that occur simultaneously with or shortly after an increase of body core temperature attributable to physical exercise or spicy food. In most patients the lesions do not occur in the face. In severely affected patients, however, the face may also be involved and swollen, simulating angioedema. In rare cases, patients may contract angioedema of the skin or mucous membranes.[23]

Factitial urticaria
Further subtypes of urticaria without angioedema include factitial urticaria (dermographic urticaria) and delayed-pressure urticaria.

Delayed-pressure urticaria

Delayed-pressure urticaria is clinically characterized by localized deep erythematous skin swellings developing 3 to 12 hours after pressure. The lesions persist for up to 2 days. Although of delayed-pressure urticaria involves deep swelling of the skin, it is not identical to angioedema.

Other subtypes of urticaria

Heat-contact urticaria and solar urticaria are usually not associated with angioedema. The same is true for aquagenic urticaria and contact urticaria elicited by contact with urticariogenic substances.

REFERENCES

1. Dejana E, Orsenigo F, Lampugnani MG. The role of adherens junctions and VE-cadherin in the control of vascular permeability. J Cell Sci 2008;121:2115–22.
2. Goddard LM, Iruela-Arispe ML. Cellular and molecular regulation of vascular permeability. Thromb Haemost 2013;109:407–15.
3. Quaranta JH, Rohr AS, Rachelefsky GS, et al. The natural history and response to therapy of chronic urticaria and angioedema. Ann Allergy 1989;62:421–4.
4. Champion RH, Roberts SO, Carpenter RG, et al. A review of 554 patients. Br J Dermatol 1969;81:588–97.
5. Sabroe RA, Seed PT, Francis DM, et al. Chronic idiopathic urticaria: comparison of the clinical features of patients with and without anti-FcepsilonRI or anti-IgE autoantibodies. J Am Acad Dermatol 1999;40:443–50.
6. Kaplan AP. Clinical practice. Chronic urticaria and angioedema. N Engl J Med 2002;346:175–9.
7. Juhlin L. Recurrent urticaria: clinical investigation of 330 patients. Br J Dermatol 1981;104:369–81.
8. Maurer M, Altrichter S, Bieber T, et al. Efficacy and safety of omalizumab in patients with chronic urticaria who exhibit IgE against thyroperoxidase. J Allergy Clin Immunol 2011;128:202–9.
9. Gleich GJ, Schroeter AL, Marcoux JP, et al. Episodic angioedema associated with eosinophilia. N Engl J Med 1984;310:1621–6.
10. Agostoni A, Cicardi M. Hereditary and acquired C1-inhibitor deficiency: biological and clinical characteristics in 235 patients. Medicine (Baltimore) 1992;71:206–15.
11. Bork K, Fischer B, Dewald G. Recurrent episodes of skin angioedema and severe attacks of abdominal pain induced by oral contraceptives or hormone replacement therapy. Am J Med 2003;114:294–8.
12. Bork K, Barnstedt SE, Koch P, et al. Hereditary angioedema with normal C1-inhibitor activity in women. Lancet 2000;356:213–7.
13. Dewald G, Bork K. Missense mutations in the coagulation factor XII (Hageman factor) gene in hereditary angioedema with normal C1 inhibitor. Biochem Biophys Res Commun 2006;343:1286–9.
14. Bork K, Wulff K, Meinke P, et al. A novel mutation in the coagulation factor 12 gene in subjects with hereditary angioedema and normal C1-inhibitor. Clin Immunol 2011;141:31–5.
15. Bork K. Diagnosis and treatment of hereditary angioedema with normal C1 inhibitor. Allergy Asthma Clin Immunol 2010;6:15.
16. Zingale LC, Castelli R, Zanichelli A, et al. Acquired deficiency of the inhibitor of the first complement component: presentation, diagnosis, course, and conventional management. Immunol Allergy Clin North Am 2006;26:669–90.

17. Alsenz J, Bork K, Loos M. Autoantibody-mediated acquired deficiency of C1 inhibitor. N Engl J Med 1987;316:1360–6.
18. Sabroe RA, Black AK. Angiotensin-converting enzyme (ACE) inhibitors and angio-oedema. Br J Dermatol 1997;136:153–8.
19. Byrd JB, Adam A, Brown NJ. Angiotensin-converting enzyme inhibitor-associated angioedema. Immunol Allergy Clin North Am 2006;26:725–37.
20. Dean DE, Schultz DL, Powers RH. Asphyxia due to angiotensin converting enzyme (ACE) inhibitor mediated angioedema of the tongue during the treatment of hypertensive heart disease. J Forensic Sci 2001;46:1239–43.
21. Frigas E, Park M. Idiopathic recurrent angioedema. Immunol Allergy Clin North Am 2006;26:739–51.
22. Zingale LC, Beltrami L, Zanichelli A, et al. Angioedema without urticaria: a large clinical survey. CMAJ 2006;175:1065–70.
23. Lawrence CM, Jorizzo JL, Kobza-Black A, et al. Cholinergic urticaria with associated angio-oedema. Br J Dermatol 1981;105:543–50.

Chronic Spontaneous Urticaria
Etiology and Pathogenesis

Sarbjit S. Saini, MD

KEYWORDS

- Chronic urticaria • Mast cells • Basophils

KEY POINTS

- Acute urticaria occurs in up to 20% of the population, and may be associated with a drug or food allergy or with infection. It is generally self-limited.
- Chronic urticaria affects up to 1% of the population, and in most cases lesions occur spontaneously without an identifiable external cause.
- Approximately 20% of patients with chronic urticaria have a reproducible physical trigger for their skin lesions, termed physical urticaria.
- There are multiple theories of pathogenesis for chronic urticaria, none of which is clearly established. One theory is that a subset has an autoantibody-mediated disease process.
- Abnormalities in skin mast cells and blood basophils have been described in chronic urticaria.

INTRODUCTION

Urticaria, also known as hives, is a very common condition thought to affect up to 20% of the population in their lifetime.[1] This skin condition is characterized by the appearance of pruritic, erythematous papules or plaques with superficial swelling of the dermis. The major complaint is the symptom of pruritus. Urticaria can be classified by both time course of symptoms and the underlying etiology. Acute urticaria is defined as having skin-symptom duration of less than 6 weeks, whereas chronic urticaria (CU) is generally defined by the presence of urticaria on most days of the week for a period of 6 weeks or longer.

CU is further classified by additional criteria. Approximately one-fifth of CU patients have a clear-cut physical trigger for their skin eruptions, therefore it is termed physical urticaria. These cases are labeled according to the nature of the inciting stimulus

Disclosure: Grant Support: Novartis, Genentech, Astra Zeneca, National Institutes of Health, Advisory Board/Consultant: Novartis, Genentech, Regeneron, MedImmune, Kendle.
Division of Allergy and Clinical Immunology, Johns Hopkins University School of Medicine, Johns Hopkins Asthma and Allergy Center, 5501 Hopkins Bayview Circle, Room 2B. 71B, Baltimore, MD 21224, USA
E-mail address: ssaini@jhmi.edu

Immunol Allergy Clin N Am 34 (2014) 33–52
http://dx.doi.org/10.1016/j.iac.2013.09.012
0889-8561/14/$ – see front matter

(**Table 1**; see also the article by Maurer and colleagues elsewhere in this issue).[2,3] Among the causative physical factors are dermographism, delayed-pressure urticaria, cholinergic urticaria, cold- and heat-contact urticaria, solar urticaria, aquagenic urticaria, exercise-induced urticaria, and vibratory urticaria. In the remaining 80% of CU, no external allergen or contributing disease process is identified and, thus, the condition is termed chronic idiopathic urticaria (CIU), which has also more recently been labeled as chronic spontaneous urticaria (CSU).[4] Approximately 40% of patients with CIU/CSU will also report accompanying episodes of angioedema or deeper swelling of dermal or mucosal tissues, whereas 10% have angioedema as their main manifestation.[5,6] In this review, the terms CSU and CIU are used synonymously. Some guidelines and experts further divide CIU/CSU patients based on serologic evidence of a presumed autoimmune etiology (observed in 30%–40% of these subjects), and call the condition chronic autoimmune urticaria (CAU). In this setting, the remaining 60% to 70% of patients are classified as CIU/CSU.[4,7]

EPIDEMIOLOGY

Given that the lifetime risk of an episode of urticaria is 20% to 25%, several conditions have been noted to be associated with urticaria. In acute urticaria, 20% of cases have

Table 1
Physical urticaria subtypes, triggers, and testing procedures

Disorder	Trigger Factor	Test Description
Dermographism (urticaria factitia)	Stroking, scratching, pressure	Mild stroking of skin with tip of pen or tongue blade, or dermatographer
Delayed-pressure urticaria	Application of pressure 30 min to 12 h before onset	Shoulder sling placed for 15 min weighing 7 kg; patient records symptoms over 24 h
Cholinergic urticaria	Elevation of body temperature with exercise, hot water, strong emotion, or spicy food	Exercise with a stationary bike for 15 min beyond sweating Passive heating of one arm to 42°C with water bath Evidence of reaction to sweat antigen
Cold-contact urticaria	Exposure of skin to cold air, cold objects, or cold liquids	Ice cube test for 5 min on arm Temperature test where available
Heat-contact urticaria	Warm object in direct contact with skin	Application of test tube containing warm water at 45°C
Aquagenic urticaria	Skin contact with water at any temperature	Application of water compress at 35°C for 30 min
Solar urticaria	Exposure of skin to sunlight of specific wavelength	Exposure of skin to ultraviolet A, ultraviolet B, or visible light
Vibratory urticaria	Lawn mowing, riding a bike, exposure to vibrating machinery	Vortex platform held to skin for 10 min

Data from Magerl M, Borzova E, Gimenez-Arnau A, et al. The definition and diagnostic testing of physical and cholinergic urticarias-EAACI/GA2LEN/EDF/UNEV consensus panel recommendations. Allergy 2009;64:1715–21.

been linked to a potential allergen, such as foods or drugs, 30% of cases are linked to infections, particularly of the respiratory tract, while the remaining 50% appear not to have a trigger.[8] These associations suggest involvement of the innate immune system via infectious triggers as well as adaptive immunity for cases involving immunoglobulin E (IgE) and allergens.

At any time, up to 1% of the North American population can be affected by CU.[9] The overall prevalence is similar in other regions.[10,11] Both children and adults can develop CU, but it appears to be more common in adults, with women affected nearly twice as often as men.[10,12–17] The average age of patients suggests that the condition typically begins in the third to fifth decades of life.[10,15,16] The coexpression of allergic disease in patients with CU appears to be slightly higher than that observed in the general population.[18]

PROGNOSIS AND RISK FACTORS

CU is a self-limited disorder in most cases, with an average duration of 2 to 5 years.[9,19] In patients in whom no trigger is identified, there is a rate of spontaneous remission at 1 year occurs in approximately 30% to 50%.[13,20–22] However, symptoms persist beyond 5 years in nearly one-fifth of patients.[13,23]

Factors that predict longer disease duration or more severe disease are limited. In a prospective study of 139 CU patients followed for 5 years, angioedema, features of severe disease, autologous serum skin test (ASST) positivity, and thyroid autoimmunity were associated with longer disease duration.[23] Hypertension and disease severity have been recently identified as a factors associated with longer disease duration.[19] However, other studies have not found an association between positive ASST and longer disease duration.[20]

Autoimmunity

Various autoimmune diseases are noted to be more prevalent in subjects with CU.[21,24] In a study involving a 13,000-patient database relative to 10,000 control subjects, the following diseases were noted to be increased among CU patients: thyroid disorders, celiac disease, Sjögren syndrome, systemic lupus erythematosus (SLE), rheumatoid arthritis, and type 1 diabetes[25]: The diagnosis of autoimmune disease most often appeared in the decade after CU occurrence.

Thyroid Disorders

A higher incidence of thyroid disease in CU patients has been long recognized[24,26] and was recently confirmed in a large study.[25] The overall incidence of hypothyroidism (9.8%) and hyperthyroidism (2.6%) is at least twice that reported in the general population.[25] There is also evidence for a higher prevalence of thyroid autoantibodies in CU subjects (antiperoxidase and antimicrosomal) than in the general population,[14,24,27] but in most CU subjects this is found with normal thyroid function. Some view the significance of a higher frequency of thyroid autoimmunity as a common underlying tendency to form autoantibodies rather than a causal link between the 2 diseases.[26,28]

Malignancy

There exist conflicting data on whether CIU patients are at increased risk for malignancies.[29,30] In one Swedish study, 1155 patients with CIU were followed in a dermatology department for an average of 8.2 years. The incidence of malignant cancer during the observation period was compared with the expected number of cancers from the Swedish Cancer Registry, yielding a relative risk of 0.88 (95% confidence interval [CI] 0.61–1.12). In the second study, a cohort of 12,720 Taiwanese patients was identified as having CU, based on the ICD-9-CM code for urticaria along with use of an antihistamine for at least 6 months over a 2-year period. The rate of malignancies diagnosed in this cohort over an average follow-up period of 5 years was compared with expected rates, obtained from the Taiwan National Cancer Registry. The standardized incidence ratio for patients with CU was 2.2 (95% CI 2.0–2.4). Younger patients appeared to be at higher risk for hematologic malignancies. At present, the identified associations warrant further evaluation.

PATHOPHYSIOLOGY
Skin Pathology

The skin pathology observed in an urticarial lesion biopsy includes degranulation of skin mast cells and a perivascular leukocyte infiltrate composed of lymphocytes, eosinophils, neutrophils, and basophils that have migrated to the skin lesion (**Fig. 1**).[31] Both mast cells and basophils release histamine and other inflammatory mediators (prostaglandins, leukotrienes, cytokines) on activation, which are capable of causing local vasodilation, itch, and swelling of the skin. In most CIU skin biopsies, there is a lack of leukocytoclasia or fibrinoid deposition such as seen in urticarial vasculitis (UV),[32,33] complement deposition, or immune deposits.[34]

Given that pruritus is the major skin symptom in CU and the overall benefits seen with antihistamine therapy, histamine appears to be a central mediator in CU. Skin-blister fluids obtained from lesional and nonlesional skin of CU subjects in a comparison with normal subjects showed greater histamine-releasing activity based on in vitro testing with healthy basophils.[35] Elevated skin histamine content was also noted in the CU lesional skin,[35,36] leading to the idea that local factors may regulate histamine release from skin mast cells in CU.[35]

The leukocyte infiltrate observed in CU skin biopsies and clinical presentation is similar to that seen in allergen-induced late-phase skin reactions. Although both feature mast-cell activation, T cells in the skin late-phase reaction express a T-helper (Th)2 cytokine pattern (interleukin [IL]-4, IL-5), whereas both Th2 cytokines (IL-4 and

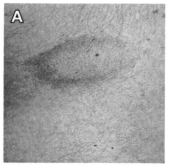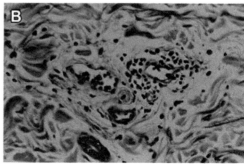

Fig. 1. (*A*) Image of skin lesion. Superficial swellings of the dermis are called wheals. Wheals are usually pale in the center with a red surrounding flare when they erupt, and become pink as they mature. (*B*) Biopsy of skin lesion. Photomicrograph of early spontaneous wheal shows perivascular lymphocytes and intraluminal and perivascular neutrophils, with perivascular and interstitial eosinophils. (*From* Grattan CE, Sabroe RA, Greaves MW. Chronic urticaria. J Am Acad Dermatol 2002;46(5):645–60. Available at: http://dx.doi.org/10.1067/mjd. 2002.122759; with permission.)

IL-5) and Th1 cytokines (interferon-γ) are noted in CU lesions.[31] Of note, little difference is found in the characteristics of skin biopsies of patients with and without serologic evidence for autoimmune urticaria.[31,37] Increased expression of IL-3 and tumor necrosis factor (TNF)-α in endothelial cells has been detected in the skin biopsies of both lesional and nonlesional skin in CU.[38]

There is limited understanding of the roles for eosinophils, lymphocytes, and neutrophils in disease pathology. A predominance of neutrophils in the skin-lesion biopsy is termed neutrophilic urticaria, and can lead to alternative disease management.[39,40] Furthermore, immune features of CIU subjects resistant to high-dose antihistamine therapy relative to antihistamine responders include greater basopenia, higher mean platelet volume, higher levels of C-reactive protein, and higher levels of serum C3, which are features of low-grade inflammation and platelet activation.[41] Other immune profiles described in CIU subjects are summarized in **Table 2**.

Pathogenesis

Although there are several theories regarding the pathogenesis of CU, none have been conclusively established.[7,52,53] Many studies have examined the autoimmune theory of disease and also the validity of serologic tests to establish an autoimmune basis. Additional theories include abnormalities of tissue mast cells and basophils as well as underlying chronic infections.

Autoimmune theory
A widely held theory is that 30% to 40% of CIU patients have an autoimmune disease, also referred to as CAU. These patients have circulating immunoglobulin G (IgG) autoantibodies to either IgE or the high-affinity IgE receptor that are believed to be pathogenic by directly activating mast cells and basophils (**Fig. 2**).[7] This theory arose from the earlier recognition of increased incidence of thyroid autoimmunity and dysfunction in patients with CU (**Fig. 3**).[24,25,54] A correlation between thyroid autoimmunity and the presence of autoimmune serum factors in CIU is often cited as evidence for a common

Table 2
Immune profiles of CIU subjects relative to controls

Immune Cell Type/Tissue	Profile
Lymphocytes	Altered signaling through the p21Ras pathway[42] Increased frequency of IL-10+ peripheral T cells[43]
Peripheral blood mononuclear cells (PBMC)	Increased stimulated production of TNF-α, IL-10, MIP-Iα, and RANTES[44] Reduced IL-4[45]
Peripheral blood dendritic cells (pDCs)	Impaired TLR9 induced interferon-α production[46]
Serum	Increased levels of TNF, IL-1β, IL-6, IL-13, IL-12p70, IL-10, and B-cell activating factor (BAFF); similar among those with CIU and CAU[47–49] Increased IL-6, CRP in CU subjects with NSAID sensitivity after aspirin challenge[50]
Coagulation	Extrinsic coagulation pathway activated with increased levels of D-dimer and prothrombin fragments[51]

Abbreviations: CAU, chronic autoimmune urticaria; CIU, chronic idiopathic urticaria; CRP, C-reactive protein; CU, chronic urticaria; IL, interleukin; MIP, macrophage inflammatory protein; NSAID, nonsteroidal anti-inflammatory drug; RANTES, regulated on activation, normal T-cell expressed and secreted (chemokine ligand 5); TNF, tumor necrosis factor.

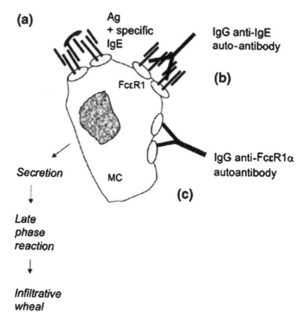

Fig. 2. Proposed pathogenic antibodies in CIU/CSU disease. Ag+, antigen-positive; Ig, immunoglobulin; MC, mast cell. (*Data from* Kaplan AP, Greaves M. Pathogenesis of chronic urticaria. Clin Exp Allergy 2009;39(6):777–87.)

underlying autoimmune diathesis in a subset of CU patients.[27,54] Furthermore, increased clustering of human leukocyte antigen (HLA) class 2 DR antigen expression is noted in subjects with CIU and, in particular, those with evidence for serum autoimmune factors.[55]

History of Autoimmunity in CIU

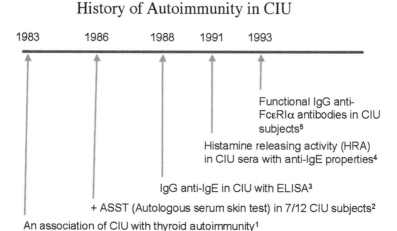

Fig. 3. Timeline for autoantibody theory. ELISA, enzyme-linked immunosorbent assay. (*Data from* Refs.[24,56,57,61,62])

The evolution of the autoimmune theory began in the 1980s when a serum factor that behaved similarly to a cross-linking anti-IgE was detected in the serum of CU patients.[56,57] At the same time a serologic factor was also identified, based on an in vivo skin-test response called the ASST (**Fig. 4**). In an early report it was noted that 7 of 12 (58%) CU patients developed wheal and flare reactions within 30 minutes at the site of intradermal injection of their own serum or ASST.[56] The serum fraction responsible for ASST positivity was originally described as being in the 10- to 15-kDa range.[58] The skin pathology of an ASST reaction resembles that of an IgE-mediated late-phase reaction, supporting the notion that mast-cell degranulation also occurs in the ASST reaction owing to a presumed CIU disease-related factor.[59] However, more recent work has shown positive ASST to occur in subjects with allergic respiratory disease and healthy controls, raising the issue of the specificity of this test to CU disease.[53,60]

In parallel with early studies of serum ASST, a report emerged that CU serum contained IgG antibodies against the Fc region of IgE, and led to a dose-dependent histamine release from the blood basophils of healthy subjects.[57] This activity was termed serum histamine-releasing activity (HRA) (**Fig. 5**). Initially, serum fractions responsible for HRA (>100 kDa) differed from those fractions described as inducing an ASST (<20 kDa).[57,58] Later, a single serum fraction (>100 kDa) was capable of inducing both a positive ASST and positive HRA.[61] These findings culminated in a landmark report identifying IgG anti-FcεRIα autoantibodies as the main serum factor responsible for HRA.[62] In this study, 26 CU subjects with a positive serum ASST were studied, and 17 of 26 also had HRA present in the IgG fraction of their serum. In a small subset of these subjects, increased serum HRA activity was seen after

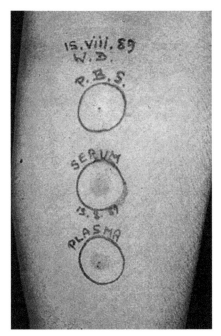

Fig. 4. An autologous serum skin test (ASST) reaction. Phosphate-buffered saline (P.B.S.), saline solution negative control, serum, and plasma are injected in a volume of 0.05 mL and the reaction read at 30 minutes. Here both serum and plasma have given positive responses. (*From* Greaves M. Chronic urticaria. J Allergy Clin Immunol 2000;105(4):664–72; with permission.)

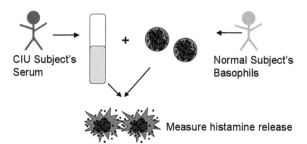

CIU Subject's
Serum

Normal Subject's
Basophils

Measure histamine release

Fig. 5. Serum histamine-releasing assays. (*Adapted from* Brodell LA, Beck LA, Saini SS. Pathophysiology of chronic urticaria. Ann Allergy Asthma Immunol 2008;100(4):294; with permission.)

stripping native IgE from the donor basophils. This finding implied that the IgE bound to the high-affinity IgE receptor (FcɛRI) inhibited the ability of some anti-FcɛRIα IgG autoantibodies to release histamine from basophils. It remained unclear as to how some of these antibodies would be functional in vivo, given the high affinity of IgE for its receptor and the overall high occupancy rate (>95%) of surface IgE receptors on basophils and mast cells.

Subsequent studies focused on describing the frequency of HRA in CU subjects, and characterized whether HRA activity targeted IgE, unoccupied IgE receptors, or occupied IgE receptors on healthy, donor basophils.[61,63–65] Although early reports suggested that HRA activity and ASST reactions decreased in disease remission,[56,65] later reports noted persistence of ASST in remission and even after IgG-depletion of the serum used in the ASST.[66,67] A direct comparison of serum ASST results with those of HRA testing in 163 CU subjects found ASST positivity in 60% of subjects, but only half of the ASST-positive sera evoked serum HRA from basophils.[68] This finding highlighted that ASST reactivity reflected skin mast-cell–specific serum factors that differed from those (IgG anti-IgE, or anti-FcɛRIα) shown to activate donor basophils.[69] HRA-defined IgG anti-FcɛRIα autoantibodies are estimated to occur in 30% to 40% of CU patients, whereas IgG anti-IgE autoantibodies occur in 10%.[7] A recent modification of the HRA assay examines CU serum for the ability to increase levels of basophil surface activation marker CD203c rather than histamine release.[64] The exact nature of CU serum factors, their role in CU disease, and the optimum test strategy for detecting such factors continues to be debated.[53,70] Concerns with the present assays are the variability of the donor basophils for both traditional and newer HRA assays, the confounding of results by other factors in serum that can trigger normal basophils (IL-3, complement), and the occurrence of positive HRA activity in the serum of healthy subjects and those with SLE.[71–73]

An enzyme-linked immunosorbent assay (ELISA) approach to detect IgG anti-FcɛRIα offered a promising alternative to the use of bioassays such as the ASST or HRA for autoantibody detection.[74] Complement-fixing subclasses IgG_1 and IgG_3 were the main subtypes found by ELISA in the serum of CU subjects. By contrast, non–complement-fixing subclasses IgG_2 and IgG_4 were detected in other autoimmune diseases (pemphigus vulgaris, dermatomyositis, SLE, and bullous pemphigoid) at a similar frequency to CU, but were nonfunctional in HRA assays. However, a later study failed to demonstrate a correlation between CU serum containing immunoreactive IgG antibodies and FcɛRIα by Western blotting and serum positive for HRA.[75] Also, broader IgG subclass anti-FcɛRIα presence in CU serum was noted in serum that possesses HRA (IgG_1, IgG_3, IgG_4)[76] and, anti-FcɛRIα was noted in serum of normal subjects.[77,78] The lack of concordance between ASST, HRA, and other detection platforms such as ELISA/Western blotting remains a problem in identifying the proper test to define the entity of CAU.[69] Furthermore, the relationship of antibody titers to CIU disease activity has not been clearly demonstrated.[79] The significance of autoimmune classification as a marker of disease severity[80,81] or predictor of response to certain therapeutic agents lacks sufficient evidence-based trials.

Summary of autoimmune theory

Summary of Points Favoring Autoimmune Hypothesis

- Functional autoantibody testing by ASST declines with effective therapies such as plasmapheresis and intravenous immunoglobulin[82,83]
- HLA-DR clustering and increased thyroid autoimmunity[24,25,54,55]
- Detection of IgG autoantibodies by HRA, Western blot, and ELISA[7]

Summary of Points Unresolved in the Autoimmune Hypothesis

- ASST lacks sensitivity and specificity for CIU[60,84]
- ASST may indicate the presence of other vasoactive factors rather than IgG autoantibodies[67]
- HRA testing results depend on the donor used for basophils and are confounded by other serum active factors[71]
- HRA positives are seen in healthy subjects and SLE subjects[72,73]
- Skin biopsies and clinical phenotype do not differ between CAU and CIU[31,37]
- Differential targeting of anti-FcεRI antibodies to occupied versus unoccupied receptors raises issues regarding functional role in disease in vivo
- It is unclear as to why IgG anti-IgE leads to only skin-limited disease and not anaphylaxis

Skin mast cells

Mast-cell degranulation is a central event in lesion development in urticaria,[31] and elevated histamine levels are noted in skin biopsies.[35,36] However, the number of skin mast cells is not increased in either lesional or nonlesional CIU skin biopsies relative to the skin of healthy controls.[85] Likewise, total serum tryptase levels, an indirect measure of total body mast-cell numbers, is only slightly elevated in CU subjects relative to healthy and atopic subjects, but well within the normal range.[86] Evidence supports that heightened histamine presence detected in CU skin lesions could be due to either enhanced quantitative release of histamine from skin mast cells or from blood basophil infiltration of CU skin tissues.[87] Elevated skin mast-cell releasability in active CU has been shown by skin challenges with compound 48/80 and codeine.[88,89] Recently, culture-derived mast cells grown from peripheral blood CD34+ cells of CU subjects showed elevated spontaneous histamine release when compared with mast cells grown from healthy donors.[90]

Recently, supernatants taken from mast cell lines (HMC-1, LUVA) after exposure to CU serum, but not to normal serum, caused increased endothelial monolayer permeability. This CU serum-evoked response was independent of IgG serum fractions or dependence on IgE receptor activation of the mast cell lines.[91] Other possible pathways that could activate mast cells, such as innate immune receptors, remain to be established. Mast-cell activation in physical urticarias has been studied using provocation challenge by a specific stimulus challenge to the skin. For example, the application of a cold-water challenge in a patient with cold urticaria showed elevations in blood histamine levels in the draining venous vessels.[92] Likewise, cold-temperature challenge of isolated skin fragments of cold urticaria subjects led to histamine release.[93] Areas of research in physical urticaria include the role of recently identified transient receptor potential channels that can be regulated via changes in temperature, pH, or osmolality, and produce calcium influx into the cell.[94] A novel familial cold urticaria syndrome with associated immunodeficiency has been described to have abnormalities in the PLCγ signaling pathway of immune cells, including mast cells.[95]

Blood basophils

Evidence that blood basophils are involved in the pathogenesis of CU has emerged over the past decades.[52,96] In the 1970s, 2 groups identified that blood basophils of CIU subjects had reduced capacity to release histamine after IgE-receptor activation.[97,98] This paradoxic reduction in histamine release was attributed to prior in vivo activation and was referred to as basophil hyporesponsiveness or hyporeleasability.[98] Basophil histamine hyporeleasability was limited to the IgE receptor pathway and was not seen with stimulation by formyl-methionyl-leucyl-phenylalanine, bradykinin, or monocyte chemoattractant protein.[99,100] Recently, blood basophil IgE receptor responses of CIU subjects were segregated into 2 basophil functional phenotypes, CIU responders (CIU-R) and CIU nonresponders (CIU-NR).[101] CIU-R basophils show a histamine degranulation profile similar to that of normal subjects, whereas basophils of CIU-NR subjects do not degranulate to ex vivo IgE-receptor activation and possess elevated levels of the IgE-receptor regulating inhibitory phosphatases, SH2-domain–containing inositol-5-phosphatase (SHIP)-1 and SHIP-2. These 2 functional phenotypes are stable in active CIU disease, are not related to the presence of autoimmune serum factors, and also reflect differences in some clinical features of subjects.[79,102] Furthermore, hyporeleasability of basophil response improves in disease remission.[79] The underlying disease mechanisms leading to these distinct basophil phenotypes remains to be elucidated, but supports the idea that basophil responsiveness is relevant to the pathogenesis of urticaria.

Blood basopenia has also been noted in CU subjects for decades, and has been linked to the presence of serum HRA.[103,104] Skin biopsy studies using basophil-specific antibodies have provided evidence for the presence of basophils in both CIU lesional sites and nonlesional skin tissues, a finding not seen in healthy skin and many other skin diseases.[31,87,105] The degree of basopenia is correlated to disease severity and appears to reflect blood basophil recruitment to the skin lesions, whereas in CIU remission basopenia improves.[41,79,98,106] Collectively this work suggests that altered basophil trafficking is present CIU.

Infections

The topic of infections and CIU was recently reviewed.[107] Among infections implicated in CU are *Helicobacter pylori*, but the data are mixed.[108–110] The role of infections and CU onset is often raised but is difficult to prove. Recent work on staphylococcal nasal carriage also revealed higher levels in CU patients than in controls.[111] In a small study, nasal carriage of *Staphylococcus aureus* was assessed in 57 CU patients and 25 controls. A positive swab was found in 32 of 57 CU subjects, and all were given empiric antistaph therapy with 28% having complete remission, 12% partial relief, and 60% no benefit from treatment.[112]

CLINICAL FEATURES

Urticarial lesions or hives are typically raised erythematous plaques that are circumscribed (**Fig. 6**). These lesions can assume a variety of sizes, and may be flattened in appearance if a patient is using antihistamines. Any area of the body can be affected, including areas where clothing may compress the skin (waistband).

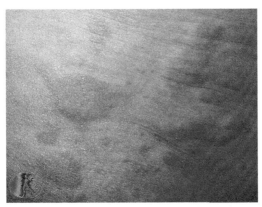

Fig. 6. Urticaria. (*Courtesy of* New Zealand Dermatological Society Incorporated. Published online at: http://www.dermnetnz.org.)

Most lesions have a life span of less than 24 hours; therefore, photographs of skin lesions are extremely useful in helping to confirm the diagnosis. Lesions with a longer life span or the occurrence of bruising may suggest the presence of vacuities. The severity of the pruritus can be disruptive of both sleep and daily activities.

Angioedema involves episodic submucosal or subcutaneous swelling that is asymmetric in distribution (**Fig. 7**). Paresthesia such as numbness or tingling is

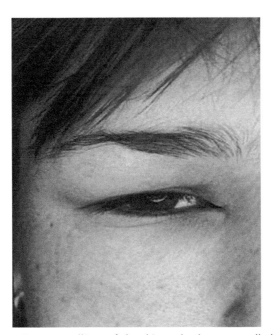

Fig. 7. Angioedema. Deeper swellings of the skin and submucosa called angioedema are less well defined and do not necessarily show any difference in color from unaffected skin. (*From* Grattan CE, Sabroe RA, Greaves MW. Chronic urticaria. J Am Acad Dermatol 2002;46(5):645–60; with permission.)

common, rather than the pruritus described in urticaria. Body areas commonly involved include the lips, eyes, cheeks, and extremities. In most cases angioedema is coexpressed with urticaria, but can be the sole feature in a limited number of cases.[113] It is important to consider other causes of isolated angioedema such as drugs (angiotensin-converting enzyme inhibitor–induced lesions), hereditary angioedema, or acquired angioedema (see the relevant article by Bork elsewhere in this issue). Among factors that are thought to contribute to disease exacerbations of urticaria are nonsteroidal anti-inflammatory medications (NSAIDs), alcohol ingestion, and stress.[21,114,115]

Table 3
Key features of diseases that are associated with urticaria

Disorder	Feature	Evaluation
Urticarial vasculitis (UV)	Painful, long-lived lesions (>48 h), bruising and pigmentation, systemic signs (fever, chills, arthralgias)	Skin biopsy
Systemic lupus erythematosus	Prolonged skin lesions, UV sensitivity, with fever, weight loss, arthritis, lymphadenopathy, other organ system	Skin biopsy and laboratory evaluation
Cryoglobulinemia	Cold-induced lesions, lesions more on extremities, arthralgias	Testing for hepatitis C, cryoglobulins
Schnitzler syndrome	Monoclonal gammopathy (IgM or IgG), fever, urticaria, bone pain, lymphadenopathy	WESR, CRP, SPEP with immunofixation
Mastocytosis	Urticaria pigmentosa, Darier's sign	Skin biopsy, tryptase
Polymorphic eruption of pregnancy (PEP) or pruritic urticarial papules and plaques of pregnancy (PUPPP)	Pruritic dermatitis, erythematous papules with striae, target-like lesions	Seen in 1 in 300 pregnancies, typically resolves postpartum, no specific laboratory abnormalities
Hypereosinophilic syndrome	Urticaria, angioedema, other organ system involvement with eosinophils	Eosinophil count
Cryopyrin-mediated periodic syndromes: familial cold autoinflammatory syndrome, Muckle-Wells syndrome	Periodic fevers, urticaria, and leukocytosis, muscle and skin tenderness post cold exposures	Early onset of symptoms, genetic
Cryopyrin-mediated periodic syndromes: Muckle-Wells syndrome	Periodic urticarial eruptions without cold sensitivity, sensorineural hearing loss, arthritis	—

Abbreviations: IgG, immunoglobulin G; IgM, immunoglobulin M; SPEP, serum protein electrophoresis; WESR, Westergren erythrocyte sedimentation rate.

DIFFERENTIAL DIAGNOSIS

Numerous disorders must be considered in the evaluation of patients with chronic idiopathic or spontaneous urticaria. Acute urticaria is often associated with viral and bacterial infections, especially in children. Some pediatric series suggest an infection to be associated with disease, or possibly related to the antibiotic used to treat the illness.[116–118] Acute urticaria can be observed in the early stages of hepatitis A, B, and C infection, but little evidence exists for hepatitis virus infection causing CU.[119] In the past, stool studies to exclude parasites as a cause of urticaria have been recommended, but are only relevant in individuals who have recently traveled to endemic areas.

It is clear that food and drug anaphylaxis often demonstrate skin symptoms within 2 hours of ingestion, and is rarely determined to be the cause of CU. The frequency of NSAID-induced exacerbations of skin disease varies form 25% to 50%.[120] In some individuals the period of aspirin sensitivity ends when the urticaria disease resolves. There is evidence for genetic variability of prostaglandin E2 receptor subtype EP4 gene in aspirin-intolerant CU.[121]

Among the systemic diseases that can be associated with CIU are several rare disorders, which are summarized in **Table 3**.

FUTURE CONSIDERATIONS AND SUMMARY

Further studies are clearly needed to advance the understanding of pathogenic factors that trigger skin symptoms in both acute and chronic urticarial disease. At present, the diverse nature of inciting factors and systemic disease that are associated with urticaria suggest that multiple pathways lead to a common pathway involving mast-cell activation, resulting in infiltration by blood leukocytes. In addition, better biomarkers to predict the course of CIU disease and assist in the selection of therapeutics are needed.

REFERENCES

1. Greaves MW. Chronic urticaria. N Engl J Med 1995;332(26):1767–72.
2. Grattan CE, Sabroe RA, Greaves MW. Chronic urticaria. J Am Acad Dermatol 2002;46(5):645–57.
3. Magerl M, Borzova E, Gimenez-Arnau A, et al. The definition and diagnostic testing of physical and cholinergic urticarias–EAACI/GA2LEN/EDF/UNEV consensus panel recommendations. Allergy 2009;64(12):1715–21. http://dx.doi.org/10.1111/j.1398-9995.2009.02177.x.
4. Zuberbier T, Asero R, Bindslev-Jensen C, et al. EAACI/GA(2)LEN/EDF/WAO guideline: definition, classification and diagnosis of urticaria. Allergy 2009; 64(10):1417–26. http://dx.doi.org/10.1111/j.1398-9995.2009.02179.x.
5. Kaplan AP. Chronic urticaria: pathogenesis and treatment. J Allergy Clin Immunol 2004;114(3):465–74.
6. Sabroe RA, Seed PT, Francis DM, et al. Chronic idiopathic urticaria: comparison of the clinical features of patients with and without anti-FcepsilonRI or anti-IgE autoantibodies. J Am Acad Dermatol 1999;40(3):443–50.
7. Kaplan AP, Greaves M. Pathogenesis of chronic urticaria. Clin Exp Allergy 2009; 39(6):777–87. http://dx.doi.org/10.1111/j.1365-2222.2009.03256.x.
8. Frigas E, Park MA. Acute urticaria and angioedema: diagnostic and treatment considerations. Am J Clin Dermatol 2009;10(4):239–50. http://dx.doi.org/10.2165/00128071-200910040-00004.

9. Greaves M. Chronic urticaria. J Allergy Clin Immunol 2000;105(4):664–72.
10. Gaig P, Olona M, Munoz Lejarazu D, et al. Epidemiology of urticaria in Spain. J Investig Allergol Clin Immunol 2004;14(3):214–20.
11. Zuberbier T, Balke M, Worm M, et al. Epidemiology of urticaria: a representative cross-sectional population survey. Clin Exp Dermatol 2010;35(8):869–73. http://dx.doi.org/10.1111/j.1365-2230.2010.03840.x.
12. Cooper KD. Urticaria and angioedema: diagnosis and evaluation. J Am Acad Dermatol 1991;25(1 Pt 2):166–74.
13. Champion RH, Roberts SO, Carpenter RG, et al. Urticaria and angio-oedema. A review of 554 patients. Br J Dermatol 1969;81(8):588–97.
14. Najib U, Bajwa ZH, Ostro MG, et al. A retrospective review of clinical presentation, thyroid autoimmunity, laboratory characteristics, and therapies used in patients with chronic idiopathic urticaria. Ann Allergy Asthma Immunol 2009; 103(6):496–501. http://dx.doi.org/10.1016/S1081-1206(10)60266-9.
15. Ferrer M. Epidemiology, healthcare, resources, use and clinical features of different types of urticaria. Alergologica 2005. J Investig Allergol Clin Immunol 2009;19(Suppl 2):21–6.
16. Juhlin L. Recurrent urticaria: clinical investigation of 330 patients. Br J Dermatol 1981;104(4):369–81.
17. Buss YA, Garrelfs UC, Sticherling M. Chronic urticaria–which clinical parameters are pathogenetically relevant? A retrospective investigation of 339 patients. J Dtsch Dermatol Ges 2007;5(1):22–9. http://dx.doi.org/10.1111/j.1610-0387. 2007.06194.x.
18. Zazzali JL, Broder MS, Chang E, et al. Cost, utilization, and patterns of medication use associated with chronic idiopathic urticaria. Ann Allergy Asthma Immunol 2012;108(2):98–102. http://dx.doi.org/10.1016/j.anai.2011.10.018.
19. Nebiolo F, Bergia R, Bommarito L, et al. Effect of arterial hypertension on chronic urticaria duration. Ann Allergy Asthma Immunol 2009;103(5):407–10. http://dx.doi.org/10.1016/S1081-1206(10)60360-2.
20. Kulthanan K, Jiamton S, Thumpimukvatana N, et al. Chronic idiopathic urticaria: prevalence and clinical course. J Dermatol 2007;34(5):294–301. http://dx.doi.org/10.1111/j.1346-8138.2007.00276.x.
21. Kozel MM, Bossuyt PM, Mekkes JR, et al. Laboratory tests and identified diagnoses in patients with physical and chronic urticaria and angioedema: a systematic review. J Am Acad Dermatol 2003;48(3):409–16. http://dx.doi.org/10.1067/mjd.2003.142.
22. Kulp-Shorten CL, Callen JP. Urticaria, angioedema, and rheumatologic disease. Rheum Dis Clin North Am 1996;22(1):95–115.
23. Toubi E, Kessel A, Avshovich N, et al. Clinical and laboratory parameters in predicting chronic urticaria duration: a prospective study of 139 patients. Allergy 2004;59(8):869–73.
24. Leznoff A, Josse RG, Denburg J, et al. Association of chronic urticaria and angioedema with thyroid autoimmunity. Arch Dermatol 1983;119(8):636–40.
25. Confino-Cohen R, Chodick G, Shalev V, et al. Chronic urticaria and autoimmunity: associations found in a large population study. J Allergy Clin Immunol 2012;129(5):1307–13. http://dx.doi.org/10.1016/j.jaci.2012.01.043.
26. Dreskin SC, Andrews KY. The thyroid and urticaria. Curr Opin Allergy Clin Immunol 2005;5(5):408–12.
27. Kikuchi Y, Fann T, Kaplan AP. Antithyroid antibodies in chronic urticaria and angioedema. J Allergy Clin Immunol 2003;112(1):218.

28. Sheikh J, Saini SS, Kulczycki A Jr, et al. A survey of allergists regarding the association of thyroid autoimmunity with chronic urticaria. J Allergy Clin Immunol 2009;123(5):1173–5. http://dx.doi.org/10.1016/j.jaci.2008.12.1130.
29. Lindelof B, Sigurgeirsson B, Wahlgren CF, et al. Chronic urticaria and cancer: an epidemiological study of 1155 patients. Br J Dermatol 1990;123(4):453–6.
30. Chen YJ, Wu CY, Shen JL, et al. Cancer risk in patients with chronic urticaria: a population-based cohort study. Arch Dermatol 2012;148(1):103–8. http://dx.doi.org/10.1001/archdermatol.2011.682.
31. Ying S, Kikuchi Y, Meng Q, et al. TH1/TH2 cytokines and inflammatory cells in skin biopsy specimens from patients with chronic idiopathic urticaria: comparison with the allergen-induced late-phase cutaneous reaction. J Allergy Clin Immunol 2002;109(4):694–700.
32. Haas N, Hermes B, Henz BM. Adhesion molecules and cellular infiltrate: histology of urticaria. J Investig Dermatol Symp Proc 2001;6(2):137–8. http://dx.doi.org/10.1046/j.0022-202x.2001.00026.x.
33. Carlson JA. The histological assessment of cutaneous vasculitis. Histopathology 2010;56(1):3–23. http://dx.doi.org/10.1111/j.1365-2559.2009.03443.x.
34. Natbony SF, Phillips ME, Elias JM, et al. Histologic studies of chronic idiopathic urticaria. J Allergy Clin Immunol 1983;71(2):177–83.
35. Claveau J, Lavoie A, Brunet C, et al. Chronic idiopathic urticaria: possible contribution of histamine-releasing factor to pathogenesis. J Allergy Clin Immunol 1993;92(1 Pt 1):132–7.
36. Kaplan AP, Horakova Z, Katz SI. Assessment of tissue fluid histamine levels in patients with urticaria. J Allergy Clin Immunol 1978;61(6):350–4.
37. Sabroe RA, Poon E, Orchard GE, et al. Cutaneous inflammatory cell infiltrate in chronic idiopathic urticaria: comparison of patients with and without anti-FcepsilonRI or anti-IgE autoantibodies. J Allergy Clin Immunol 1999;103(3 Pt 1):484–93.
38. Hermes B, Prochazka AK, Haas N, et al. Upregulation of TNF-alpha and IL-3 expression in lesional and uninvolved skin in different types of urticaria. J Allergy Clin Immunol 1999;103(2 Pt 1):307–14.
39. Peters MS, Winkelmann RK. Neutrophilic urticaria. Br J Dermatol 1985;113(1):25–30.
40. Kieffer C, Cribier B, Lipsker D. Neutrophilic urticarial dermatosis: a variant of neutrophilic urticaria strongly associated with systemic disease. Report of 9 new cases and review of the literature. Medicine 2009;88(1):23–31. http://dx.doi.org/10.1097/MD.0b013e3181943f5e.
41. Magen E, Mishal J, Zeldin Y, et al. Clinical and laboratory features of antihistamine-resistant chronic idiopathic urticaria. Allergy Asthma Proc 2011;32(6):460–6. http://dx.doi.org/10.2500/aap.2011.32.3483.
42. Confino-Cohen R, Aharoni D, Goldberg A, et al. Evidence for aberrant regulation of the p21Ras pathway in PBMCs of patients with chronic idiopathic urticaria. J Allergy Clin Immunol 2002;109(2):349–56.
43. Irinyi B, Aleksza M, Antal-Szalmas P, et al. Cytokine production of CD4+ and CD8+ peripheral T lymphocytes in patients with chronic idiopathic urticaria. Acta Derm Venereol 2002;82(4):249–53.
44. Piconi S, Trabattoni D, Iemoli E, et al. Immune profiles of patients with chronic idiopathic urticaria. Int Arch Allergy Immunol 2002;128(1):59–66.
45. Confino-Cohen R, Goldberg A, Aharoni D, et al. Low stimulated IL-4 secretion in PBMC from patients with chronic idiopathic urticaria. Cytokine 2004;27(2–3):74–80.

46. Futata E, Azor M, Dos Santos J, et al. Impaired IFN-alpha secretion by plasma-cytoid dendritic cells induced by TLR9 activation in chronic idiopathic urticaria. Br J Dermatol 2011;164(6):1271–9. http://dx.doi.org/10.1111/j.1365-2133.2010. 10198.x.

47. Dos Santos JC, Azor MH, Nojima VY, et al. Increased circulating pro-inflammatory cytokines and imbalanced regulatory T-cell cytokines production in chronic idiopathic urticaria. Int Immunopharmacol 2008;8(10):1433–40.

48. Caproni M, Volpi W, Giomi B, et al. Chronic idiopathic and chronic autoimmune urticaria: clinical and immunopathological features of 68 subjects. Acta Derm Venereol 2004;84(4):288–90.

49. Kessel A, Yaacoby-Bianu K, Vadasz Z, et al. Elevated serum B-cell activating factor in patients with chronic urticaria. Hum Immunol 2012;73(6):620–2. http://dx.doi.org/10.1016/j.humimm.2012.03.016.

50. Kasperska-Zajac A, Grzanka A, Czecior E, et al. Acute phase inflammatory markers in patients with non-steroidal anti-inflammatory drugs (NSAIDs)-induced acute urticaria/angioedema and after aspirin challenge. J Eur Acad Dermatol Venereol 2012. http://dx.doi.org/10.1111/j.1468–3083.2012.04486.x.

51. Asero R, Tedeschi A, Coppola R, et al. Activation of the tissue factor pathway of blood coagulation in patients with chronic urticaria. J Allergy Clin Immunol 2007; 119(3):705–10.

52. Vonakis BM, Saini SS. New concepts in chronic urticaria. Curr Opin Immunol 2008;20(6):709–16.

53. Brodell LA, Beck LA, Saini SS. Pathophysiology of chronic urticaria. Ann Allergy Asthma Immunol 2008;100(4):291–7.

54. O'Donnell BF, Francis DM, Swana GT, et al. Thyroid autoimmunity in chronic ur-ticaria. Br J Dermatol 2005;153(2):331–5. http://dx.doi.org/10.1111/j.1365-2133. 2005.06646.x.

55. O'Donnell BF, O'Neill CM, Francis DM, et al. Human leucocyte antigen class II associations in chronic idiopathic urticaria. Br J Dermatol 1999;140(5):853–8.

56. Grattan CE, Wallington TB, Warin RP, et al. A serological mediator in chronic idiopathic urticaria–a clinical, immunological and histological evaluation. Br J Dermatol 1986;114(5):583–90.

57. Gruber BL, Baeza ML, Marchese MJ, et al. Prevalence and functional role of anti-IgE autoantibodies in urticarial syndromes. J Invest Dermatol 1988;90(2): 213–7.

58. Grattan CE, Hamon CG, Cowan MA, et al. Preliminary identification of a low mo-lecular weight serological mediator in chronic idiopathic urticaria. Br J Dermatol 1988;119(2):179–83.

59. Grattan CE, Boon AP, Eady RA, et al. The pathology of the autologous serum skin test response in chronic urticaria resembles IgE-mediated late-phase reac-tions. Int Arch Allergy Appl Immunol 1990;93(2–3):198–204.

60. Guttman-Yassky E, Bergman R, Maor C, et al. The autologous serum skin test in a cohort of chronic idiopathic urticaria patients compared to respiratory allergy patients and healthy individuals. J Eur Acad Dermatol Venereol 2007;21(1): 35–9.

61. Grattan CE, Francis DM, Hide M, et al. Detection of circulating histamine releasing autoantibodies with functional properties of anti-IgE in chronic urti-caria. Clin Exp Allergy 1991;21(6):695–704.

62. Hide M, Francis DM, Grattan CE, et al. Autoantibodies against the high-affinity IgE receptor as a cause of histamine release in chronic urticaria. N Engl J Med 1993;328(22):1599–604.

63. Tong LJ, Balakrishnan G, Kochan JP, et al. Assessment of autoimmunity in patients with chronic urticaria. J Allergy Clin Immunol 1997;99(4):461–5.
64. Yasnowsky KM, Dreskin SC, Efaw B, et al. Chronic urticaria sera increase basophil CD203c expression. J Allergy Clin Immunol 2006;117(6):1430–4.
65. Zweiman B, Valenzano M, Atkins PC, et al. Characteristics of histamine-releasing activity in the sera of patients with chronic idiopathic urticaria. J Allergy Clin Immunol 1996;98(1):89–98.
66. Fusari A, Colangelo C, Bonifazi F, et al. The autologous serum skin test in the follow-up of patients with chronic urticaria. Allergy 2005;60(2):256–8.
67. Fagiolo U, Kricek F, Ruf C, et al. Effects of complement inactivation and IgG depletion on skin reactivity to autologous serum in chronic idiopathic urticaria. J Allergy Clin Immunol 2000;106(3):567–72.
68. Niimi N, Francis DM, Kermani F, et al. Dermal mast cell activation by autoantibodies against the high affinity IgE receptor in chronic urticaria. J Invest Dermatol 1996;106(5):1001–6.
69. Sabroe RA, Greaves MW. Chronic idiopathic urticaria with functional autoantibodies: 12 years on. Br J Dermatol 2006;154(5):813–9.
70. Sheikh J. Autoantibodies to the high-affinity IgE receptor in chronic urticaria: how important are they? Curr Opin Allergy Clin Immunol 2005;5(5):403–7.
71. Vasagar K, Vonakis BM, Gober LM, et al. Evidence of in vivo basophil activation in chronic idiopathic urticaria. Clin Exp Allergy 2006;36(6):770–6. http://dx.doi.org/10.1111/j.1365-2222.2006.02494.x.
72. Eckman JA, Hamilton RG, Saini SS. Independent evaluation of a commercial test for "autoimmune" urticaria in normal and chronic urticaria subjects. J Invest Dermatol 2009;129(6):1584–6.
73. Cho CB, Stutes SA, Altrich ML, et al. Autoantibodies in chronic idiopathic urticaria and nonurticarial systemic autoimmune disorders. Ann Allergy Asthma Immunol 2013;110(1):29–33. http://dx.doi.org/10.1016/j.anai.2012.10.020.
74. Fiebiger E, Hammerschmid F, Stingl G, et al. Anti-FcepsilonRIalpha autoantibodies in autoimmune-mediated disorders. Identification of a structure-function relationship. J Clin Invest 1998;101(1):243–51.
75. Kikuchi Y, Kaplan AP. Mechanisms of autoimmune activation of basophils in chronic urticaria. J Allergy Clin Immunol 2001;107(6):1056–62.
76. Soundararajan S, Kikuchi Y, Joseph K, et al. Functional assessment of pathogenic IgG subclasses in chronic autoimmune urticaria. J Allergy Clin Immunol 2005;115(4):815–21.
77. Horn MP, Pachlopnik JM, Vogel M, et al. Conditional autoimmunity mediated by human natural anti-Fc(epsilon)RIalpha autoantibodies? FASEB J 2001;15(12):2268–74.
78. Horn MP, Gerster T, Ochensberger B, et al. Human anti-FcepsilonRIalpha autoantibodies isolated from healthy donors cross-react with tetanus toxoid. Eur J Immunol 1999;29(4):1139–48.
79. Eckman JA, Hamilton RG, Gober LM, et al. Basophil phenotypes in chronic idiopathic urticaria in relation to disease activity and autoantibodies. J Invest Dermatol 2008;128(8):1956–63. http://dx.doi.org/10.1038/jid.2008.55.
80. Viswanathan RK, Biagtan MJ, Mathur SK. The role of autoimmune testing in chronic idiopathic urticaria. Ann Allergy Asthma Immunol 2012;108(5):337–41.e1. http://dx.doi.org/10.1016/j.anai.2012.02.018.
81. Lapolla W, Desai N, English JC 3rd. Clinical utility of testing for autoimmunity in chronic idiopathic urticaria. J Am Acad Dermatol 2012;66(3):e83–8. http://dx.doi.org/10.1016/j.jaad.2010.11.030.

82. Grattan CE, Francis DM, Slater NG, et al. Plasmapheresis for severe, unremitting, chronic urticaria. Lancet 1992;339(8801):1078–80.
83. O'Donnell BF, Barr RM, Black AK, et al. Intravenous immunoglobulin in autoimmune chronic urticaria. Br J Dermatol 1998;138(1):101–6.
84. Konstantinou GN, Asero R, Maurer M, et al. EAACI/GA(2)LEN task force consensus report: the autologous serum skin test in urticaria. Allergy 2009;64(9):1256–68. http://dx.doi.org/10.1111/j.1398-9995.2009.02132.x.
85. Smith CH, Kepley C, Schwartz LB, et al. Mast cell number and phenotype in chronic idiopathic urticaria. J Allergy Clin Immunol 1995;96(3):360–4.
86. Ferrer M, Nunez-Cordoba JM, Luquin E, et al. Serum total tryptase levels are increased in patients with active chronic urticaria. Clin Exp Allergy 2010. http://dx.doi.org/10.1111/j.1365-2222.2010.03582.x.
87. Ito Y, Satoh T, Takayama K, et al. Basophil recruitment and activation in inflammatory skin diseases. Allergy 2011;66(8):1107–13. http://dx.doi.org/10.1111/j.1398-9995.2011.02570.x.
88. Jacques P, Lavoie A, Bedard PM, et al. Chronic idiopathic urticaria: profiles of skin mast cell histamine release during active disease and remission. J Allergy Clin Immunol 1992;89(6):1139–43.
89. Cohen RW, Rosenstreich DL. Discrimination between urticaria-prone and other allergic patients by intradermal skin testing with codeine. J Allergy Clin Immunol 1986;77(6):802–7.
90. Saini SS, Paterniti M, Vasagar K, et al. Cultured peripheral blood mast cells from chronic idiopathic urticaria patients spontaneously degranulate upon IgE sensitization: relationship to expression of Syk and SHIP-2. Clin Immunol 2009;132(3):342–8. http://dx.doi.org/10.1016/j.clim.2009.05.003.
91. Bossi F, Frossi B, Radillo O, et al. Mast cells are critically involved in serum-mediated vascular leakage in chronic urticaria beyond high-affinity IgE receptor stimulation. Allergy 2011;66(12):1538–45. http://dx.doi.org/10.1111/j.1398-9995.2011.02704.x.
92. Kaplan AP, Gray L, Shaff RE, et al. In vivo studies of mediator release in cold urticaria and cholinergic urticaria. J Allergy Clin Immunol 1975;55(6):394–402.
93. Kaplan AP, Garofalo J, Sigler R, et al. Idiopathic cold urticaria: in vitro demonstration of histamine release upon challenge of skin biopsies. N Engl J Med 1981;305:1074–7.
94. Freichel M, Almering J, Tsvilovskyy V. The role of TRP proteins in mast cells. Frontiers in Immunology 2012;3:150. http://dx.doi.org/10.3389/fimmu.2012.00150.
95. Ombrello MJ, Remmers EF, Sun G, et al. Cold urticaria, immunodeficiency, and autoimmunity related to PLCG2 deletions. N Engl J Med 2012;366(4):330–8. http://dx.doi.org/10.1056/NEJMoa1102140.
96. Saini SS. Basophil responsiveness in chronic urticaria. Curr Allergy Asthma Rep 2009;9(4):286–90.
97. Greaves MW, Plummer VM, McLaughlan P, et al. Serum and cell bound IgE in chronic urticaria. Clin Allergy 1974;4(3):265–71.
98. Kern F, Lichtenstein LM. Defective histamine release in chronic urticaria. J Clin Invest 1976;57(5):1369–77.
99. Sabroe RA, Francis DM, Barr RM, et al. Anti-Fc(epsilon)RI auto antibodies and basophil histamine releasability in chronic idiopathic urticaria. J Allergy Clin Immunol 1998;102(4 Pt 1):651–8.
100. Luquin E, Kaplan AP, Ferrer M. Increased responsiveness of basophils of patients with chronic urticaria to sera but hypo-responsiveness to other stimuli. Clin Exp Allergy 2005;35(4):456–60.

101. Vonakis BM, Vasagar K, Gibbons SP, et al. Basophil FceRI histamine release parallels expression of Src-homology2-containing inositol phosphatases in chronic idiopathic urticaria. J Allergy Clin Immunol 2007;119:441–8.
102. Baker R, Vasagar K, Ohameje N, et al. Basophil histamine release activity and disease severity in chronic idiopathic urticaria. Ann Allergy Asthma Immunol 2008;100:244–9.
103. Rorsman H. Basophilic leucopenia in different forms of urticaria. Acta Allergol 1962;17:168–84.
104. Grattan CE, Walpole D, Francis DM, et al. Flow cytometric analysis of basophil numbers in chronic urticaria: basopenia is related to serum histamine releasing activity. Clin Exp Allergy 1997;27(12):1417–24.
105. Caproni M, Volpi W, Macchia D, et al. Infiltrating cells and related cytokines in lesional skin of patients with chronic idiopathic urticaria and positive autologous serum skin test. Exp Dermatol 2003;12(5):621–8.
106. Grattan CE, Dawn G, Gibbs S, et al. Blood basophil numbers in chronic ordinary urticaria and healthy controls: diurnal variation, influence of loratadine and prednisolone and relationship to disease activity. Clin Exp Allergy 2003;33(3):337–41.
107. Wedi B, Raap U, Wieczorek D, et al. Urticaria and infections. Allergy Asthma Clin Immunol 2009;5(1):10. http://dx.doi.org/10.1186/1710-1492-5-10.
108. Liutu M, Kalimo K, Uksila J, et al. Etiologic aspects of chronic urticaria. Int J Dermatol 1998;37(7):515–9.
109. Di Campli C, Gasbarrini A, Nucera E, et al. Beneficial effects of *Helicobacter pylori* eradication on idiopathic chronic urticaria. Dig Dis Sci 1998;43:1226–9.
110. Baskan EB, Turker T, Gulten M, et al. Lack of correlation between *Helicobacter pylori* infection and autologous serum skin test in chronic idiopathic urticaria. Int J Dermatol 2005;44(12):993–5.
111. Ertam I, Biyikli SE, Yazkan FA, et al. The frequency of nasal carriage in chronic urticaria patients. J Eur Acad Dermatol Venereol 2007;21(6):777–80. http://dx.doi.org/10.1111/j.1468-3083.2006.02083.x.
112. Sharma AD. Role of nasal carriage of *Staphylococcus aureus* in chronic urticaria. Indian J Dermatol 2012;57(3):233–6. http://dx.doi.org/10.4103/0019-5154.96211.
113. Zingale LC, Beltrami L, Zanichelli A, et al. Angioedema without urticaria: a large clinical survey. CMAJ 2006;175(9):1065–70. http://dx.doi.org/10.1503/cmaj.060535.
114. Ozkan M, Oflaz SB, Kocaman N, et al. Psychiatric morbidity and quality of life in patients with chronic idiopathic urticaria. Ann Allergy Asthma Immunol 2007;99(1):29–33. http://dx.doi.org/10.1016/S1081-1206(10)60617-5.
115. Ben-Shoshan M, Blinderman I, Raz A. Psychosocial factors and chronic spontaneous urticaria: a systematic review. Allergy 2013;68(2):131 41. http://dx.doi.org/10.1111/all.12068.
116. Sackesen C, Sekerel BE, Orhan F, et al. The etiology of different forms of urticaria in childhood. Pediatr Dermatol 2004;21(2):102–8. http://dx.doi.org/10.1111/j.0736-8046.2004.21202.x.
117. Mortureux P, Leaute-Labreze C, Legrain-Lifermann V, et al. Acute urticaria in infancy and early childhood: a prospective study. Arch Dermatol 1998;134(3):319–23.
118. Plumb J, Norlin C, Young PC. Exposures and outcomes of children with urticaria seen in a pediatric practice-based research network: a case-control study. Arch Pediatr Adolesc Med 2001;155(9):1017–21.

119. Cribier B. Urticaria and hepatitis. Clin Rev Allergy Immunol 2006;30(1):25–9. http://dx.doi.org/10.1385/CRIAI:30:1:025.
120. Grattan CE. Aspirin sensitivity and urticaria. Clin Exp Dermatol 2003;28(2): 123–7.
121. Palikhe NS, Sin HJ, Kim SH, et al. Genetic variability of prostaglandin E2 receptor subtype EP4 gene in aspirin-intolerant chronic urticaria. J Hum Genet 2012. http://dx.doi.org/10.1038/jhg.2012.55.

Diagnostic Tests for Urticaria

Michihiro Hide, MD, PhD*, Makiko Hiragun, MD,
Takaaki Hiragun, MD, PhD

KEYWORDS

- Diagnosis • Differential diagnosis • Subtypes • Severity • Underground disease
- Complementation • Threshold

KEY POINTS

- Asking adequate clinical questions is essential and an important step in the diagnosis of urticaria and subtypes of urticaria.
- The aims of clinical examinations are to confirm the diagnosis of urticaria subtypes, evaluate disease severity/threshold, and/or find or rule out underlying causes or diseases.
- Provocation tests may be performed for the diagnosis and threshold evaluation of inducible types of urticaria.
- Severity and disease activities of urticaria may be evaluated by questionnaire-based scores, such as UAS-7 (urticaria activity score over 7 consecutive days), AAS (Angioedema Activity Score), CU-Q2oL (Chronic Urticaria Quality of Life Questionnaire), and AE-QoL (Angioedema Quality of Life Questionnaire).
- Certain biomarkers for inflammation, such as serum C-reactive protein and interleukin-6, and blood coagulation/fibrinolysis, such as fibrin degradation products, D-dimer, and prothrombin fragment F1 + 2, may reflect disease severity and activity of chronic spontaneous urticaria.

INTRODUCTION

The manifestation of individual skin symptoms of urticaria is a simple wheal and flare, which, although itchy, disappear without residual signs. On the other hand, the pathogenesis of urticaria is highly heterogeneous. Therefore, there is no single clinical examination commonly required for all patients with urticaria. Moreover, the aims of clinical examinations for urticaria may be variable on a case by case basis. They include confirmation of urticaria subtype, differential diagnoses, threshold determinations, the evaluation of disease activities, and/or to find underlying causes. Thus, the proper performance of diagnostic tests for urticaria is important not only for efficient

Conflicts of Interest: The authors declared no conflict of interest in relation to this work.
Department of Dermatology, Integrated Health Sciences, Institute of Biomedical and Health Sciences, Hiroshima University, Hiroshima 734-8551, Japan
* Corresponding author. 1-2-3 Kasumi, Minami-ku, Hiroshima 734-8551, Japan.
E-mail address: ed1h-w1de-road@hiroshima-u.ac.jp

Immunol Allergy Clin N Am 34 (2014) 53–72
http://dx.doi.org/10.1016/j.iac.2013.09.009
immunology.theclinics.com

clinical practice for individual patients but also to reduce the socioeconomic problems of urticaria.

CLASSIFICATION OF URTICARIA

Proper diagnosis of the urticaria subtype is important for adequate management of urticaria. At present, the classification proposed by the EAACI (European Academy of Allergology and Clinical Immunology), GA[2]LEN (Global Allergy and Asthma European Network), EDF (European Dermatology Forum), and WAO (World Allergy Organization) (**Table 1**) is probably the most widely accepted classification in the world for the management of urticaria.[1–4] This classification was further clarified by the definition of chronic urticaria[5] and supplemented by a classification of angioedema in other publications (**Table 2**).[6]

DIAGNOSIS OF URTICARIA SUBTYPES

A diagnosis of urticaria can be made based on the confirmed appearance of a transient and local skin edema with flare that disappears within a few hours or a day at the most. The skin surface should be smooth and intact, but the size, shape, and color of the eruptions are largely variable and not considered important for determining whether the condition does or does not represent urticaria. This stage of the diagnosis should be completed by careful history taking and clinical examination, especially by inspection.

For the diagnosis of urticaria subtypes, however, various provocation tests and blood examinations may be necessary. All medications for urticaria, especially antihistamines, should be withdrawn; antihistamines should be withdrawn for at least 48 hours before the provocation test, if possible, because they may lead to false-negative results. For this stage of the diagnosis, careful and thorough history taking is again important and information regarding the urticaria eruptions may help in the diagnosis of urticaria subtypes (**Table 3**). It is important to keep in mind that the same patient may concurrently have multiple urticaria subtypes. In addition, provocation tests should be performed with potential emergency treatment in mind, because

Table 1 Classification of urticaria subtypes proposed by the EAACI/GA²LEN/EDF/WAO guidelines in 2009	
Types	**Subtypes**
Spontaneous urticaria	Acute spontaneous urticaria Chronic spontaneous urticaria
Physical urticaria	Cold contact urticaria Delayed pressure urticaria Heat contact urticaria Solar urticaria Urticaria factitia/dermographic urticaria Vibratory urticaria/angioedema
Other urticaria types	Aquagenic urticaria Cholinergic urticaria Contact urticaria Exercise-induced anaphylaxis/urticaria

From Zuberbier T, Asero R, Bindslev-Jensen C, et al. EAACI/GA²LEN/EDF/WAO guideline: definition, classification and diagnosis of urticaria. Allergy 2009;64:1419; with permission.

Table 2
Classification of angioedema

Category	Disease	Notes
Bradykinin-mediated		Not responsive to antihistamines
C1-INH deficient/defect		
Positive inheritance	HAE-1, HAE-2	
Negative inheritance	ACID	Possibly caused by lymphoproliferative disorders, or autoantibody against C1-INH
	Sporadic HAE-1	Both protein and function are low
	Sporadic HAE-2	Only activity is low
Normal C1-INH		
Positive inheritance	HAE with normal C1-INH (type 3)	
Negative inheritance	Drug-induced AE (eg, ACEI)	
Mast cell–mediated		Normal C1-INH
IgE-mediated	Anaphylaxis, IgE-mediated urticaria	
Non–IgE-mediated	Chronic spontaneous urticaria, inducible urticarias, unclassified angioedema	
Idiopathic	Nonclassified angioedema	Normal C1-INH, negative inheritance

Abbreviations: ACEI, angiotensin-converting enzyme inhibitor; ACID, acquired angioedema as a result of C1 inhibitor deficiency; C1-INH, C1-esterase inhibitor; HAE, hereditary angioedema; HAE-1, HAE type 1; HAE-2, HAE type 2.

Modified from Lang DM, Aberer W, Bernstein JA, et al. International consensus on hereditary and acquired angioedema. Ann Allergy Asthma Immunol 2012;109:396; with permission.

the patient may develop systemic symptoms including shock. Specific examinations for the diagnosis of urticaria subtypes are summarized in **Table 4**.

Physical Urticarias

The diagnosis of physical urticarias is made mainly by careful history taking and confirmed by positive physical provocation testing.[18,19] Because patients with a predominantly nonphysical urticaria may also have 1 or more physical urticarias, all physical triggers that seem to be relevant from the medical history should be tested. Provocation by physical triggers should be performed using adequate strengths of the triggers at appropriate skin sites that have not been recently affected by urticaria. These sites may be refractory for hours or a day after urticarial reactions.[18] Recommended methods for provocation testing for each of the physical urticarias and cholinergic urticaria were described in 2009 by EAACI, GA²LEN, and the urticaria network e.V. (UNEV).[18]

Urticaria factitia/dermatographic urticaria/mechanical urticaria

Dermographic urticaria is a common subtype of physical urticaria, and its symptoms appear in response to lightly stroking the skin. Several instruments for testing this have been developed and used to determine the threshold of individual patients.[19–21] The forearm is more suitable for this test than the abdomen, back, and shin areas.[20]

Table 3
Questions for making urticaria and its subtype diagnosis

Common characteristics of urticaria (to make a diagnosis of urticaria)
1. Flare (reddish eruption)
2. Wheal (hive; local swelling or superficial skin swelling)
3. Duration of individual eruptions (commonly less than 24 hours except for delayed pressure urticaria and angioedema)

Specific characteristics of urticaria subtypes (to determine the subtype of urticaria)

Categories to be Clarified	Corresponding Subtypes of Urticaria
Size	
<~5 mm	Cholinergic urticaria, adrenergic urticaria, aquagenic urticaria
>~5 mm	Any other subtypes
Shape	
Linear	Mechanical urticaria
Geographic	Mostly spontaneous urticaria, urticarial vasculitis
Area	
Limited to or mostly in exposed body surfaces	Cold contact urticaria, solar urticaria, heat contact urticaria, contact urticaria
Limited to the face	Angioedema, oral allergy syndrome
Duration	
>12 h	Spontaneous urticaria (acute or chronic), delayed pressure urticaria, angioedema, mostly not cholinergic urticaria and the other physical urticarias
Directly related eliciting stimuli	
None	Spontaneous urticaria (acute or chronic)
Friction, shear	Mechanical urticaria
Cold	Cold urticaria
Sun exposure	Solar urticaria, possibly cholinergic urticaria due to sweating
Heat	Heat urticaria, possibly cholinergic urticaria due to sweating
Pressure	Delayed pressure urticaria
Perspiration (sweating), increase of body core temperature	Cholinergic urticaria
Particular substance (intake; foods, drugs)	Allergic urticaria, intolerance, urticaria due to radiographic contrast media, and so forth
Particular substance (contact; plant, chemicals, foods, and so forth)	Contact urticaria
Exercise	Exercise-induced anaphylaxis, cholinergic urticaria due to sweating
Psychological tension	Adrenergic urticaria, cholinergic urticaria due to sweating

The reaction should be evaluated 10 minutes after testing. It is considered positive if the patient shows a wheal and reports itching at the site of provocation at 36 g/mm^2 (353 kPa) or less. A wheal response without itching on provocation at 60 g/mm^2 (589 kPa) or higher indicates the less clinically significant simple dermographism.[18]

Table 4
Specific examinations for diagnosis of urticaria subtypes. All examinations should be performed based on careful history taking and general physical examinations

Subtypes of Urticaria	Types of Examinations	Aims of Examination	Notes
Acute spontaneous urticaria	Blood examinations	To look for possible underlying causes, such as infections	Not mandatory. CBC, CRP and other serum biochemical tests, as necessary, based on the detailed medical history and physical examinations
Chronic spontaneous urticaria	Blood examinations	To look for possible underlying causes, such as infections, thyroid autoimmunity, autoinflammatory diseases	Not mandatory. CBC, CRP and other serum biochemical tests, as necessary, based on the detailed medical history and physical examinations. Thyroid functions and antithyroid autoantibodies may be examined for thyroid autoimmunity. Increase of monoclonal IgM or IgG in addition to recurrent bouts of unexplained fever and pain in the joints, muscles, and/or bones suggest Schnitzler syndrome
		To evaluate disease severity/activity	D-dimer, FDP, prothrombin fragment F1+2, CRP, and serum levels of several proinflammatory cytokines may reflect disease severity and/or activity, but their sensitivities are low.[7,8] Peripheral blood basopenia and low release of histamine from basophils may also be associated with disease activity.[9,10]
	Autologous serum skin test (ASST)	Screening of histamine-releasing autoantibodies against IgE or the high-affinity IgE receptor (FcεRI)	The presence of functional and specific autoantibodies may be verified by a positive bioassay using basophils (the histamine release assay or cell surface expression of activation marker) and a positive immunoassay (Western blotting or ELISA).[11] A protocol for ASST is shown in **Fig. 4**.[12]
	Skin biopsy	To differentiate from other diseases, such as urticarial vasculitis and erythema multiforme	Histopathology of urticaria lesions typically shows edema of the upper and mid dermis and dilatation of the postcapillary venules and lymphatic vessels. A small to intermediate infiltration of lymphocytes with or without granulocytes around small blood vessels and edema is commonly observed in the upper dermis. Histopathology does not show interface dermatitis observed in erythema multiforme, or apparent leukocytoklastic vasculitis observed in Schönlein-Henoch purpura and urticarial vasculitis
	Provocation and elimination test	To test the involvement of dietary pseudoallergens	For a diagnosis of food pseudoallergy, a 3-week pseudoallergen-free diet is recommended[13]

(continued on next page)

Table 4
(continued)

Subtypes of Urticaria	Types of Examinations	Aims of Examination	Notes
Cold contact urticaria	Provocation test	To confirm the diagnosis by testing skin reactivity for low temperature	Ice cube, cool packs, cold water, or special instruments may be applied on the volar forearm for 5 min. Thresholds may be determined by temperature and/or time of provocation
	Blood examinations	To rule out the involvement of cryoprotein	Plasma cryoglobulin may be measured to rule out cryoglobulinemia as an underlying cause
Delayed pressure urticaria	Provocation test	To confirm the diagnosis by testing skin reactivity for physical pressure	A weight bag or special instruments may be loaded on the shoulder, upper back, thighs, or volar forearm. Thresholds may be determined by the level of pressure (area and weight) and/or time of provocation
	Skin biopsy		In addition to changes observed in other subtypes of urticaria, moderate infiltrations of eosinophils and upregulation of several adhesion molecules may be observed in the mid to lower dermis
Heat contact urticaria	Provocation test	To confirm the diagnosis by testing skin reactivity for high temperature	Metal or glass cylinders filled with hot water, or special instruments may be loaded on the volar forearm for 5 min. Thresholds may be determined by temperature and/or time of provocation
Solar urticaria		To confirm the diagnosis by testing skin reactivity for sunlight	Sunlight, solar simulators with filters, or a monochromator may be irradiated to the buttock area. Thresholds may be determined by the time of provocation. The specific wavelength for provocation may be determined. The suppressive wavelength may also be determined in some patients
Urticaria factitia/ dermographic urticaria/ mechanical urticaria		To confirm the diagnosis by testing skin reactivity for scratching or shear forces	A smooth blunt object, such as the tip of a closed ball point pen or a wooden spatula, or special instruments may be applied on the volar forearm or upper back. Thresholds may be determined by the level of pressure using a special instrument
Vibratory urticaria/ angioedema		To confirm the diagnosis by testing skin reactivity for vibration	The volar forearm may be attached to a laboratory vortex mixer for 10 min at 1000 rpm
Aquagenic urticaria	Provocation test	To confirm the diagnosis by testing skin reactivity for contact with water	Attaching compresses with water or 5% saline on the back or volar forearm at body temperature for 20 min. Wiping the test area with an organic solvent such as acetone may increase the reactivity

Condition	Test	Purpose	Description
Cholinergic urticaria	Provocation test	To confirm the diagnosis by testing skin reactivity for sweating	Perform an appropriate physical exercise to the point of sweating and up to 15 min beyond (eg, on a treadmill or stationary bicycle). The age and general condition of the patient should be considered before exercising. Wearing warm clothing in a warm room facilitates the provocation tests
	Skin test	To test the increase in reactivity to acetylcholine	Wheal and flare with satellite wheal formation in response to 20 μg or less of acetylcholine in 20 μL of saline injected into the dermis are evaluated as positive. Only one-third to one-half of patients show positive reactions[14,15]
Adrenergic urticaria	Skin test	To confirm the diagnosis by testing skin reactivity for adrenaline	Wheal and flare with a halo of blanched skin in response to 10–20 ng of noradrenaline or 5 ng of adrenaline in 20 μL of saline injected into the dermis are evaluated as positive
Contact urticaria	Skin test	To confirm the diagnosis by testing skin reactivity for a suspected substance	Open test with original or adequately diluted suspected substance should be taken first. Prick test may be performed if the open test is negative. An intradermal skin test may be performed only for limited cases when strongly suspected from the history and the other skin tests are negative
Exercise-induced anaphylaxis/ urticaria	Provocation test	To confirm the diagnosis by testing sensitivity to exercise, certain foods, and their combinations in vivo	Exercise should be undertaken in a controlled setting, such as the Bruce method,[16] with a continuous cardiac monitor and emergency equipment. For the diagnosis of food-dependent exercise-induced anaphylaxis, both exercise and food challenges are taken separately and in combination. If both challenges are negative, 100–500 mg of aspirin may be added for provocation[16]
	Tests for type I allergy	To confirm the sensitivity against a suspected food antigen	General examinations for type I allergy: binding of circulating IgE, such as ImmunoCAP, the prick test, and the basophil activating test. In case of wheat-dependent exercise-induced anaphylaxis, detection of serum IgE against ω-5 gliadin is valuable[17]
Urticaria evoked by particular substances	Tests for type I allergy	To confirm the sensitivity against a suspected food antigen	General examinations for type I allergy: binding of circulating IgE, such as ImmunoCAP, the prick test, and the basophil activating test
	Provocation test	To confirm the diagnosis by testing local skin or whole body reactivity for a suspected substance	Challenge with suspected substances. Tests should begin with a small amount of suspected substance to avoid serious reactions, such as anaphylactic shock. No reliable in vitro test is available for nonallergic anaphylactic reactions, such as NSAID-induced urticaria/anaphylaxis
Angioedema	Blood test	To determine the involvement of C1-INH	C3, C4, CH50, C1-INH (amount of protein and activity), C1q
	Gene analysis	To determine the presence or absence of a gene disorder in C1-INH and/or factor XII	Gene sequences for C1-INH and/or factor XII

All provocation tests and skin tests should be performed without the effect of medications. Antihistamines should be discontinued for at least 2 to 3 days.
Abbreviations: C1-INH, C1-inhibitor; CBC, complete blood count; CRP, C-reactive protein; ELISA, enzyme-linked immunosorbent assay; FDP, fibrin degradation products.

Cold contact urticaria/acquired cold urticaria

Symptoms of cold contact urticaria appear on exposure of the skin to cold fluids or cold surfaces. Provocation testing should be performed by applying a cold stimulus to the skin of a volar forearm, abdomen, or a hand. The stimulus may be a melting ice cube with a thin plastic bag, a cool pack, or a cold water bath. If the skin is directly in contact with water, symptoms due to aquagenic urticaria should be differentiated. Ice cube testing should be performed for 5 minutes. The time of contact may be shortened if the patient's history suggests that the patient is very sensitive and may develop massive reactions. If patients do not develop wheals after provocation for 5 minutes, the ice cube may be applied for up to 20 minutes. Patients may be tested further by immersing an arm in cold water at 5 to 10°C for 10 minutes. Test sites should be assessed 10 minutes after the end of the provocation step.[18]

The test should be considered positive if the skin site exposed to the cold shows a palpable and clearly visible wheal and flare. A special instrument, Temp *Test* 3.0 (EMO Systems GmbH, Berlin, Germany), developed for the diagnostic evaluation of cold contact urticaria, may be used to determine the threshold, in addition to making a diagnosis.[22]

Delayed pressure urticaria

Patients with this subtype of urticaria develop a skin swelling on the site of sustained pressure often with pain or burning sensations with or without itching. Whealing occurs after a latent period, typically 2 to 4 hours after the pressure stimulus has been applied. The resulting swelling is deep and large compared with most other urticaria subtypes. Moreover, unlike angioedema, this urticaria subtype is not associated with mucosal symptoms.[19] Skin biopsies reveal an inflammatory infiltrate with prominent eosinophils, but no vasculitis. Provocation may be performed by suspending a 7 kg weight on a 3 cm shoulder strap for 15 minutes, or applying rods supported in a frame to the back, thighs, or forearm, or using a calibrated dermographometer on the upper back. Regarding rod weight application, Lawlor and colleagues[23] used a 1.5-cm diameter rod with a weight of 2.29 kg (127 kPa) to 4.79 kg (266 kPa) for up to 15 minutes on the back. Barlow and colleagues[24] used 1.5-cm diameter rods with 2.5 kg (139 kPa) and 3.5 kg (194 kPa) for 20 minutes on the anterior thighs. In our clinical practice, we use a 1.4-cm diameter rod with a weight of 4.0 kg (255 kPa) for 15 minutes on the back (**Fig. 1**).[25] The approach recommended by a EAACI/GA²LEN/UNEV panel is to apply a 2.5-kg weight with a 1.5-cm diameter rod, or a 5-kg weight with 6.5-cm diameter rod for 15 minutes.[18] When using a dermographometer, the device should be applied at 100 g/m² (981 kPa) for 70 seconds on the upper back.[18,26]

Heat contact urticaria

Heat contact urticaria is rare and is characterized by the appearance of a wheal and flare on the skin area locally heated to a certain temperature. Provocation is performed by applying hot metal or glass cylinders filled with hot water to the skin of the volar forearm. The Temp *Test* described for cold contact urticaria may also be used for this type of urticaria.[22] The temperature for provocation should be 45°C, but may be higher. A standard time for provocation is 5 minutes, but shorter or longer times may be appropriate in some patients.[18] The area exposed to heat should be inspected 10 minutes after the provocation. The test should be considered positive if the test site shows a palpable and clearly visible wheal-and-flare type skin reaction.[18]

Solar urticaria

Wheal-and-flare reactions of solar urticaria appear in response to the exposure of skin to sunlight. Ideally, provocation testing should be done on the buttock skin, but the

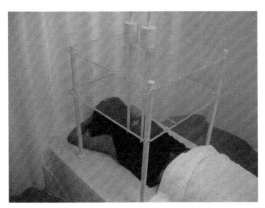

Fig. 1. Device for a pressure challenge test (4 kg/1.5 cm², for 15 minutes). (*Adapted from* Morioke S, Takahagi S, Iwamoto K, et al. Pressure challenge test and histopathological inspections for 17 Japanese cases with clinically diagnosed delayed pressure urticaria. Arch Dermatol Res 2010;302:614; with permission.)

parts of the trunk that are usually covered by clothes can also be tested (**Fig. 2**). The light source may be sunlight or a slide projector from 10 cm distance with or without filters, or a monochromator (UV-A, UV-B, visible light).[18,27] The test site should be inspected 10 minutes after the irradiation. The provocation time may be shortened or prolonged based on the severity of the symptoms predicted by the patient's history.

The action wavelength spectrum of each patient may be determined by using either light filters or monochromator(s). In some patients, the development of a wheal by an action wavelength may be suppressed by exposure to other wavelengths.[28] Patients with solar urticaria reported from Europe and North America tend to be sensitive to ultraviolet part of the spectrum rather than visible part of the spectrum, whereas patients from Japan and Singapore tend to be more sensitive to visible light than ultraviolet light (**Fig. 3**).[14,27–32]

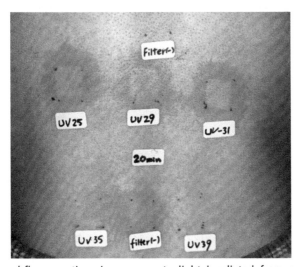

Fig. 2. Wheal-and-flare reactions in response to light irradiated from a slide projector through various filters. (*Adapted from* Kawai M, Hide M, Okabe T, et al. A case of solar urticaria induced by UVA. Nishinihon J Dermatol 2000;62:299; with permission.)

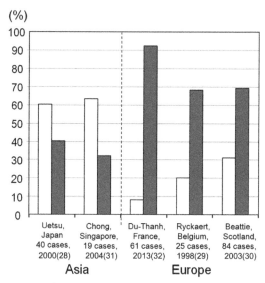

Fig. 3. Action wavelengths for patients with solar urticaria reported in various countries. Patients with solar urticaria reported in Japan and Singapore are more susceptible to visible light than to ultraviolet light, whereas the pattern is the other way round for patients in Europe. Open bar, sensitive to visible light only; filled bar, sensitive to ultraviolet light.

Vibratory urticaria/angioedema

Vibratory urticaria/angioedema is characterized by itching and swelling of the skin exposed to vibration. For provocation, the forearm is held on a flat plate placed on a vortex mixer that is run at between 780 rpm and 1380 rpm for 10 minutes. The site of application should be assessed for swelling 10 minutes after testing. The measurement of the circumference of the arm before and after the provocation at 3 points (wrist, midforearm, and elbow) can help with evaluation of swelling.[18]

Aquagenic Urticaria

Aquagenic urticaria is a relatively rare subtype of urticaria, characterized by small follicular wheals and flare on exposure to aqueous solutions. Provocation is performed by attaching wet cloths at body temperature for 20 minutes.[18] Wiping the test area with an organic solvent, such as acetone or ethanol, and challenging with saline instead of tap water may increase the reactivity (**Fig. 4**).[33]

Cholinergic Urticaria

Cholinergic urticaria is a subtype of urticaria common in children and young adults.[34] Symptoms of cholinergic urticaria develop in conditions causing sweating, such as exercise, taking a hot bath, or emotional stimuli.[18] It may be accompanied by angioedema and systemic symptoms including wheezing or, rarely, anaphylaxis. Cholinergic urticaria must be differentiated from exercise-induced urticaria/anaphylaxis, which is induced by exercise but not by passive warming. The diagnosis is established by an appropriate provocation test and/or skin test with acetylcholine.[14,15,18]

Provocation is performed by physical exercise appropriate for the patient's age and general condition (eg, on a treadmill or stationary bicycle). The exercise should be performed to the point of sweating and up to 15 minutes beyond this point. To differentiate from exercise-induced anaphylaxis, a passive warming test should done,

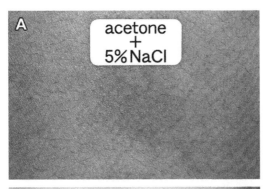

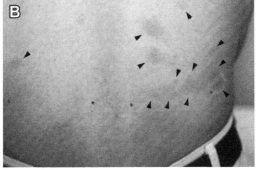

Fig. 4. Wheal-and-flare reactions induced by contact with 5% saline on the back for 15 minutes. (*A*) A wheal with flare appeared at a hair follicle. (*B*) Pretreatment with acetone induced more wheals and flares indicated by *arrowheads* (*right*) than in the control (*left*). (*From* Hide M, Yamamura Y, Sanada S, et al. Aquagenic urticaria: a case report. Acta Derm Venereol 2000;80:148; with permission.)

recording core body temperature to achieve an increase of 1.0°C or more. The skin should be inspected immediately and 10 minutes after the end of the test.[18]

Skin testing with intradermal injection of 0.1 mL of acetylcholine at 100 μg/mL may reinforce the diagnosis of cholinergic urticaria (**Fig. 5**). The test should be considered positive if the test site shows satellite wheals around the injection site. The specificity of this test seems to be high, but the sensitivity is approximately 30% to 50%.[14,15]

Adrenergic Urticaria

Adrenergic urticaria has been reported to be a rare subtype of urticaria. Patients develop small maculopapular lesions with a halo of blanched skin in association with psychological tension.[35–39] Wheal and flare may be reproduced by a skin test with 5 ng of adrenaline or 10 to 20 ng of noradrenaline in 20 μL of saline (**Fig. 6**). Although the independence of this disease entity is controversial, symptoms improved in all cases treated with propranolol reported so far.[35–39]

Contact Urticaria

Contact urticaria (see the article by McFadden in this issue for a detailed review) is characterized by immediate development of a wheal and flare with itching at the site of contact with specific substances and may be immunologic (IgE-mediated) or less commonly nonimmunologic. The wheal and flare usually appears within

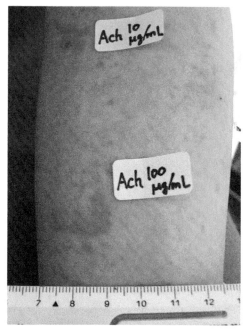

Fig. 5. Wheal-and-flare reactions induced by intradermal injections of 20 µL of acetylcholine at 10 µg/mL and 100 µg/mL.

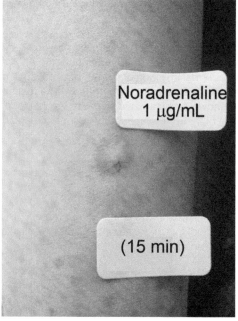

Fig. 6. A pale wheal and surrounding flare induce by injection of 20 µL of noradrenaline at 1 µg/mL.

30 minutes and completely disappears within a few hours and may also develop into generalized urticaria and even anaphylaxis.[40]

The suspected substance is applied in its original form or as an extract on a normal-looking 3×3 cm area of the volar forearm or the upper back for 15 to 20 minutes.[40] The EAACI/GA^{2}LEN/EDF/UNEV consensus panel recommends reading the reaction 20 minutes after the provocation (open test).[18] If this test is negative, the next step is occlusive application. We use chambers for closed patch testing for this purpose. For patients with a history of severe symptoms, tests should be started with sufficiently diluted suspected substances. If no itchy wheal and flare appears in these tests, a prick test may be performed.[40,41] The performance of intradermal skin tests should be limited to patients for whom contact urticaria is strongly suggested by the history but negative results are obtained for both the open test and the skin prick test. In vitro tests may also be used for contact urticaria by type I allergy, such as latex allergy.[40]

Exercise-Induced Anaphylaxis/Urticaria

Exercise may result in anaphylaxis with an urticarial eruption in patients with this category. Some patients may develop urticaria and anaphylaxis regardless of food intake (EIA), but other patients develop anaphylaxis only when they exercise after partaking of a food (FDEIA). The diagnosis of EIA and FDEIA is based on the detailed history and adequate provocation testing performed as necessary. The demonstration of specific food allergen-reactive IgE in the serum may help, but may not be sufficient for the diagnosis of FDEIA in some cases. Some patients may develop anaphylaxis by exercise after intake of any food but, in others, IgE-mediated allergy to 1 or more specific food allergens is involved.[42] The presence of anti-ω5-gliadin IgE in adults has been reported to be an exceptionally good marker for FDEIA caused by wheat with regard to sensitivity and specificity.[16]

The exercise challenge test is typically performed according to the protocol of Bruce and colleagues[43] with a continuous cardiac monitor and emergency equipment. In cases of FDEIA, the provocation test should include the food challenge alone, exercise alone, and a combination of food ingestion and exercise. The amounts of food and exercise required to cause symptoms to develop are largely variable not only among patients but also vary depending on the different circumstances in which the same patient is tested. Other conditions, such as fatigue, lack of sleep, or low temperature may affect the threshold for developing anaphylaxis.[17] Aspirin intake is a well-documented augmenting factor for FDEIA. To provoke or exacerbate symptoms, 500 mg of aspirin may be taken together with the suspected food.[44] In some cases, the combination of only aspirin and a culprit diet may result in anaphylaxis.[45] The sensitivity of provocation testing for FDEIA was reported to be up to 70%.[16]

Urticaria Induced by Particular Substances

Acute urticaria may develop in response to the intake of particular substances as a result of a specific hypersensitivity. The mechanism could be either type I IgE-mediated or nonimmunologic. In cases of type I allergy, hypersensitivities of individual patients should be proved by serum tests, such as ImmunoCAP, and IMMULITE 3gAllergy or basophil activating tests (BAT), such as the histamine release test and CD203c expression on the surface of basophils, or skin testing, such as the prick test as described earlier.[16,17,46] In cases of urticaria induced by nonimmunologic mechanisms, such as those from radiographic contrast media or nonsteroidal antiinflammatory drugs (NSAIDs), provocation is the only examination for a definitive diagnosis. The provocation test may be appropriate in selected patients and should begin with sufficiently small amounts of suspected substances under careful observation and with emergency equipment readily available.

Angioedema

Angioedema is a common complicating feature of some subtypes of urticaria and, like urticaria, is usually taken to be mast cell mediated. Cases where angioedema appears by itself may also be mast cell mediated. However, a bradykinin-mediated mechanism should be excluded. It is important to ask patients if they use an angiotensin-converting enzyme inhibitor, which inhibits bradykinin degradation and may elicit bradykinin-mediated angioedema. Hereditary angioedema cannot be ruled out if the patient developed the first symptoms of angioedema by adolescence, and/or a sibling has the same condition. For the screening of bradykinin-mediated angioedema, blood levels of C3, C4, C1-inhibitor (C1-INH) (protein concentration and activity), and C1q are informative. If an acquired form of C1-INH is suspected, lymphoproliferative diseases should be ruled out (see **Tables 2** and **4**).[6]

DIAGNOSIS OF UNDERLYING CAUSES OR DISEASES

Several factors, diseases, and/or conditions have been reported as underlying causes of urticaria. Frequently suspected factors in relation to spontaneous urticaria are listed in **Box 1**. However, a systematic review of the laboratory investigations for chronic urticaria revealed that the number of diagnoses identified varied from 1% to 84%, and was not related to the number of laboratory tests performed.[47] Therefore, intensive programs of clinical examinations are not recommended for routine screening of the causes of urticarias, unless suggested by the medical history and/or physical examination.[1,4,47]

Infections

Acute infections by viruses and bacteria are known to be often associated with the onset of acute urticaria and transient aggravation of chronic spontaneous urticaria. Many studies have suggested chronic persistent infection by *Helicobacter pylori* as an important cause of chronic spontaneous urticaria. However, its significance is disputed.[1,4,48] The relationship between many other kinds of infections and urticaria have not been substantiated.

Stress and Fatigue

Many investigators have suggested a relationship between stress and/or fatigue and aggravation and/or elicitation of urticaria.[4,48] However, urticaria itself induces stress and impairs the quality of life of patients.[49,50] Therefore, it is largely controversial if stress and fatigue should be included as underlying causes of urticaria. Moreover,

---

Box 1
Factors suggested as underlying causes of urticaria

1. Infection (acute, chronic)
2. Stress, fatigue
3. Autoimmunity against thyroid
4. Autoimmunity against IgE/FcεRI
5. Pseudoallergy (food, drug)
6. Other organ disorders

no diagnostic test for these factors has been established. Nevertheless, with respect to quality of life assessments, it is good clinical practice to ask patients with urticaria about their psychosomatic and psychiatric conditions.

Autoimmunity Against the Thyroid

Autoantibodies against thyroglobulin, thyroid microsomal antigen, and thyroid peroxidase may be detected in patients with chronic spontaneous urticaria, regardless of an apparent disorder of thyroid function.[51–53] However, results from recent studies conducted on a large scale do not support the therapeutic effect of thyroxin on urticaria.[54,55]

Autoimmunity Against IgE/High-Affinity IgE Receptor (FcεRI)

Approximately 30% to 50% of patients with chronic spontaneous urticaria have IgG autoantibodies that activate mast cells and basophils by crosslinking of IgE and/or the high-affinity IgE receptor (FcεRI).[19,56,57] The presence of such autoantibodies should be demonstrated by a histamine release assay using the patient's serum and basophils from healthy donors.[56,57] However, this assay is somewhat cumbersome and requires special equipment, which has therefore limited its application across the world. A solid phase assay, such as enzyme-linked immunosorbent assay, is relatively easy and quantitative, but not specific.[11] Alternatively, skin reactions evoked by intradermal injection of autologous serum (autologous serum skin test [ASST]) have been widely used as a screening test because of their relative simplicity and high sensitivity.[11,12,58,59] So far, various modifications of the ASST have been made but its specificity has not been solidly established for use in clinical practice. The EAACI task force reviewed the evidence regarding ASST for best practice for chronic spontaneous urticaria in 2009 and 2013.[11,12] Their recommended procedure for ASST is shown in **Fig. 7**.

The ASST should be performed at least 2 to 3 days after the last dose of H1 antihistamine. Patients should have also ceased using systemic corticosteroids, equivalent to or more than 15 mg prednisolone, heparin and antileukotrienes before performing the ASST. Standard precautions for handling blood products are required to protect both the patient and the operator.[12]

Pseudoallergy

Nonallergic hypersensitivity to dietary pseudoallergens, including naturally occurring food ingredients, such as salicylates and biogenous amines, food additives, and continuous use of oral or topical NSAIDs may be relevant as a cause and/or precipitating or aggravating factor for chronic spontaneous urticaria. Because the mechanism of pseudoallergen provocation of urticaria remains unclear, strict exclusion and subsequent provocation testing with a suspected substance are necessary for the diagnosis.[13] For a diagnosis of food pseudoallergy, a 3-weeks pseudoallergen-free diet is recommended.[13]

Other Organ Disorders

Many diseases or disorders, including malignancies, have been reported to underlie spontaneous urticaria. In some cases, the treatment of these disorders resulted in the remission of the urticaria. With respect to physical urticaria, cryoglobulinemia was identified in several patients with cold contact urticaria.[18,60] However, in other cases, the relationship between these disorders and the pathogenesis of urticaria is largely unknown. Moreover, screening for malignant neoplasms as a routine in urticaria is no longer recommended, because the incidence of neoplasms in patients

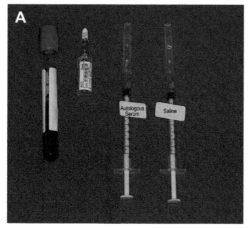
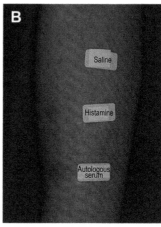

C

Collect blood into sterile (no additive) glass tubes without additives.

(Red-topped 7 mL BD Vacutainer® [Becton, Dickinson and Company, Franklin Lakes, NJ, USA] blood collection tubes is recommended)
↓
Allow blood to clot at room temperature for 30 min.
Centrifuge sample at 450-500 g for 10 min.
↓
Clean the volar forearm skin with antiseptic.
Perform intradermal injections of 0.05 mL of normal saline as a negative control and the same amount of autologous serum. Skin prick with 10 mg/mL histamine solution or intradermal injection of 0.05 mL of 0.5 to 1.0 μg histamine as a positive control.
↓
Wait 30 min
↓
Ensure a positive histamine reaction, and measure the two longest perpendicular diameters of any red wheal reactions to the ASST and the normal saline skin test.

Fig. 7. The autologous serum skin test (ASST) and devices for the test. (*A*) The identity of the blood donor and the labeling of samples should be verified to avoid any risk of skin testing with the wrong serum. (*B*) Fifty microliters of autologous serum, saline, and 10 μg/mL histamine are injected, respectively. (*C*) Flowchart for ASST procedure recommended by the EAACI/GA²LEN/EDF/WAO task force. (*Adapted from* Konstantinou GN, Asero R, Maure M, et al. EAACI/GA(2)LEN task force consensus report: the autologous serum skin test in urticaria. Allergy 2009;64:1257 and 1261; with permission.)

with urticaria and that in the general population have been found to be similar.[1,61] If any symptoms different from urticaria are recognized, clinical examinations should be undertaken as necessary.

EVALUATION OF THE SEVERITY OF URTICARIA

The evaluation of disease severity of inducible urticarias may be performed according to the threshold for eliciting factors. For spontaneous urticarias and angioedema, questionnaire-based scores may be used.[1,62] The urticaria activity score over 7 consecutive days (UAS7) is a unified and simple scoring system, validated in comparison with the Dermatology Life Quality Index (DLQI).[63] The quality of life of patients with superficial urticaria and that of patients with angioedema may be evaluated using the Chronic Urticaria Quality of Life Questionnaire (CU-Q2oL)[50] and Angioedema Quality of Life Questionnaire (AE-QoL),[64] respectively.

Coagulation/fibrinolysis markers, such as D-dimer, fibrin degradation products, prothrombin fragment F1+2, and C-reactive protein have been reported to reflect disease severity and/or activity, but their sensitivities are low.[7,65] Serum levels of proinflammatory cytokines, such as interleukin (IL)-6, tumor necrosis factor (TNF), and IL-23, may also reflect disease activity in certain patients,[7,66] but are of doubtful usefulness.[8] Peripheral blood basopenia and low release of histamine from basophils may also be associated with disease activity,[9,10] but their value is at present confined to the research laboratory.

SUMMARY

Diagnostic tests for urticaria should be performed based on the detailed history of the patient and physical examination. The definitive diagnosis of urticaria subtypes, which may be complicated in the individual patient, is important for both adequate treatment and further detailed examinations specific for individual subtypes. Disease severity and activity of spontaneous urticaria and angioedema are evaluated by questionnaire-based scoring systems. The establishment of more sensitive and specific biomarkers is a major aspiration in the future management of spontaneous urticaria and angioedema.

REFERENCES

1. Zuberbier T, Asero R, Bindslev-Jensen C, et al. EAACI/GA^{2}LEN/EDF/WAO guideline: definition, classification and diagnosis of urticaria. Allergy 2009;64: 1417–26.
2. Sánchez-Borges M, Asero R, Ansotegui IJ, et al. Diagnosis and treatment of urticaria and angioedema: a worldwide perspective. World Allergy Organ J 2012; 5:125–47.
3. Chow SK. Management of chronic urticaria in Asia: 2010 AADV consensus guidelines. Asia Pac Allergy 2012;2:149–60.
4. Hide M, Hiragun T, Japanese Dermatological Association. Japanese guidelines for diagnosis and treatment of urticaria in comparison with other countries. Allergol Int 2012;61:517–27.
5. Maurer M, Bindslev-Jensen C, Gimenez-Arnau A, et al. Chronic idiopathic urticaria (CIU) is no longer idiopathic: time for an update. Br J Dermatol 2013;168:455–6.
6. Lang DM, Aberer W, Bernstein JA, et al. International consensus on hereditary and acquired angioedema. Ann Allergy Asthma Immunol 2012;109:395–402.
7. Rabelo-Filardi R, Daltro-Oliveira R, Campos RA. Parameters associated with chronic spontaneous urticaria duration and severity: a systematic review. Int Arch Allergy Immunol 2013;161:197–204.
8. Metz M, Krull C, Maurer M. Histamine, TNF, C5a, IL-6, -9, -18, -31, -33, TSLP, Neopterin, and VEGF are not elevated in chronic spontaneous urticaria. J Dermatol Sci 2013;70:222–5.
9. Grattan CE, Dawn G, Gibbs S, et al. Blood basophil numbers in chronic ordinary urticaria and healthy controls: diurnal variation, influence of loratadine and prednisolone and relationship to disease activity. Clin Exp Allergy 2003;33:337–41.
10. Eckman JA, Hamilton RG, Gober LM, et al. Basophil phenotypes in chronic idiopathic urticaria in relation to disease activity and autoantibodies. J Invest Dermatol 2008;128:1956–63.

11. Konstantinou GN, Asero R, Ferrer M, et al. EAACI taskforce position paper: evidence for autoimmune urticaria and proposal for defining diagnostic criteria. Allergy 2013;68:27–36.
12. Konstantinou GN, Asero R, Maure M, et al. EAACI/GA^{2}LEN task force consensus report: the autologous serum skin test in urticaria. Allergy 2009;64:1256–68.
13. Zuberbier T, Chantraine-Hess S, Hartmann K, et al. Pseudoallergen-free diet in the treatment of chronic urticaria. A prospective study. Acta Derm Venereol 1995;75:484–7.
14. Fukunaga A, Bito T, Tsuru K, et al. Responsiveness to autologous sweat and serum in cholinergic urticaria classifies its clinical subtypes. J Allergy Clin Immunol 2005;116:397–402.
15. Commens CA, Greaves MW. Test to establish the diagnosis in cholinergic urticaria. Br J Dermatol 1978;98:47–51.
16. Morita E, Kunie K, Matsuo H. Food-dependent exercise-induced anaphylaxis. J Dermatol Sci 2007;47:109–17.
17. Morita E, Chinuki Y, Takahashi H. Recent advances of in vitro tests for the diagnosis of food-dependent exercise-induced anaphylaxis. J Dermatol Sci 2013;71:155–9.
18. Magerl M, Borzova E, Giménez-Arnau A, et al. The definition and diagnostic testing of physical and cholinergic urticarias–EAACI/GA2LEN/EDF/UNEV consensus panel recommendations. Allergy 2009;64:1715–21.
19. Hide M, Greaves MW. Chronic urticaria as an autoimmune disease. In: Hertl M, editor. Autoimmune diseases of the skin, Pathogenesis, diagnosis, management. 2nd edition. Vienna, New York: Springer; 2005. p. 309–32.
20. Termklinchan V, Kulthanan K, Bunyaratavej S. Assessment of dermographism at different anatomical regions by dermographometer. J Med Assoc Thai 2006;89:992–6.
21. Mlynek A, Vieira dos Santos R, Ardelean E, et al. A novel, simple, validated and reproducible instrument for assessing provocation threshold levels in patients with symptomatic dermographism. Clin Exp Dermatol 2013;38:360–6.
22. Siebenhaar F, Weller K, Mlynek A, et al. Acquired cold urticaria: clinical picture and update on diagnosis and treatment. Br J Dermatol 2010;162:198–200.
23. Lawlor F, Barr R, Kobza-Black A, et al. Arachidonic acid transformation is not stimulated in delayed pressure urticaria. Br J Dermatol 1989;121:317–21.
24. Barlow RJ, Warburton F, Watson K, et al. Diagnosis and incidence of delayed pressure urticaria in patients with chronic urticaria. J Am Acad Dermatol 1993;29:954–8.
25. Morioke S, Takahagi S, Iwamoto K, et al. Pressure challenge test and histopathological inspections for 17 Japanese cases with clinically diagnosed delayed pressure urticaria. Arch Dermatol Res 2010;302:613–7.
26. Lawlor F, Black AK, Ward AM, et al. Delayed pressure urticaria, objective evaluation of a variable disease using a dermographometer and assessment of treatment using colchicine. Br J Dermatol 1989;120:403–8.
27. Kawai M, Hide M, Okabe T, et al. A case of solar urticaria induced by UVA. Nishinihon Journal of Dermatol 2000;62:298–301.
28. Uetsu N, Miyauchi-Hashimoto H, Okamoto H, et al. The clinical and photobiological characteristics of solar urticaria in 40 patients. Br J Dermatol 2000;142:32–8.
29. Ryckaert S, Roelandts R. Solar urticaria. A report of 25 cases and difficulties in phototesting. Arch Dermatol 1998;134:71–4.

30. Beattie PE, Dawe RS, Ibbotson SH, et al. Characteristics and prognosis of idiopathic solar urticaria: a cohort of 87 cases. Arch Dermatol 2003;139:1149–54.
31. Chong WS, Khoo SW. Solar urticaria in Singapore: an uncommon photodermatosis seen in a tertiary dermatology center over a 10-year period. Photodermatol Photoimmunol Photomed 2004;20:101–4.
32. Du-Thanh A, Debu A, Lalheve P, et al. Solar urticaria: a time-extended retrospective series of 61 patients and review of literature. Eur J Dermatol 2013; 23:202–7.
33. Hide M, Yamamura Y, Sanada S, et al. Aquagenic urticaria: a case report. Acta Derm Venereol 2000;80:148–9.
34. Hirschmann JV, Lawlor F, English JS, et al. Cholinergic urticaria. A clinical and histologic study. Arch Dermatol 1987;123:462–7.
35. Shelley WB, Shelley ED. Adrenergic urticaria: a new form of stress-induced hives. Lancet 1985;2:1031–3.
36. Mihara S, Hide M. Adrenergic urticaria in a patient with cholinergic urticaria. Br J Dermatol 2008;158:629–31.
37. Wang Y, Yu J, Tu P. Adrenergic urticaria in a patient with atopic skin reaction and thyroid autoantibody. J Dermatol 2013;40:131–2.
38. Chedraoui A, Uthman I, Abbas O, et al. Adrenergic urticaria in a patient with anti-double-stranded DNA antibodies. Acta Derm Venereol 2008;88:263–6.
39. Capella GL. Adrenergic urticaria and rheumatoid arthritis in a patient with melanoma: an intricate medical management. J Drugs Dermatol 2012;11: 409–12.
40. Gimenez-Arnau A, Maurer M, De La Cuadra J. Immediate contact skin reactions, an update of Contact Urticaria, Contact Urticaria Syndrome and Protein Contact Dermatitis – "A Never Ending Story". Eur J Dermatol 2010;20:552–62.
41. Heinzerling L, Mari A, Bergmann KC, et al. The skin prick test - European standards. Clin Transl Allergy 2013;3:3.
42. Dohi M, Suko M, Sugiyama H, et al. Food-dependent, exercise-induced anaphylaxis: a study on 11 Japanese cases. J Allergy Clin Immunol 1991;87:34–40.
43. Bruce RA, Blackmon JR, Jones JW, et al. Exercising testing in adult normal subjects and cardiac patients. Pediatrics 1963;32(Suppl):742–56.
44. Aihara M, Miyazawa M, Osuna H, et al. Food-dependent exercise-induced anaphylaxis: influence of concurrent aspirin administration on skin testing and provocation. Br J Dermatol 2002;146:466–72.
45. Matsukura S, Aihara M, Sugawara M, et al. Two cases of wheat-dependent anaphylaxis induced by aspirin administration but not by exercise. Clin Exp Dermatol 2010;35:233–7.
46. Hiragun T, Ishii K, Hiragun M, et al. Fungal protein MGL_1304 in sweat is an allergen for atopic dermatitis patients. J Allergy Clin Immunol 2013;132:608–15.
47. Kozel MM, Bossuyt PM, Mekkes JR, et al. Laboratory tests and identified diagnoses in patients with physical and chronic urticaria and angioedema: a systematic review. J Am Acad Dermatol 2003;48:409–16.
48. Maurer M, Weller K, Bindslev-Jensen C, et al. Unmet clinical needs in chronic spontaneous urticaria. A GA^{2}LEN task force report. Allergy 2011;66:317–30.
49. O'Donnell BF, Lawlor F, Simpson J, et al. The impact of chronic urticaria on the quality of life. Br J Dermatol 1997;136:197–201.
50. Baiardini I, Giardini A, Pasquali M, et al. Quality of life and patients' satisfaction in chronic urticaria and respiratory allergy. Allergy 2003;58:621–3.
51. Leznoff A, Josse RG, Denburg J, et al. Association of chronic urticaria and angioedema with thyroid autoimmunity. Arch Dermatol 1983;119:636–40.

52. Verneuil L, Leconte C, Ballet JJ, et al. Association between chronic urticaria and thyroid autoimmunity: a prospective study involving 99 patients. Dermatology 2004;208:98–103.
53. Cebeci F, Tanrikut A, Topcu E, et al. Association between chronic urticaria and thyroid autoimmunity. Eur J Dermatol 2005;16:402–5.
54. Kiyici S, Gul OO, Baskan EB, et al. Effect of levothyroxine treatment on clinical symptoms and serum cytokine levels in euthyroid patients with chronic idiopathic urticaria and thyroid autoimmunity. Clin Exp Dermatol 2010;35:603–7.
55. Magen E, Mishal J. The effect of L-thyroxine treatment on chronic idiopathic urticaria and autoimmune thyroiditis. Int J Dermatol 2012;51:94–7.
56. Grattan CE, Francis DM, Hide M, et al. Detection of circulating histamine releasing autoantibodies with functional properties of anti-IgE in chronic urticaria. Clin Exp Allergy 1991;21:695–704.
57. Hide M, Francis DM, Grattan CE, et al. Autoantibodies against the high-affinity IgE receptor as a cause of histamine release in chronic urticaria. N Engl J Med 1993;328:1599–604.
58. Grattan CE, Wallington TB, Warin RP, et al. A serological mediator in chronic idiopathic urticaria–a clinical, immunological and histological evaluation. Br J Dermatol 1986;114:583–90.
59. Sabroe RA, Grattan CE, Francis DM, et al. The autologous serum skin test: a screening test for autoantibodies in chronic idiopathic urticaria. Br J Dermatol 1999;140:446–52.
60. Ito A, Kazama T, Ito K, et al. Purpura with cold urticaria in a patient with hepatitis C virus infection-associated mixed cryoglobulinemia type III: successful treatment with interferon-β. J Dermatol 2003;30:321–5.
61. Lindelöf B, Sigurgeirsson B, Wahlgren CF, et al. Chronic urticaria and cancer: an epidemiological study of 1155 patients. Br J Dermatol 1990;123:453–6.
62. Weller K, Groffik A, Magerl M, et al. Development, validation, and initial results of the Angioedema Activity Score. Allergy 2013;68(9):1185–92.
63. Młynek A, Zalewska-Janowska A, Martus P, et al. How to assess disease activity in patients with chronic urticaria? Allergy 2008;63:777–80.
64. Weller K, Groffik A, Magerl M, et al. Development and construct validation of the angioedema quality of life questionnaire. Allergy 2012;67:1289–98.
65. Takahagi S, Mihara S, Iwamoto K, et al. Coagulation/fibrinolysis and inflammation markers are associated with disease activity in patients with chronic urticaria. Allergy 2010;65:649–56.
66. Atwa MA, Emara AS, Youssef N, et al. Serum concentration of IL-17, IL-23 and TNF-α among patients with chronic spontaneous urticaria: association with disease activity and autologous serum skin test. J Eur Acad Dermatol Venereol 2013. [Epub ahead of print]. http://dx.doi.org/10.1111/jdv.12124.

Physical Urticarias and Cholinergic Urticaria

Marina Abajian, Nicole Schoepke, MD, Sabine Altrichter, MD,
H.C. Torsten Zuberbier, MD, Marcus Maurer, MD*

KEYWORDS

- Physical urticaria • Urticaria factitia • Pressure urticaria • Cold urticaria
- Heat urticaria • Solar urticaria • Vibratory urticaria/angioedema
- Cholinergic urticaria

KEY POINTS

- Physical urticarias and cholinergic urticaria are more frequent, chronic, and debilitating than commonly thought.
- Many patients are severely impaired in their quality of life, but disease-specific instruments to measure this are missing.
- The signs and symptoms of physical urticarias and cholinergic urticaria are known to be mast cell-mediated, but their underlying causes remain to be identified and characterized.
- Trigger threshold measurements are important to inform patients and physicians about disease severity and to monitor its course over time as well as treatment responses.
- As of yet, validated protocols and instruments to measure trigger thresholds are available only for urticaria factitia/symptomatic dermographism, cold contact urticaria, heat contact urticaria and solar urticaria, but not for the other physical urticarias and cholinergic urticaria.
- Treatment choices include trigger avoidance and second-generation nonsedating H1-antihistamines in all physical urticarias and cholinergic urticaria.
- Future research efforts will need to focus on the identification of underlying causes and associated mast cell secretagogues, because this will allow for the development of curative, rather than symptomatic, therapies.

INTRODUCTION

Physical urticarias (PhysU) are characterized by itchy wheal and flare-type skin reactions and/or angioedema induced by external physical factors, which include mechanical (friction, pressure, and vibration), thermal (cold, heat) stimuli, and electromagnetic radiation (solar radiation).[1] Thus, characterized by the nature of the eliciting factor

Department of Dermatology and Allergy, Allergie – Centrum Charité/ECARF, Charité – Universitätsmedizin Berlin, Charitéplatz 1, Berlin 10117, Germany
* Corresponding author.
E-mail address: marcus.maurer@charite.de

acting on the skin, physU encompass several distinct subtypes: urticaria factitia/symptomatic dermographism (UF/SD), delayed pressure urticaria (DPU), vibratory urticaria/angioedema, cold contact urticaria (ColdU), heat contact urticaria (HeatU), and solar urticaria (SolU).[2] Cholinergic urticaria (CholU), which is also an inducible form of urticaria, is not classified as a PhysU, because its symptoms occur as a response to a rise in body temperature. The signs and symptoms of CholU are typically provoked by exercise or hot showers or baths and not by exogenous physical triggers acting on the skin.[2] PhysU need to be accurately distinguished from other inducible forms of urticaria as well as from chronic spontaneous urticaria (**Table 1**).

In CholU and in all PhysU subtypes except for DPU, wheal and flare responses, or angioedema, appear rapidly (ie, within minutes) after exposure to the relevant trigger and they last for a short time (several minutes to hours). However, systemic reactions with generalized urticaria and variable extracutaneous manifestations can also occur.[3,4] PhysU and CholU are chronic conditions and comprise up to 25% and 5% of cases of chronic urticaria, respectively. They occur most frequently in young adults.[5–7] Some patients exhibit more than one physical or other subtype of chronic urticaria simultaneously.[8–10]

The underlying causes of PhysU and CholU remain poorly understood. Pathogenetically, the activation of skin mast cells and their release of histamine and other proinflammatory mediators are the most relevant factors.[11] However, it is largely unknown how and why physical stimuli or the increase of body temperature activate skin mast cells.

PhysU and CholU are usually diagnosed from patients' case histories and the results of provocation testing. Patients who are suspected to have more than one PhysU should be tested for every potentially relevant trigger.[2] Furthermore, measurements of individual trigger thresholds should be done. This allows both patients and physicians to evaluate disease activity and response to the treatment.[12] The treatment of inducible urticarias including PhysU and CholU relies on 2 basic principles: avoidance of eliciting stimuli and inhibition of mast cell mediators, such as histamine. However,

Table 1
Classification of inducible forms of urticaria

Types of Inducible Urticaria	Type of Stimuli	Subtypes of Inducible Urticaria	Relevant Trigger
Physical Urticarias	Mechanic	Symptomatic dermographism[a]	Friction, rubbing
		DPU	Static pressure
		Vibratory urticaria/angioedema	Vibration
	Thermal	Cold contact urticaria	Cold contact
		Heat contact urticaria	Heat contact
	Electromagnetic waves	Solar urticaria	UV/visible light
Other inducible urticarias	—	Cholinergic urticaria	Increase in body temperature due to exercises, warmth, emotional distress
		Aquagenic urticaria	Water contact
		Contact urticaria	Contact with urticariogenic substances

[a] Also called urticaria factitia.

complete avoidance of relevant triggers is often impossible or associated with unbearable impairment of daily activities. Therefore, second-generation nonsedating H1-antihistamines are recommended as a first-line symptomatic treatment.[13] However, in most patients, higher than standard dosing is required to control the symptoms. In addition, desensitization to triggers is possible and helpful in some PhysU, such as SolU and ColdU and in CholU.

The aim of this review is to discuss the current diagnostic and therapeutic possibilities for each form of PhysU and for CholU.

URTICARIA FACTITIA/SYMPTOMATIC DERMOGRAPHISM: THE MOST COMMON PHYSICAL URTICARIAS

UF/SD is the most common form of PhysU (about 50% of PhysU) with an estimated prevalence of up to 5% of the general human population.[5] In accordance with the word dermographism, which means writing on the skin, the disease is characterized by itching and/or burning skin and strip-shaped wheals due to shear force acting on the skin (eg, by scratching or rubbing; **Fig. 1**).[1,14] Symptoms typically persist for 1.5 to 2 hours.[1,15,16] In most patients, symptoms substantially influence everyday life, for instance, the choice of clothes or engaging in physical activity.[1,17] According to the literature, the average duration of the disease is 6.5 years, with great variance.[1,15,16] UF/SD is different from other forms of urticarial dermographism including simple dermographism (red dermographic wheal with no itching or axon flare), which affects about 5% of otherwise normal young adults.[18,19] Cholinergic dermographism, associated with CholU, delayed dermographism, and localized dermographism, which is restricted to the sites of insect bites, tattoo marks, and so on, are rare forms of urticarial dermographism.[20,21]

Although the disease has been known for many years,[22] its cause is largely unknown. Reports in the older literature indicate that, in some patients, the injection of their serum into healthy volunteers induces wheals after scratching.[19,23,24] Possibly specific immunoglobulin (Ig) E to autoallergens generated by exposing the skin to shear force could play a role in the pathomechanism in some UF/SD patients.

Patients who, based on their history, are suspected to have UF/SD should be subjected to provocation tests, which should include the assessment of their thresholds—the lowest shear force needed for causing wheals. Evaluation of thresholds should be

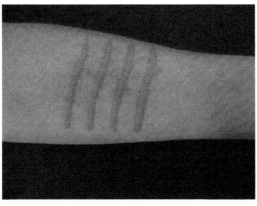

Fig. 1. Marked symptomatic dermographism with strip-shaped wheals after provocation with FricTest 4.0. Positive reaction for all trigger strengths.

performed initially, as well as during follow-up visits to monitor disease progression and to assess the efficacy of therapy. Skin provocation tests should be done on the volar forearm or the upper back by rubbing of the skin. A wooden spatula or the end of a ballpoint pen can be used. For optimal results, special dermographometers should be used. One example of such a dermographometer is FricTest (Moxie GmbH, Berlin, Germany) (**Fig. 2**). This instrument allows for simultaneous testing of 4 different strengths of shear force, which is ideal for threshold testing. Another example is a pen-shaped dermographic tester with a spring-loaded tip that can be adjusted to exert different strengths of shear force (HTZ Limited, New Addington, Croydon, Surrey, United Kingdom). Both dermographometers are placed vertically on the skin, and the shear force is caused by their movement across the skin with a predetermined pressure. UF/SD provocation tests are positive when a wheal occurs at the provocation site after 10 minutes.[2,25]

The aim of treatment in UF/SD and in all other chronic urticarias is the absence of symptoms and could be achieved by avoiding exposure of the skin to rubbing, scratching, and shear force–inducing situations. However, avoidance is difficult, if not impossible, for patients. Symptomatic treatment, therefore, is the therapy of choice and SD/UF patients should receive, as first-line therapy, a nonsedating second-generation H1-antihistamine at standard dose. Some patients will not experience complete protection with this approach, in which case increasing the dose to up to 4 times the standard dose is recommended.[1,13,14] Third-line treatment options include omalizumab,[26,27] cyclosporine A,[28] and leukotriene antagonists such as montelukast. Ultraviolet (UV) B light therapy has also been reported to be effective.[29] However, controlled studies are missing.

DELAYED PRESSURE URTICARIA: THE ONLY PHYSICAL URTICARIAS THAT COMES WITHOUT WHEALS

DPU is characterized by erythematous angioedema–like swellings. These swellings are typically located at skin sites exposed to pressure but can also occur on mucous membranes (eg, of the upper airways and oropharynx). Swellings are induced by vertical pressure and can be associated with itching, burning, or pain. Systemic symptoms such as flulike symptoms, arthralgia, or malaise can occur. Typical situations that elicit swellings in DPU patients are carrying objects (shoulder strap of bags and backpacks), walking in tight shoes, standing (eg, barefoot on a ladder), or prolonged

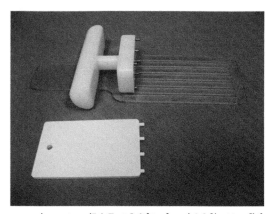

Fig. 2. Special dermographometers (FricTest 3.0 [*top*] and 4.0 [*bottom*]) for skin provocation.

sitting on uncushioned chairs. Typically, swellings occur after exposure to pressure with a delay of 4 to 8 hours and they usually persist for several hours (in some patients more than 24 hours). The average duration of DPU is 6 to 9 years. DPU often impairs quality of life markedly. DPU patients frequently also have chronic spontaneous urticaria and/or other forms of PhysU. Up to one-third of patients with chronic spontaneous urticaria report aggravation of symptoms at skin sites exposed to pressure (belt, bra). In these patients it is important (but sometimes difficult) to clarify whether they have DPU and chronic spontaneous urticaria or if their chronic spontaneous urticaria is exacerbated by pressure. Pressure-induced skin lesions in patients with chronic spontaneous urticaria are usually of shorter duration and more superficial than the angioedema-like swellings in DPU.

For the diagnosis of DPU, different provocation test methods are available: ideally, weighted rods or dermographometers are used and test readings are done after 30 minutes and after 4, 6, 8, and 24 hours. Tests are positive if a red swelling is palpable 6 hours after provocation.

DPU patients should be educated on the benefits of avoiding exposure to vertical pressure. Recommended drug therapy regimens include second-generation nonsedating H1-antihistamines; however, often higher than standard doses are needed. Other possible treatment options include montelukast, dapson, sulfasalazine, omalizumab, and anti-tumor necrosis factor (TNF).[1,5,15,16,30,31]

COLD CONTACT URTICARIA

ColdU, also called acquired cold urticaria, is a common subtype of PhysU, characterized by itchy wheal and flare-type skin reactions or angioedema after exposure to cold. Typically, symptoms occur within minutes after cold contact (cold air, cold liquids, or objects) and are restricted to the skin areas exposed to cold. However, extensive cold contact (eg, swimming in cold water) may lead to systemic reactions accompanied by hypotension and loss of consciousness.[3] Several cases of death have been reported because of anaphylaxis while swimming in cold water.[32] Up to 72% of ColdU patients experience at least one systemic reaction after extensive cold exposure.[3,32–34] Besides aquatic activities, patients should avoid ice-cold drinks and food to prevent oropharyngeal edema. ColdU may occur at any age but shows a peak in young adults and a weak predominance in women.[3,33,35] The mean duration of symptoms ranges between 4.8 and 7.9 years.[3,33,35] Up to one-third of all PhysU cases are ColdU.[36]

Atypical, rare forms of ColdU are also described.[36,37] These conditions include delayed ColdU, where localized whealing develops up to 24 hours after cold exposure; cold-dependent dermographism, which is characterized by the occurrence of urticarial lesions restricted to cold-exposed and mechanically stimulated skin, cold-induced cholinergic urticaria, which is induced by exercising in cold environments, systemic atypical acquired cold urticaria elicited by specific or unique stimuli (eg, cold wind). In contrast to ColdU, atypical forms show negative results in standard cold provocation tests. Some extremely rare hereditary (autosomal-dominant) conditions such as familial delayed cold urticaria, familial cold auto-inflammatory syndrome, and familial atypical cold urticaria also present with cold-induced wheals. Pathogenetically, these hereditary diseases are characterized by an activation of the NLRP/3 inflammasome complex due to a mutation of CIAS1/NLRP3 and the release of interleukin-1ß.[38] The central role of interleukin-1ß is demonstrated by the exceptionally good response of disease-specific symptoms to interleukin-1ß antagonists.[39]

In contrast, ColdU signs and symptoms are induced by histamine and other proinflammatory mast cell mediators, such as TNF, leukotrienes, prostaglandin D_2, and platelet-activating factor released in response to cold exposure.[40–42] The exact mechanism of mast cell activation, however, still remains unknown. In a recent study, 5 of 9 ColdU patients were found to exhibit antibodies against IgE or against high-affinity receptor for IgE.[43] It has been hypothesized that autoimmune mechanisms (eg, IgE Antibodies to cold-dependent skin antigens) could be involved in the pathogenesis of ColdU, because it can be adoptively transferred to healthy individuals by intracutaneous injection of the serum of some ColdU patients.[44]

In patients with a history of cold-induced whealing or angioedema, a cold stimulation test should be performed. The traditional method is to place a melting ice cube in a thin plastic bag (to avoid cold damage of the skin) on the volar forearm for 5 minutes. The test response should be assessed 10 minutes after removing the ice cube. It is held to be positive if the test site shows a palpable and clearly visible wheal, which is usually associated with a pruritic or burning sensation.[37] A positive ice cube cold stimulation test confirms the diagnosis of ColdU. Patients with a positive reaction to the ice cube test should be evaluated for individual temperature and/or stimulation time thresholds (**Fig. 3**).[2] For this purpose, a Peltier element-based electronic provocation device (TempTest, Moxie GmbH) has been developed, which simultaneously tests temperatures from 4°C to 44°C in a standardized and reproducible way (**Fig. 4**).[45] Determination of thresholds by TempTest allows both patients and physicians to evaluate disease activity and therapy response.[46] Laboratory tests are of limited value in most cases of cold urticaria and should be restricted to cases in which the patient's history suggests existence of an underlying disease.[47]

ColdU patients are often severely impaired in their daily lives, especially those with high temperature thresholds who live in countries with a cold climate. Also, ColdU patients are at risk of suffering fatal anaphylactic reactions. Effective therapeutic measures are, therefore, important and needed.[37] The underlying causes of ColdU remain unknown, but some patients show remission after antibiotic treatment with doxycycline or penicillin given for several weeks.[35,48] All patients should be counseled

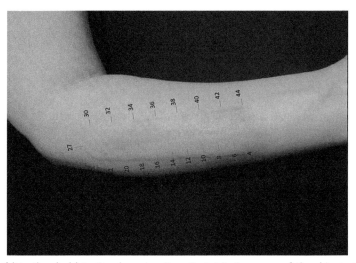

Fig. 3. ColdU—threshold testing by using TempTest 4.0. Exposure of the skin to temperatures from 4°C to 44°C over 5 minutes. Response assessment 10 minutes after provocation. Cold temperature threshold = highest temperature sufficient to induce a positive reaction, in this case 27°C.

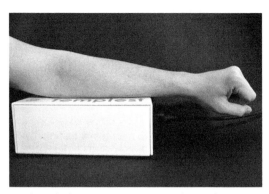

Fig. 4. Peltier element-based electronic provocation device (TempTest 4.0, Moxie GmbH) with temperatures from 4°C to 44°C to confirm cold urticaria and heat urticaria and to determine individual temperature thresholds.

on the importance of avoiding cold, especially patients with higher temperature thresholds. The symptomatic treatment of choice in ColdU is second-generation nonsedating H1-antihistamines. They have been shown to be effective, safe, and well tolerated in several controlled studies and are recommended by the EAACI/ GA[2]LEN/EDF/WAO (European Academy of Allergology and Clinical Immunology/ Global Allergy and Asthma European Network/ European Dermatology Forum/World Allergy Organization) guidelines as first-line therapy.[13,49] In many patients, however, standard treatment with antihistamines is insufficient. Recent data have shown that the use of high doses of H1-antihistamines is significantly more effective in ColdU than standard doses.[50–54] Treatment options for antihistamine-resistant ColdU patients include cold desensitization[55] and omalizumab (anti-IgE) treatment.[26,56,57] Desensitization, where skin sensitivity to cold is diminished by repeated cold exposure, involves the risk of anaphylactic shock during induction and requires daily cold showers to maintain the protective effect.[55,58,59] ColdU patients may also benefit from anakinra (anti-interleukin-1) or etanercept (TNF inhibitor) treatment, as shown by recent case reports.[60,61] However, controlled studies are missing.

HEAT CONTACT URTICARIA

HeatU, also called localized heat urticaria, is a rare PhysU characterized by the appearance of wheal and flare-type skin reaction after heat exposure of the skin. Less than 100 cases of HeatU have been reported in the literature including cases in children and atypical familial localized delayed heat urticaria.[1]

As in all other PhysU, skin mast cell activation is held to be critically involved in the pathogenesis, and this is supported by the demonstration of increased plasma histamine levels after exposing HeatU patients to warm water testing.[62] The relevance of a previously described temperature-activated serum factor remains unknown.[63]

HeatU wheals are usually well-defined, limited to the area of heat exposure; they typically develop within a few minutes after heat contact and resolve after 1 to 3 hours. Suspicion of HeatU from the case history should be confirmed by local heat testing. Heat should be applied for 5 minutes (metal/glass cylinders, filled with water, hot water bath, TempTest) at a temperature of up to 45°C. Test responses should be assessed 10 minutes after provocation. In patients with a positive response, temperature and/or stimulation time thresholds should be performed.[2]

Treatment options for HeatU are limited and variably effective. Second-generation nonsedating H1-antihistamines are the first choice for symptomatic therapy.[13] Some case reports suggest that omalizumab (anti-IgE) may be beneficial in difficult-to-treat patients.[26,64]

SOLAR URTICARIA

SolU is a rare type of PhysU characterized by urticarial lesions (mostly itchy wheals) that occur immediately (usually within 5–15 minutes) after light (UV and/or visible light) exposure and resolve within less than 24 hours. SolU must be discriminated from the much commoner polymorphic light eruption, which differs from SolU in that sunlight-evoked inflammatory rashes in the former are prolonged and persistent, whereas the wheals in the latter are transitory. A few case reports have reported SolU cases with unusual clinical features such as delayed onset (more that 1 hour), delayed resolution (more than 24 hours), and solar angioedema. A retrospective study from Singapore evaluated 21,974 patients with urticaria over a 10-year period and detected SolU in 0.08% of these patients.[65] In patients who consult a hospital because of sunlight-related skin problems, the prevalence of SolU was reported to be 2.3%[66] and 17.8%.[67] Epidemiologic analyses showed a female preponderance and a peak age onset between 20 and 40 years for both genders, but no influence of the Fitzpatrick skin type on the occurrence or severity of disease.[66] Atopy is common in SolU patients (up to 48%[68]), and combinations with other PhysU forms are frequent (up to 28%).[65,69]

UVA is the most frequent action spectrum to elicit skin reactions, followed by visible light and UVB light. Generally, SolU patients have very diverse action spectra. Horio[70] postulated that this is due to the heterogeneous nature of chromophores or photosensitizers involved as well as ethnic and geographic differences. The results of serum transfer test studies led to the hypothesis of circulating serum factors that cause mast cell degranulation in SolU patients. Based on these studies done in the 1960s and 1970s,[71–73] distinct subtypes of SolU were postulated, implicating abnormal serum and/or dermal factors. In vitro studies led to the classification of type I SolU (IgE antibodies against an abnormal chromophore) and type II SolU (IgE antibodies against a normal chromophore).[74] Interestingly, in some cases anti-IgE therapy can completely protect from SolU symptoms[75] while in others it did not,[76] which indicates that IgE plays a central role in the pathophysiology of the disease in some but not all patients. Further studies are needed to identify and characterize in detail the pathogenic principles in SolU.

For the diagnosis of SolU, a detailed history and provocation tests are needed. Solar simulators with filters (UVA and UVB) or monochromators (UVA and UVB, visible light) should be used for provocation testing (preferably on the buttocks). UVA should be tested at 6 J/cm^2 and UVB at 60 mJ/cm^2. Visible light can also be tested by using a projector (eg, slide projector, 10 cm distance). Positive provocation leads to a rapid urticarial response at the site of exposure within 10 minutes. The test is positive if the test site shows a palpable and clearly visible wheal and flare type skin reaction that is itchy and/or burns.[2] Threshold testing (minimal urticarial dose) should be performed by varying the radiation dose, which allows the determination of disease activity and response to therapy.[68]

Standard treatment options include avoidance of sunlight, protective clothing, broadband sunscreens, and second-generation nonsedating H1-antihistamines. Unfortunately, exposure to sunlight is hard to avoid, and antihistamines, even at higher than standard doses, provide incomplete protection in most cases. Tolerance can be induced by "light hardening," usually in rush hardening protocols that required a hospital setting.[77,78] Anti-IgE treatment[26,75] and intravenous immunoglobulin treat-ment[79,80] were reported to be effective in some cases, whereas in others these treat-ments failed.[76,81] Recently, afamelanotide, an α-MSH alfa-melanocyte stimulating hormone analogue and melanocortin receptor agonist, was demonstrated to increase melanization and effectively protect from urticarial symptoms in SolU patients.[82]

VIBRATORY ANGIOEDEMA

Vibratory angioedema (VA) is a very rare PhysU characterized by cutaneous swellings immediately (usually within 10 minutes) after exposure to vibration at contact sites. Single case reports described atypical VA subform (delayed VA[83] and hereditary VA[84]). Little is known about its cause. In one case, lesion development was not found to be associated with mast cell degranulation,[85] whereas in other cases, mast cell degranulation and a raise in histamine levels were detected.[83,86] VA diagnosis can be confirmed by provocation tests (eg, done with a laboratory vortex mixer).[16,85] Inter-estingly, one report demonstrated cutaneous swellings in 35% of the healthy volun-teers after provocation testing, which raises the question of the specificity of the test.[87] Treatment options are limited and consist mainly of avoidance of exposure to vibratory stimulation (eg, use of power tools) and the use of second-generation nonsedating H1-antihistamines.[16] Anti-IgE treatment failed to improve VA in one case report.[88]

CHOLINERGIC URTICARIA

CholU is a very frequent inducible urticaria[7,89] that is defined by itching and whealing following a rise in body temperature—induced actively (eg, exercise) or passively (eg, hot bath). Angioedema development is very rare.[2] CholU must be differentiated from exercise-induced urticaria/anaphylaxis, which is induced by exercise but not passive warming and is more often associated with systemic symptoms.

CholU is a disorder of young adults and has a high prevalence in this age group (up to 20%).[7] In most patients the symptoms get milder with age until they eventually cease to occur completely. It was reported that the severity of the disease shows sea-sonal changes, with milder symptoms in the summer.[90] CholU patients typically develop itchy pinpoint-sized short-lived wheals with large flare reactions commonly localized to the limbs and the trunk a few minutes after exercise or passive warming. In some patients, emotional stress or hot and spicy food or beverages can also elicit symptoms. Usually, skin lesions last for 15 to 60 minutes. Atopy[7] and bronchial hyper-responsiveness[91] seem to be more frequent in CholU patients. Some CholU patients exhibit generalized hypohidrosis.[92] Japanese studies suggest several distinct CholU subclasses: (1) CholU with poral occlusion, (2) CholU with hypohidrosis, (3) CholU with allergy against sweat, and (4) idiopathic CholU.[92,93]

There are several reports of cases that suggest that CholU could be caused by poral occlusion, which then leads to the leakage of sweat from sweat glands. Sweat con-tains numerous enzymes, such as renin-like substances, secretory IgA, IgE, and cyto-kines, including interleukin 1a and b, and interleukin-8 that, in turn, can induce local inflammation and may cause wheals. Symptoms in CholU patients with poral occlu-sion reportedly exacerbate in winter and resolve in the summer, suggesting that daily sweating in summer may inhibit the formation of keratotic plugs to prevent the occur-rence of CholU.[94]

It is well known that acquired generalized hypohidrosis (AGH) can be accompanied by CholU. A variety of causes, including autoimmunity to sweat glands or to acetylcho-line receptors, degeneration of post-ganglionic sympathetic skin nerve fibers, and poral occlusion (see above) have been proposed as causes of AGH.[95] CholU in AGH patients may be due to elevated local acetylcholine levels induced by their impaired sweat production. Consequently, excess acetylcholine may activate muscarinic CHRM3 on mast cells in the vicinity of sweat glands to cause wheals.[96] Acetylcholine is a mast cell degranulator,[97] and previous reports have demonstrated that subcutaneous injections of cholinergic agents induce sweating and the development of pin-point-sized hives in patients with CholU.

Several recent studies indicate that CholU can be due to an allergy to components of human sweat. Some CholU patients show immediate-type hypersensitivity reactions to their own diluted sweat after intradermal injections, and basophils from these patients react to autologous sweat and release high amounts of histamine in vitro.[98,99] In addition, CholU patients, but not healthy controls, reportedly express IgE to sweat antigens. Very recently, a new allergen component from a fungus was identified in human sweat.[100]

To diagnose CholU and to differentiate CholU from exercise-induced urticaria/anaphylaxis, provocation testing should be performed in a 2-step approach. As a first step, moderate physical exercise appropriate to the patients' age and general condition is recommended (eg, on a treadmill or stationary bicycle wearing warm clothing in a warm room). Exercise should be performed to the point of sweating and up to 15 minutes beyond. The test is positive if the typical urticarial rash is seen 10 minutes after exercise challenge. In this case, a passive warming test should be done (at least 24 hours later, 42°C full bath for up to 15 minutes while recording body core temperature to achieve a rise of +1.0°C).[2] A positive test reaction is seen in CholU, but not exercise-induced urticaria/anaphylaxis patients. These tests are not suited to determine trigger thresholds or to determine and monitor disease activity.

The first-line treatment options in CholU are avoidance of eliciting triggers and second-generation nonsedating H1-antihistamines.[16] Desensitization protocols involving regular physical exercise or treatment with autologous sweat may be useful in some patients,[101,102] and the same is true for omalizumab,[26,103,104] scopolamine butylbromide,[105] combinations of propanolol, antihistamines, and montelukast[106] treatments, and injections with botulinumtoxin.[107]

SUMMARY

PhysU and CholU are more frequent, chronic, and debilitating than commonly thought. Many patients are severely impaired in their quality of life, but disease-specific instruments to measure this are missing. The signs and symptoms of PhysU and CholU are known to be mast cell-mediated, but their underlying causes remain to be identified and characterized. Trigger threshold measurements are important to inform patients and physicians about disease severity and to monitor its course over time as well as treatment responses. As of yet, validated protocols and instruments to measure trigger thresholds are available only for UF/SD, ColdU, HeatU and SolU, but not for the other PhysU and CholU. Treatment choices include trigger avoidance and second-generation nonsedating H1-antihistamines in all PhysU and CholU. Future research efforts will need to focus on the identification of underlying causes and associated mast cell secretagogues, because this will allow for the development of curative, rather than symptomatic, therapies.

REFERENCES

1. Abajian M, Mlynek A, Maurer M. Physical urticaria. Curr Allergy Asthma Rep 2012;12(4):281–7.

2. Magerl M, Borzova E, Gimenez-Arnau A, et al. The definition and diagnostic testing of physical and cholinergic urticarias–EAACI/GA2LEN/EDF/UNEV consensus panel recommendations. Allergy 2009;64(12):1715–21.
3. Wanderer AA, Grandel KE, Wasserman SI, et al. Clinical characteristics of cold-induced systemic reactions in acquired cold urticaria syndromes: recommendations for prevention of this complication and a proposal for a diagnostic classification of cold urticaria. J Allergy Clin Immunol 1986;78(3 Pt 1):417–23.
4. Nichols AW. Exercise-induced anaphylaxis and urticaria. Clin Sports Med 1992; 11(2):303–12.
5. Kontou-Fili K, Borici-Mazi R, Kapp A, et al. Physical urticaria: classification and diagnostic guidelines. An EAACI position paper. Allergy 1997;52(5):504–13.
6. Dice JP. Physical urticaria. Immunol Allergy Clin North Am 2004;24(2):225–46, vi.
7. Zuberbier T, Althaus C, Chantraine-Hess S, et al. Prevalence of cholinergic urticaria in young adults. J Am Acad Dermatol 1994;31(6):978–81.
8. Torchia D, Francalanci S, Bellandi S, et al. Multiple physical urticarias. Postgrad Med J 2008;84(987):e1–2.
9. Arikan-Ayyildiz Z, Isik S, Caglayan-Sozmen S, et al. Cold, cholinergic and aquagenic urticaria in children: presentation of three cases and review of the literature. Turk J Pediatr 2013;55(1):94–8.
10. Cheon HW, Han SJ, Yeo SJ, et al. A case of combined cholinergic and cold urticaria. Korean J Intern Med 2012;27(4):478–9.
11. Cohen RW, Rosenstreich DL. Discrimination between urticaria-prone and other allergic patients by intradermal skin testing with codeine. J Allergy Clin Immunol 1986;77(6):802–7.
12. Zuberbier T, Asero R, Bindslev-Jensen C, et al. EAACI/GA(2)LEN/EDF/WAO guideline: definition, classification and diagnosis of urticaria. Allergy 2009; 64(10):1417–26.
13. Zuberbier T, Asero R, Bindslev-Jensen C, et al. EAACI/GA(2)LEN/EDF/WAO guideline: management of urticaria. Allergy 2009;64(10):1427–43.
14. Magerl M, Schmolke J, Metz M, et al. Prevention of signs and symptoms of dermographic urticaria by single-dose ebastine 20 mg. Clin Exp Dermatol 2009; 34(5):e137–40.
15. Fleischer M, Grabbe J. Physical urticaria. Hautarzt 2004;55(4):344–9 [in German].
16. Zuberbier T, Maurer M. Urticaria: current opinions about etiology, diagnosis and therapy. Acta Derm Venereol 2007;87(3):196–205.
17. Wallengren J, Isaksson A. Urticarial dermographism: clinical features and response to psychosocial stress. Acta Derm Venereol 2007;87(6):493–8.
18. Lewis T. Vascular reactions of the skin to injury - 1. Reactions to stroking. Urticaria factita. Heart 1924;11:119–39.
19. Breathnach SM, Allen R, Ward AM, et al. Symptomatic dermographism: natural history, clinical features laboratory investigations and response to therapy. Clin Exp Dermatol 1983;8(5):463–76.
20. Mayou SC, Kobza Black A, Eady RA, et al. Cholinergic dermographism. Br J Dermatol 1986;115(3):371–7.
21. Warin RP. Clinical observations on delayed pressure urticaria. Br J Dermatol 1989;121(2):225–8.
22. Schmidt CC. Schmidt's Jahrbücher der in- und ausländischen gesammten Medizin. Otto Wigand; 1860.
23. Horiko T, Aoki T. Dermographism (mechanical urticaria) mediated by IgM. Br J Dermatol 1984;111(5):545–50.

24. Newcomb RW, Nelson H. Dermographia mediated by immunoglobulin E. Am J Med 1973;54(2):174–80.

25. Bettley FR. A device for the measurement of factitious urticaria. J Invest Dermatol 1962;39:1.

26. Metz M, Altrichter S, Ardelean E, et al. Anti-immunoglobulin E treatment of patients with recalcitrant physical urticaria. Int Arch Allergy Immunol 2011;154(2): 177–80.

27. Krause K, Degener F, Altrichter S, et al. Cold-induced urticaria and angioedema. Classification, diagnosis and therapy. Hautarzt 2010;61(9):743–9 [in German].

28. Toda S, Takahagi S, Mihara S, et al. Six cases of antihistamine-resistant dermographic urticaria treated with oral ciclosporin. Allergol Int 2011;60(4):547–50.

29. Borzova E, Rutherford A, Konstantinou GN, et al. Narrowband ultraviolet B phototherapy is beneficial in antihistamine-resistant symptomatic dermographism: a pilot study. J Am Acad Dermatol 2008;59(5):752–7.

30. Kobza-Black A. Delayed pressure urticaria. J Investig Dermatol Symp Proc 2001;6(2):148–9.

31. Magerl M, Philipp S, Manasterski M, et al. Successful treatment of delayed pressure urticaria with anti-TNF-alpha. J Allergy Clin Immunol 2007;119(3):752–4.

32. Alangari AA, Twarog FJ, Shih MC, et al. Clinical features and anaphylaxis in children with cold urticaria. Pediatrics 2004;113(4):e313–7.

33. Neittaanmaki H. Cold urticaria. Clinical findings in 220 patients. J Am Acad Dermatol 1985;13(4):636–44.

34. Katsarou-Katsari A, Makris M, Lagogianni E, et al. Clinical features and natural history of acquired cold urticaria in a tertiary referral hospital: a 10-year prospective study. J Eur Acad Dermatol Venereol 2008;22(12):1405–11.

35. Moller A, Henning M, Zuberbier T, et al. Epidemiology and clinical aspects of cold urticaria. Hautarzt 1996;47(7):510–4 [in German].

36. Siebenhaar F, Weller K, Mlynek A, et al. Acquired cold urticaria: clinical picture and update on diagnosis and treatment. Clin Exp Dermatol 2007;32(3):241–5.

37. Krause K, Zuberbier T, Maurer M. Modern approaches to the diagnosis and treatment of cold contact urticaria. Curr Allergy Asthma Rep 2010;10(4):243–9.

38. Nakamura Y, Kambe N, Saito M, et al. Mast cells mediate neutrophil recruitment and vascular leakage through the NLRP3 inflammasome in histamine-independent urticaria. J Exp Med 2009;206(5):1037–46.

39. Lachmann HJ, Kone-Paut I, Kuemmerle-Deschner JB, et al. Use of canakinumab in the cryopyrin-associated periodic syndrome. N Engl J Med 2009; 360(23):2416–25.

40. Andersson T, Wardell K, Anderson C. Human in vivo cutaneous microdialysis: estimation of histamine release in cold urticaria. Acta Derm Venereol 1995; 75(5):343–7.

41. Wasserman SI, Ginsberg MH. Release of platelet factor 4 into the blood after cold challenge of patients with cold urticaria. J Allergy Clin Immunol 1984; 74(3 Pt 1):275–9.

42. Hermes B, Prochazka AK, Haas N, et al. Upregulation of TNF-alpha and IL-3 expression in lesional and uninvolved skin in different types of urticaria. J Allergy Clin Immunol 1999;103(2 Pt 1):307–14.

43. Gruber BL, Baeza ML, Marchese MJ, et al. Prevalence and functional role of anti-IgE autoantibodies in urticarial syndromes. J Invest Dermatol 1988;90(2):213–7.

44. Kaplan AP, Garofalo J, Sigler R, et al. Idiopathic cold urticaria: in vitro demonstration of histamine release upon challenge of skin biopsies. N Engl J Med 1981;305(18):1074–7.

45. Siebenhaar F, Staubach P, Metz M, et al. Peltier effect-based temperature challenge: an improved method for diagnosing cold urticaria. J Allergy Clin Immunol 2004;114(5):1224–5.
46. Mlynek A, Magerl M, Siebenhaar F, et al. Results and relevance of critical temperature threshold testing in patients with acquired cold urticaria. Br J Dermatol 2010;162(1):198–200.
47. Kozel MM, Bossuyt PM, Mekkes JR, et al. Laboratory tests and identified diagnoses in patients with physical and chronic urticaria and angioedema: a systematic review. J Am Acad Dermatol 2003;48(3):409–16.
48. Illig L. Positive side-effects of antibiotic and antimicrobial drugs in therapy (author's transl). Infection 1979;7(Suppl 6):584–8 [in German].
49. Weinstein ME, Wolff AH, Bielory L. Efficacy and tolerability of second- and third-generation antihistamines in the treatment of acquired cold urticaria: a meta-analysis. Ann Allergy Asthma Immunol 2010;104(6):518–22.
50. Siebenhaar F, Degener F, Zuberbier T, et al. High-dose desloratadine decreases wheal volume and improves cold provocation thresholds compared with standard-dose treatment in patients with acquired cold urticaria: a randomized, placebo-controlled, crossover study. J Allergy Clin Immunol 2009;123(3):672–9.
51. Magerl M, Schmolke J, Siebenhaar F, et al. Acquired cold urticaria symptoms can be safely prevented by ebastine. Allergy 2007;62(12):1465–8.
52. Metz M, Scholz E, Ferran M, et al. Rupatadine and its effects on symptom control, stimulation time, and temperature thresholds in patients with acquired cold urticaria. Ann Allergy Asthma Immunol 2010;104(1):86–92.
53. Magerl M, Pisarevskaja D, Staubach P, et al. Critical temperature threshold measurement for cold urticaria: a randomised controlled trial of H1-antihistamine up-dosing. Br J Dermatol 2012;166:1095–9.
54. Krause K, Spohr A, Zuberbier T, et al. Up-dosing with bilastine results in improved effectiveness in cold contact urticaria. Allergy 2013;68(7):921–8.
55. Kring Tannert L, Stahl Skov P, Bjerremann Jensen L, et al. Cold urticaria patients exhibit normal skin levels of functional mast cells and histamine after tolerance induction. Dermatology 2012;224(2):101–5.
56. Boyce JA. Successful treatment of cold-induced urticaria/anaphylaxis with anti-IgE. J Allergy Clin Immunol 2006;117(6):1415–8.
57. Brodska P, Schmid-Grendelmeier P. Treatment of severe cold contact urticaria with omalizumab: case reports. Case Rep Dermatol 2012;4(3):275–80.
58. Black AK, Sibbald RG, Greaves MW. Cold urticaria treated by induction of tolerance. Lancet 1979;2(8149):964.
59. von Mackensen YA, Sticherling M. Cold urticaria: tolerance induction with cold baths. Br J Dermatol 2007;157(4):835–6.
60. Bodar EJ, Simon A, de Visser M, et al. Complete remission of severe idiopathic cold urticaria on interleukin-1 receptor antagonist (anakinra). Neth J Med 2009;67(9):302–5.
61. Gualdi G, Monari P, Rossi MT, et al. Successful treatment of systemic cold contact urticaria with etanercept in a patient with psoriasis. Br J Dermatol 2012;166(6):1373–4.
62. Irwin RB, Lieberman P, Friedman MM, et al. Mediator release in local heat urticaria: protection with combined H1 and H2 antagonists. J Allergy Clin Immunol 1985;76(1):35–9.
63. Fukunaga A, Shimoura S, Fukunaga M, et al. Localized heat urticaria in a patient is associated with a wealing response to heated autologous serum. Br J Dermatol 2002;147(5):994–7.

64. Bullerkotte U, Wieczorek D, Kapp A, et al. Effective treatment of refractory severe heat urticaria with omalizumab. Allergy 2010;65(7):931–2.
65. Chong WS, Khoo SW. Solar urticaria in Singapore: an uncommon photodermatosis seen in a tertiary dermatology center over a 10-year period. Photodermatol Photoimmunol Photomed 2004;20(2):101–4.
66. Du-Thanh A, Debu A, Lalheve P, et al. Solar urticaria: a time-extended retrospective series of 61 patients and review of literature. Eur J Dermatol 2013; 23(2):202–7.
67. Stratigos AJ, Antoniou C, Papathanakou E, et al. Spectrum of idiopathic photodermatoses in a Mediterranean country. Int J Dermatol 2003;42(6):449–54.
68. Ryckaert S, Roelandts R. Solar urticaria. A report of 25 cases and difficulties in phototesting. Arch Dermatol 1998;134(1):71–4.
69. Monfrecola G, Masturzo E, Riccardo AM, et al. Solar urticaria: a report on 57 cases. Am J Contact Dermat 2000;11(2):89–94.
70. Horio T. Solar urticaria-idiopathic? Photodermatol Photoimmunol Photomed 2003;19(3):147–54.
71. Harber LC, Holloway RM, Wheatley VR, et al. Immunologic and biophysical studies in solar urticaria. J Invest Dermatol 1963;41:439–43.
72. Horio T, Minami K. Solar uticaria. Photoallergen in a patient's serum. Arch Dermatol 1977;113(2):157–60.
73. Horio T. Photoallergic urticaria induced by visible light. Additional cases and further studies. Arch Dermatol 1978;114(12):1761–4.
74. Leenutaphong V, Holzle E, Plewig G. Pathogenesis and classification of solar urticaria: a new concept. J Am Acad Dermatol 1989;21(2 Pt 1):237–40.
75. Guzelbey O, Ardelean E, Magerl M, et al. Successful treatment of solar urticaria with anti-immunoglobulin E therapy. Allergy 2008;63(11):1563–5.
76. Duchini G, Baumler W, Bircher AJ, et al. Failure of omalizumab (Xolair(R)) in the treatment of a case of solar urticaria caused by ultraviolet A and visible light. Photodermatol Photoimmunol Photomed 2011;27(6):336–7.
77. Masuoka E, Fukunaga A, Kishigami K, et al. Successful and long-lasting treatment of solar urticaria with ultraviolet A rush hardening therapy. Br J Dermatol 2012;167(1):198–201.
78. Wolf R, Herzinger T, Grahovac M, et al. Solar urticaria: long-term rush hardening by inhibition spectrum narrow-band UVB 311 nm. Clin Exp Dermatol 2013;38(4):446–7.
79. Hughes R, Cusack C, Murphy GM, et al. Solar urticaria successfully treated with intravenous immunoglobulin. Clin Exp Dermatol 2009;34(8):e660–2.
80. Correia I, Silva J, Filipe P, et al. Solar urticaria treated successfully with intravenous high-dose immunoglobulin: a case report. Photodermatol Photoimmunol Photomed 2008;24(6):330–1.
81. Llamas-Velasco M, Argila DD, Eguren C, et al. Solar urticaria unresponsive to intravenous immunoglobulins. Photodermatol Photoimmunol Photomed 2011; 27(1):53–4.
82. Haylett AK, Nie Z, Brownrigg M, et al. Systemic photoprotection in solar urticaria with alpha-melanocyte-stimulating hormone analogue [Nle4-D-Phe7]-alpha-MSH. Br J Dermatol 2011;164(2):407–14.
83. Keahey TM, Indrisano J, Lavker RM, et al. Delayed vibratory angioedema: insights into pathophysiologic mechanisms. J Allergy Clin Immunol 1987;80(6):831–8.
84. Metzger WJ, Kaplan AP, Beaven MA, et al. Hereditary vibratory angioedema: confirmation of histamine release in a type of physical hypersensitivity. J Allergy Clin Immunol 1976;57(6):605–8.

85. Lawlor F, Black AK, Breathnach AS, et al. Vibratory angioedema: lesion induction, clinical features, laboratory and ultrastructural findings and response to therapy. Br J Dermatol 1989;120(1):93–9.
86. Ting S, Reimann BE, Rauls DO, et al. Nonfamilial, vibration-induced angioedema. J Allergy Clin Immunol 1983;71(6):546–51.
87. Mathelier-Fusade P, Vermeulen C, Leynadier F. Vibratory angioedema. Ann Dermatol Venereol 2001;128(6–7):750–2 [in French].
88. Pressler A, Grosber M, Halle M, et al. Failure of omalizumab and successful control with ketotifen in a patient with vibratory angio-oedema. Clin Exp Dermatol 2013;38(2):151–3.
89. Godse K, Farooqui S, Nadkarni N, et al. Prevalence of cholinergic urticaria in Indian adults. Indian Dermatol Online J 2013;4(1):62–3.
90. Ramam M, Pahwa P. Is cholinergic urticaria a seasonal disorder in some patients? Indian J Dermatol Venereol Leprol 2012;78(2):190–1.
91. Petalas K, Kontou-Fili K, Gratziou C. Bronchial hyperresponsiveness in patients with cholinergic urticaria. Ann Allergy Asthma Immunol 2009;102(5):416–21.
92. Bito T, Sawada Y, Tokura Y. Pathogenesis of cholinergic urticaria in relation to sweating. Allergol Int 2012;61(4):539–44.
93. Horikawa T, Fukunaga A, Nishigori C. New concepts of hive formation in cholinergic urticaria. Curr Allergy Asthma Rep 2009;9(4):273–9.
94. Kobayashi H, Aiba S, Yamagishi T, et al. Cholinergic urticaria, a new pathogenic concept: hypohidrosis due to interference with the delivery of sweat to the skin surface. Dermatology 2002;204(3):173–8.
95. Nakamizo S, Kurosawa M, Sawada Y, et al. A case of cholinergic urticaria associated with acquired generalized hypohidrosis and reduced acetylcholine receptors: cause and effect? Clin Exp Dermatol 2011;36(5):559–60.
96. Sawada Y, Nakamura M, Bito T, et al. Cholinergic urticaria: studies on the muscarinic cholinergic receptor M3 in anhidrotic and hypohidrotic skin. J Invest Dermatol 2010;130(11):2683–6.
97. Fantozzi R, Masini E, Blandina P, et al. Release of histamine from rat mast cells by acetylcholine. Nature 1978;273(5662):473–4.
98. Adachi J, Aoki T, Yamatodani A. Demonstration of sweat allergy in cholinergic urticaria. J Dermatol Sci 1994;7(2):142–9.
99. Takahagi S, Tanaka T, Ishii K, et al. Sweat antigen induces histamine release from basophils of patients with cholinergic urticaria associated with atopic diathesis. Br J Dermatol 2009;160(2):426–8.
100. Hiragun T, Ishii K, Hiragun M, et al. Fungal protein MGL_1304 in sweat is an allergen for atopic dermatitis patients. J Allergy Clin Immunol 2013;132:608–15.e4.
101. Nakamizo S, Egawa G, Miyachi Y, et al. Cholinergic urticaria: pathogenesis-based categorization and its treatment options. J Eur Acad Dermatol Venereol 2012;26(1):114–6.
102. Kozaru T, Fukunaga A, Taguchi K, et al. Rapid desensitization with autologous sweat in cholinergic urticaria. Allergol Int 2011;60(3):277–81.
103. Metz M, Bergmann P, Zuberbier T, et al. Successful treatment of cholinergic urticaria with anti-immunoglobulin E therapy. Allergy 2008;63(2):247–9.
104. Sabroe RA. Failure of omalizumab in cholinergic urticaria. Clin Exp Dermatol 2010;35(4):e127–9.
105. Ujiie H, Shimizu T, Natsuga K, et al. Severe cholinergic urticaria successfully treated with scopolamine butylbromide in addition to antihistamines. Clin Exp Dermatol 2006;31(4):588–9.

106. Feinberg JH, Toner CB. Successful treatment of disabling cholinergic urticaria. Mil Med 2008;173(2):217–20.
107. Sheraz A, Halpern S. Cholinergic urticaria responding to botulinum toxin injection for axillary hyperhidrosis. Br J Dermatol 2013;168:1369–70.

Urticaria

Impact on Quality of Life and Economic Cost

Brigid F. O'Donnell, MD, MRCPI, DCH[a,b],*

KEYWORDS

- Urticaria • Angioedema • Health-related quality of life • Patient-reported outcomes
- Psychiatric comorbidity • Cost

KEY POINTS

- The QoL impairment of patients with chronic urticaria attending a tertiary referral center is comparable with that experienced by a group of older patients with severe, ischemic heart disease.
- The severe impairment of QoL in chronic urticaria is often underestimated, and in several dimensions is comparable with the impairment suffered by patients with atopic dermatitis (AD) and psoriasis (PSO).
- A systematic search of medical databases (PubMed and OVID/Medline) revealed a high prevalence (46.09%) of psychosocial factors in patients with chronic spontaneous urticaria.

URTICARIA

Urticaria describes short-lived erythematous swellings caused by local, transient dermal edema and vasodilatation. Individual lesions are usually intensely itchy and vary from red weals and papules to larger plaques (**Fig. 1**). Despite the itch, excoriation is exceptional, because patients tend to rub rather than scratch.[1] Crops of weals appear suddenly and resolve completely in 12 to 24 hours. However, fresh lesions may continue to appear almost indefinitely, and more patients have symptoms that are worst in the evening[2] or at night.[3]

ANGIOEDEMA

Angioedema, caused by edema of the subcutaneous tissue and mucous membranes causing deeper swellings, may occur alone or in association with urticaria. Some 30% to 50% of patients with urticaria develop recurrent angioedema.[4] These swellings are sudden in onset and disappear completely in 24 to 72 hours. Angioedema is

Disclosures: No conflicts of interest.
[a] Department of Dermatology, Children's University Hospital, Temple Street, Dublin 1, Ireland;
[b] Department of Dermatology, Mater Misericordiae Hospital, Eccles Street, Dublin 7, Ireland
* Children's University Hospital, Temple Street, Dublin 1, Ireland.
E-mail address: brid.odonnell@cuh.ie

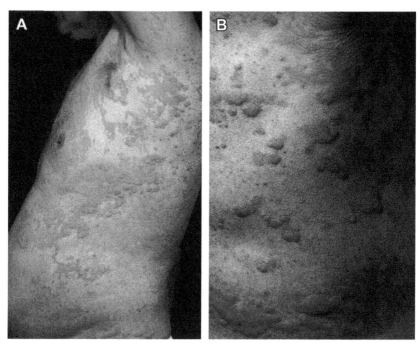

Fig. 1. (*A*) Urticarial weals on the lateral aspect of the trunk. (*B*) Close-up view emphasizes the edematous nature of individual weals. (*Courtesy of* the Illustrations Department, St John's Institute of Dermatology, London.)

cosmetically distressing because of the swelling of the eyelids, lips, and face. Swelling of the hands and feet may make movement more difficult, and swelling of the lips, tongue, and throat cause fear and problems with speech, swallowing, and breathing.

CLASSIFICATION OF URTICARIA

Urticaria, a heterogeneous group of diseases, has been classified into 3 groups: spontaneous urticaria (acute <6 weeks, chronic >6 weeks), physical urticaria, and other urticaria types (**Table 1**).[5] However, the authors point out some inconsistencies

Table 1 Urticaria classification	
Spontaneous urticaria	Acute spontaneous urticaria Chronic spontaneous urticaria
Physical urticaria	Cold contact urticaria Delayed pressure urticaria Heat contact urticaria Solar urticaria Urticaria factitia/dermographic urticaria Vibratory urticaria/angioedema
Other urticaria types	Aquagenic urticaria Cholinergic urticaria Contact urticaria Exercise-induced anaphylaxis/urticaria

Adapted from Zuberbier T, Asero R, Bindslev-Jensen C, et al. EAACI/GA(2)LEN/EDF/WAO guideline: definition, classification and diagnosis of urticaria. Allergy 2009;64(10):1419; with permission.

in the classification, for example physical urticarias are also chronic but are grouped separately, because of the special nature of their eliciting factors.[5] The guideline also suggests that to avoid confusion, the commonly used term for chronic urticaria remains chronic urticaria, even if the full term for classification purposes is chronic spontaneous urticaria.[5] A further issue is that 2 or more different subtypes of urticaria can coexist in an individual patient.[5] Reports of the prevalence of chronic spontaneous urticaria occurring in combination with physical urticaria, most commonly symptomatic dermographism and delayed pressure urticaria (DPU) vary from 10% to 50%.[4] In 1 study (n = 135)[6] in which formal pressure testing was carried out on all patients, 37% of patients with chronic urticaria had concurrent DPU (**Fig. 2**). There is a trend to classify patients with combinations of chronic spontaneous urticaria and physical urticaria or cholinergic urticaria as chronic spontaneous urticaria.[4] This trend has implications for study comparisons and for quality-of-life (QoL) assessments in urticaria and subsets of urticaria.

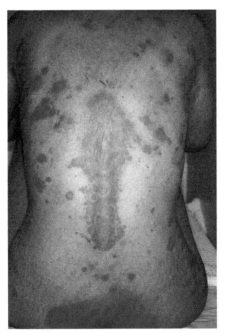

Fig. 2. DPU over the spine and sacrum provoked by lying on a hard surface. Spontaneous weals are seen at nonpressure sites. (*Courtesy of* the Illustrations Department, St John's Institute of Dermatology, London.)

QOL

QoL, or more specifically health-related QoL, is not simply a measure of health status, but more particularly the individual's perception of the impact of an illness or its treatment on their life.[7] It embraces physical and emotional well-being and satisfaction with social functioning.[8] It is a uniquely personal experience, not easily evaluated by clinicians. It has been known for some time that patients who have cancer[9] and more recently patients with urticaria[10] assess QoL differently from their doctors. The importance of considering the subjective dimension of diseases is increasingly recognized.[11]

QoL is a personal matter to be assessed by the individual, and the development of measures to evaluate it meaningfully is a challenge for the clinician. In addition to health-related QoL, the broader term patient-reported outcome (PRO) (which embraces health-related QoL) is increasingly being used.

PROS

PROs include all health reports coming from the patient, without involvement or interpretation by physicians or others, such as symptoms, health-related QoL, illness perception, satisfaction, or adherence to treatment.[11,12] PRO assessment should be carried out using tools validated to ensure responsiveness, construct validity, reliability, internal consistency and acceptability.[13] The Global Allergy and Asthma European Network (GA²LEN) position paper provides information on available instruments for PRO assessments in urticaria and gives recommendations for PRO assessments in clinical trials and routine patient care.[14] The taskforce recommends that PRO should be used in clinical trials as a primary outcome, coprimary outcome, and in some cases, as a secondary outcome.[14]

MEASURES TO EVALUATE QOL

Generic QoL tools, for example, the Medical Outcome Survey Short Form 36 (SF-36) or the Nottingham Health Profile (NHP), provide an overall assessment of patient perceived well-being and allow comparisons with general medical conditions. However, not all the items may be relevant to patients with skin disease and issues largely pertaining to skin disorders may be missing. A dermatology-specific measure, for example the Dermatology Life Quality Index (DLQI) or the Skindex, may be more appropriate. In order to encapsulate all relevant patient factors, which would also be sensitive to changes in the patient's condition, a disease-specific tool is required. Health-related QoL instruments in dermatology have been comprehensively and critically reviewed.[15] **Table 2** summarizes some health outcome measures referred to in this article and commonly used[14] to evaluate QoL in urticaria.

DLQI

DLQI, the first dermatology-specific QoL instrument,[16] is the most commonly and widely used. It has been used to assess QoL in 33 different skin conditions and there were 272 published articles up to 2007.[17] It is a 10-question instrument covering

Table 2
QoL measures in chronic urticaria

Type	QoL Instrument	Reference
Generic	SF-36	26,41
	World Health Organization QoL Assessment-Brief	47,51
	NHP	21,52
Dermatology specific	DLQI	16–19,27–29,31–33,35,52
	Skindex	10,29–32,45,50
	VQ-Dermato	25
Disease specific	Chronic urticaria–quality of life questionnaire	26,27,29–33

Adapted from Baiardini I, Braido F, Bindslev-Jensen C, et al. Recommendations for assessing patient-reported outcomes and health-related quality of life in patients with urticaria: a GA(2) LEN taskforce position paper. Allergy 2011;66(7):841; with permission.

symptoms and feelings, daily activities, leisure, work/school, personal relationships, and treatment.[16] Because it is simple and short, taking on average 126 seconds to complete,[18] it is popular in clinical practice and research.[17] Scores range from 0 to 30. Higher scores mean greater QoL impairment. Banding of the scores allows clinical interpretation of the score,[19] as follows:

DLQI Score	Clinical Interpretation
0–1	No effect on patient's life
2–5	Small effect
6–10	Moderate effect
11–20	Very large effect
21–30	Extremely large effect

Up to 2007, DLQI has been used in 12 studies of urticaria, involving a total of 3027 patients.[17]

IMPORTANCE OF QOL ASSESSMENTS IN URTICARIA

Chronic urticaria is largely non–life-threatening, its symptoms are transitory, and any disfigurement is temporary. Therefore, its impact on patients may not be appreciated. Such patients suffer in silence, and their predicament and needs are underestimated[20] and perhaps poorly understood by their medical carers.[2,10] QoL assessments are needed to better understand the impact of urticaria on affected patients and obtain patients' views of their disease and its consequences.[14] The effects of medications and other interventions on the QoL of patients need to be consistently assessed in routine patient care and in clinical research.[14] Of course, robust QoL data are essential in influencing decisions regarding the allocation of resources.

EARLY STUDY ON THE IMPACT OF CHRONIC URTICARIA ON THE QOL

An early study by Greaves' group in London signposted the negative impact of chronic urticaria on the QoL of affected patients.[21] A disease-specific, purpose-designed questionnaire highlighted the problems experienced by patients in 7 areas of interest (domains). Between 49% and 71% of patients had problems with aspects of home management, normally taken for granted. Many patients experienced problems in the areas of personal care (10%–70%), recreation and social interaction (73%–84%), mobility (45%–60%), and emotional factors (16%–86%). Thirty-eight per cent reported marked sleep disruption, and a further 54% had some sleep interference. More than half of the patients had missed at least 1 day from work in the preceding 4 weeks, because of their urticaria.[21]

A second questionnaire,[21] the NHP, is a well-validated,[22] reliable health status measure.[23] Part I of the NHP measures subjective health status with statements relating to limitations in activity in 6 dimensions: physical mobility, pain, sleep, energy, social isolation, and emotional reactions. **Fig. 3** compares the NHP scores (part I) of the cohort of 142 (45 male, 97 female) patients with urticaria (mean age 39.7 years, range 14–71 years) with the results of a previous study of 98 men with ischemic heart disease (mean age 51 years, range 37–59 years), awaiting coronary artery bypass grafting, most of whom had triple vessel coronary artery disease.[24] Comparison of the scores shows that sleep disruption was a greater problem for patients with chronic urticaria. The scores for energy, social isolation, and emotional reactions were similarly impaired in the 2 patient

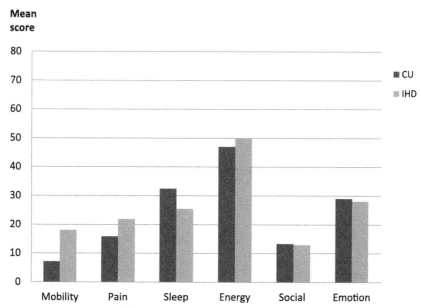

Fig. 3. Comparison of the NHP (part I) scores in patients with chronic urticaria (CU, n = 134)[21] and in patients with ischemic heart disease (IHD, n = 98)[24] awaiting coronary artery bypass grafting. (*From* O'Donnell BF, Lawlor F, Simpson J, et al. The impact of chronic urticaria on the quality of life. Br J Dermatol 1997;136(2):200; with permission.)

groups, suggesting that patients with chronic urticaria feel similarly lacking in energy, socially isolated, and emotionally upset as the patients with heart disease (see **Fig. 3**).[21]

> The QoL impairment of patients with chronic urticaria (mean age 39.7 years) attending a tertiary referral center is comparable with that experienced by a group of older patients (mean age 51 years) with severe, ischemic heart disease.

COMPARISON OF THE QOL OF PATIENTS WITH CHRONIC URTICARIA AND THE QOL OF PATIENTS WITH OTHER SKIN DISEASES

DLQI scores summarized in 12 studies of urticaria[17] show a range of 7.16 to 13.4 (moderate effect to very large effect on patient's life), with a mean of mean scores of 9.8. The mean of mean DLQI scores for psoriasis (PSO) and atopic dermatitis (AD) was 10.53 and 11.2, respectively. The DLQI score for urticaria was lower than the score for hidradenitis suppurativa but higher (ie, worse impairment) than the scores for acne, alopecia, Behçet syndrome, Darier disease, pyoderma gangrenosum, and vitiligo.[17]

Grob and colleagues[25] prospectively examined a large cohort of patients with chronic urticaria (n = 466), PSO (n = 464), and AD (n = 426) using the VQ-Dermato, a validated, French dermatology-specific tool. These investigators reported that the 3 conditions are characterized by completely different profiles of impact on health-related QoL. The physical discomfort dimension was more impaired in AD and chronic urticaria than in PSO (P<.001). The daily living activities scores were significantly higher (higher score indicates worse QoL, P<.001) in chronic urticaria and AD than in PSO, suggesting that pruritus is the dominant factor that interferes with everyday life in the former 2 skin diseases. Self-perception and treatment-induced restrictions were less affected in chronic urticaria than in AD and PSO ($P<.001$). The dimension scores for mood state, chronic urticaria (50.3), AD (49.3), and PSO (50.1) were remarkably similar in the 3 conditions.

Although it is widely accepted that AD and PSO may severely affect QoL, the severe impairment of QoL in chronic urticaria is often underestimated, and in several dimensions is comparable with the impairment suffered by patients with AD and PSO and significantly worse than many dermatoses.

DEVELOPMENT OF A DISEASE-SPECIFIC QOL MEASURE FOR CHRONIC URTICARIA
Chronic Urticaria–Quality of Life Questionnaire

Baiardini and colleagues[26] developed a new questionnaire specifically designed for the assessment of QoL in chronic urticaria. In the development phase, items were generated from a panel of experts in immunology, dermatology, and allergy and using exploratory semistructured interviews with 60 patients suffering from chronic urticaria. After the elimination of those items that were ambiguous, a list of 37 items was administered to 80 consecutive patients with chronic urticaria. An overall importance score was generated based on the percentage of patients who indicated each item as a consequence of their disease and the importance attributed by the patient to each item. This procedure generated a 23-item questionnaire. This questionnaire was subsequently tested on a different set of patients with chronic urticaria for validation.

For the validation phase, in addition to the Chronic Urticaria–Quality of Life Questionnaire (CU-Q_2oL), 125 patients completed the SF-36 health survey, to evaluate the properties of validity, internal consistency, reliability, and responsiveness of the new instrument.

The investigators reported that the new CU-Q_2oL satisfies the criteria for validity.[26] Factor analysis revealed a 6-dimensional structure and good levels of internal consistency for the extracted factors: pruritus, swelling, impact on life activities, sleep problems, looks, and limits.[26] This finding makes it a most useful tool for evaluating the specific burden of chronic urticaria on health-related QoL and also for documenting the changes induced by therapy.[27] It is quick to complete (5 minutes), well received by patients, and the scores are easily evaluated with the appropriate software.[26]

The German Version of the CU-Q_2oL

Translated questionnaires always need to be revalidated in the new language/culture/setting.[28] Mlynek and colleagues[29] successfully presented factor analysis of a German version of the CU-Q_2oL, yielding 6 scales. Correlation with the DLQI and Skindex-29 confirmed robust validation. On a percentile scale, the median CU-Q_2oL scores were as follows: functioning, 29; sleep, 44; itching/embarrassment, 50; mental status, 50; swelling/eating, 31; limits looks, 31. The scores from this German population indicate that the greatest burden of QoL impairment were in the areas of sleep, itching/embarrassment, and mental status.

Scale VI (limits looks), with a total of 2 items pertaining to clothing choices and cosmetics, had the lowest consistency (Cronbach $\alpha = 0.52$) and was retained because it was just above the standard set in the previous Italian study (Cronbach $\alpha = 0.5$). As a revision option for future studies and in view of the known psychological problems associated with chronic urticaria, the investigators suggested including the item on anxiety ("I feel anxious about my health condition"), assigned a mean importance of

3.12 on a scale of 0 to 4 in the original Italian study,[26] and the next item due for inclusion in CU-Q$_2$oL if the arbitrary cutoff on the overall impact score had been set at 1.0 rather than at 1.5.

Mlynek and colleagues[29] recommended that the minimal important difference (the smallest difference in scores considered clinically meaningful) of CU-Q$_2$oL scores be determined. This strategy would enhance understanding of translating a score on paper to meaningful changes in the patient's life. Although both the Italian[26] and the German studies[29] used the same 23-item questionnaire, the 23 items are assigned differently, creating 6 different scales in each version.

CU-Q$_2$oL has been adapted and validated across languages and cultures. The Spanish[30] and Turkish[31] versions have the same 6-scale structure as the original Italian questionnaire.[26] The Polish version has 6 scales: itching, swelling/mental status, functioning, sleep, eating/limits, and embarrassment.[32] The Brazilian-Portuguese version has a three-dimensional structure: sleep/mental status/eating, pruritus/impact on life activities, and swelling/limits/look.[33] Because the items in the scales in the various versions are assigned differently in some versions of the CU-Q$_2$oL, only the scale results from the Italian, Spanish, and Turkish versions can be directly compared. Of course, the scores of the 23 individual items from the international versions could be compared, one by one.[29]

HOW TO MEASURE DISEASE ACTIVITY IN CHRONIC URTICARIA?

Urticaria activity scores (UAS), originally developed an as outpatient diary sheet,[34] documenting the number of weals (score 0–3) and the severity of itch (0–3) daily, to give a maximum total weekly score of 42 (UAS7), has been used in clinical studies for some time. The recent European Academy of Allergy and Clinical Immunology (EAACI)/GA^{2}LEN/European Dermatology Forum (EDF)/World Allergy Organization (WAO) guidelines recommended its use.[5] It has more recently been proved a valid tool for measuring and monitoring disease activity in patients with chronic urticaria.[35] UAS has proved to be as good as more complex scores. Patients were more likely to document the 2 symptom qualities that comprise the UAS (the number of weals and intensity of itch) than other urticaria symptoms.[35]

HOW TO ASSESS PROS AND HEALTH-RELATED QOL IN PATIENTS WITH URTICARIA?

The GA^{2}LEN taskforce position paper recommends the UAS and CU-Q$_2$oL in routine clinical practice to determine urticaria disease activity.[14] It is recommended that both the UAS and CU-Q$_2$oL should also be used routinely for assessing patient responses to treatment.[14,27] More generic instruments like those adopted for chronic skin diseases may also be used.[14] SF-36 and the Skindex have been recommended as the health-related QoL instruments of choice and the runner-up measures are the World Health Organization QoL Assessment (WHOQOL) and the Skindex-17.[15]

THE WORST ASPECT OF URTICARIA

A wide range of factors affect patients, because of their urticaria. An open-ended question "What is the worst aspect of your urticaria?" yielded insightful replies[21] (most patients gave >1 answer), as follows: the swellings (59%), itch (42%), pain (22%), and feelings of being tired, irritable, weak or a feeling of loss of control over their lives (22%). The unpredictability of attacks upset 20%. Other problems were the social restrictions (18%), feeling embarrassed (13%), time off work (7%), restriction of food or clothing (7%), side effects of drugs (5%), and being unable to relax or sit (3.6%).

In Baiardini and colleagues' study,[26] the 12 most important issues, ranked in descending order based on their overall impact were, pruritus, wheals, embarrassment from urticaria signs on body, feeling nervous, swelling of eyes, embarrassment in going to public places, interference with sleep, interference with eating, swelling of the lips, interference with work, bad mood, and interference with sporting activities.

EMOTIONS IN CHRONIC URTICARIA

Fears loom large for patients with chronic urticaria.[21,36] Many suffer nonspecific anxiety. They also have specific worries, for example that their urticaria is caused by an underlying more serious disease.[21] Patients with urticaria score lower than the 20th percentile for items indexing psychological health.[37] They experience higher emotional distress, anxiety, anger, and depression compared with controls.[36] Patients with chronic urticaria may have difficulty dealing with these emotions, because they are not adequately able to identify, express, and communicate their feelings, a personality trait described as alexithymia, (literally, no words for emotions).[36] Formal studies using the Toronto Alexithymia Scale confirmed that patients with chronic urticaria showed higher alexithymia compared with healthy controls.[36,38]

There is a strong correlation between depression and pruritus severity.[39] For those patients with chronic urticaria who are depressed, their itch scores are significantly higher than those of patients with urticaria who are normothymic.[40] Anger has also been shown to be a significant predictor of pruritus severity in chronic urticaria.[36] There is a direct correlation between itch intensity and stress.[40]

STRESS IN CHRONIC URTICARIA

Many patients believe that their illness is caused by stress[41] or aggravated by stress,[4] as do their attending allergists.[42] The role of stress in precipitating, maintaining, or flaring chronic urticaria is unclear.[4] Urticaria itself is apparently and understandably a major cause of stress. The pathophysiology of stress in chronic urticaria remains unclear.[4] Work from human in vitro studies showed that the basophils in patients with urticaria have heightened response to corticotropin-releasing factor and patients with urticaria have higher levels of serum cortisol.[43] Patients with urticaria have also been shown to have lower serum concentrations of dehydroepiandrosterone sulfate (DHEA-S), lower level of the sense of coherence, higher level of anxiety as a state and as a trait, and higher level of depression, which suggests that the DHEA-S decline is secondary to psychological disturbances.[44] There is an unmet need for well-controlled studies on the role of stress and its treatment in chronic urticaria.[4]

PSYCHIATRIC COMORBIDITY IN CHRONIC URTICARIA

Dermatology outpatients in general have a high prevalence of psychiatric morbidity, with approximately 25% of patients having significant psychiatric problems,[45] a prevalence 2 to 3 times higher than the 1-month or point prevalence estimates of psychiatric disorders in Western countries.[46] The psychological well-being of patients with skin disease in this large Italian cohort (n = 2579) was examined using the Skindex-29 and the General Health Questionnaire.[45] The latter is a 12-item questionnaire designed to detect minor, nonpsychotic psychiatric disorders. The prevalence of psychiatric morbidity in patients with urticaria at 34.5% was higher than the overall prevalence of 25% and also higher than in psoriatic patients (26%) or in those with various dermatitides (27.3%). Health-related QoL was a stronger predictor of psychiatric morbidity than physician-rated clinical severity,[45] underscoring the importance of QoL measures in the holistic management of patients.

Uguz and colleagues[47] studied the impact of Axis I (includes all diagnostic categories except mental retardation and personality disorder) and Axis II psychiatric disorders (personality disorders and intellectual disabilities) on QoL in subsets of 100 patients with chronic idiopathic urticaria (CIU). Significant differences were shown among the groups with respect to all the WHOQOL-Brief subscale scores (physical health, psychological health, social relationships, and environment). QoL levels were similarly impaired ($P<.0001$) among patients with CIU with an Axis I diagnosis, an Axis II diagnosis, and with both Axis I and Axis II diagnoses compared with patients with CIU without an Axis I or Axis II diagnosis and healthy controls.[47] Obsessive-compulsive disorder, major depression, obsessive-compulsive, and avoidant personality disorders were more frequent in patients with chronic urticaria than in control individuals.[48]

A high prevalence of mental disorders, as assessed by diagnostic interviews and mini-DIPS (diagnostic interview for mental disorders), was noted in 48 of 100 patients with chronic urticaria, most commonly anxiety disorders (30%), depressive disorders (17%), and somatoform disorders (17%).[49] Agoraphobia was found to be the most frequent (15%) anxiety disorder in patients with chronic urticaria.[49] Increased scores for anxiety as measured by the Hospital Anxiety and Depression Scale (HADS), depression (HADS), and somatization, as measured by Symptom Check List-90 Revisited (SCL-90R), were found in 30%, 21%, and 23% of patients, respectively.[49] All 3 scores were found to be significantly higher and to be increased more often in patients with chronic urticaria diagnosed with a mental disorder.[50] In addition, patients with urticaria with mental disorder showed significantly higher levels of emotional distress as assessed by Global Severity Index of psychological distress of SCL-90R.[49]

Psychiatric comorbidity (depression, anxiety, somatoform disorders) was associated with a more pronounced reduction of QoL compared with patients with chronic urticaria without a psychiatric diagnosis.[50] The severity of psychiatric disease correlates with QoL impairment,[50,51] and not with other factors like the presence or absence of angioedema or the course or cause of chronic urticaria.[50] Despite the psychiatric morbidity associated with chronic urticaria, many patients were reluctant to undergo formal psychological treatment.[52] However, if the physician enquired from the patient how they were feeling and discussed the emotional impact of urticaria, this improved the patient's satisfaction with treatment and with their physician.[10]

PSYCHIATRIC COMORBIDITY IN CHRONIC URTICARIA
The Bottom Line

A recent meta-analysis[42] of psychosocial factors and chronic spontaneous urticaria, involving 22 studies, concluded that the pooled prevalence of psychosocial factors among patients with urticaria was 46.09%. (There was high heterogeneity among the studies.) A comprehensive table provides a summary list of the studies reporting that compared with a healthy control group, patients with urticaria had significantly higher scores on measures of somatization, obsessive-compulsive disorder, interpersonal sensitivity and depression, anxiety, insomnia, and stressful life events.[42]

A systematic search of medical databases (PubMed and OVID/Medline) revealed a high prevalence (46.09%) of psychosocial factors in patients with chronic spontaneous urticaria.

EFFECT OF CHRONIC URTICARIA ON SEXUAL LIFE

In the 4 weeks before completing the urticaria questionnaire, the presence of chronic urticaria had a minor (39%) or major (34%) impact on patient's sexual relationships.[21] The presence of cholinergic urticaria or DPU had a significantly greater impact.[53] In the Turkish validation (CU-Q$_2$oL) study, based on the Skindex-29 and the DLQI question-naires, 40% of patients indicated impairment in their sexual life, because of urticaria.[21] The Italian study showed that although 31.58% of patients experienced problems in their sexual lives, the overall impact at 0.77 was less than the arbitrary cutoff value of 1.5, and this item was removed at the item reduction phase in the development of the CU-Q$_2$oL.[26]

QOL IN SUBSETS OF CHRONIC URTICARIA

CU-Q$_2$oL has been validated and is suited for investigation of patients with chronic spontaneous urticaria. Disease-specific instruments need to be developed and vali-dated for QoL assessments in patients with a subset of chronic urticaria.[14]

DPU

As evaluated by DLQI, patients with chronic urticaria and concurrent DPU (n = 26) suf-fered significantly higher QoL impairment (43 ± 23%, DLQI mean ± standard deviation [SD]) than patients with urticaria without a concurrent physical urticaria (n = 47) (25 ± 24%, DLQI mean ± SD).[53]

Cholinergic Urticaria

Patient with cholinergic urticaria (n = 9), attending a tertiary referral center recorded a high DLQI score (50 ± 34%, mean ± SD), largely in relation to sporting activities. This finding may not be representative of the morbidity seen in a community population with cholinergic urticaria.[53]

Cold Urticaria

Patients with cold urticaria (n = 8) suffered moderate levels of QoL impairment (28 ± 20%, DLQI mean ± SD), during autumn.[53]

The presence of dermographism in addition to chronic urticaria did not confer addi-tional impairment. Patients with acute/intermittent urticaria suffered little disability, as evaluated by DLQI.[53]

QOL IN ANGIOEDEMA

As evaluated by DLQI, for patients with chronic urticaria ± angioedema, the presence of angioedema did not confer additional QoL impairment.[53] However, DLQI may not have been an adequately sensitive tool. A disease-specific angioedema QoL ques-tionnaire has been developed with 4 domains (functioning, fatigue/mood, fears/shame, food) and is a short, valid, and reliable instrument.[54]

IMPACT OF CHRONIC URTICARIA ON THE MENTAL HEALTH OF CHILDREN

Chronic urticaria is less common in children than in adults (0.1%–3% of children), and there are few studies of the impact of the disease in this age group. A study involving 27 children with chronic urticaria and 27 age-matched and gender-matched controls showed that the children with urticaria had more frequent psychi-atric diagnoses (70% vs 30%), most commonly social anxiety, separation anxiety disorder, and specific phobia.[55] Depression, trait anxiety, internalizing problems, somatic complaints, and anxiety/depressed scores were significantly higher in children with chronic urticaria.[55]

ECONOMIC COST

Delong and colleagues[56] estimated the annual direct and indirect health care costs of 50 patients with chronic urticaria, who had not been taking systemic corticosteroids or other immunosuppressants in the preceding month. The 4 direct health care costs estimated (medication usage, outpatient visits, emergency department/hospital costs and laboratory tests) and 2 indirect costs (loss of earnings because of travel to outpatient visits and absenteeism caused by the urticaria), accrued a mean total cost of $2048.[56]

The mean primary direct cost of $1280 was for medications (largely nonsedating antihistamines but also sedating antihistamines, corticosteroid taper, doxepin, epinephrine hydrochloride autoinjector [16%], histamine 2 blockers, and antileukotrienes). The mean annual cost of outpatient visits was $280, emergency department visits was $148, and for laboratory tests was $17. The mean annual earnings lost because of work absences was $252, and costs because of travel time for outpatient visits was $70. The mean annual cost of medication at $1280 resulted in highest economic burden (62.5%).[56]

Evaluation of insurance claims to estimate the cost of chronic urticaria showed that although the patients are relatively young (mean age 36 years) and otherwise healthy, their health care charges are substantial, with approximately $1700 per year related directly to care and treatment of urticaria.[57]

The costs are almost certainly an underestimate because over-the-counter medications, particularly antihistamines, are not included. Patients on immunosuppressive medications have the added expense of increased laboratory tests and outpatient visits in addition to possible inpatient treatment. Because chronic urticaria is such a difficult management problem, patients at the severe end of the spectrum require specialized treatments. For example, intravenous immunoglobulin induced prolonged complete remissions (3-year follow-up) in 30% of patients with recalcitrant, autoimmune chronic urticaria,[58] a finding recently confirmed by others.[59] Further treatments justified in selected patients and recommended in the EAACI/GA²LEN/EDF/WAO guideline[60] are cyclosporin, dapsone, and omalizumab. Immunomodulatory therapies for which less evidence is available include methotrexate, azathioprine, mycophenolate mofetil, cyclophosphamide, and tacrolimus.[60] Plasmapheresis has been used successfully in a specialized center.[61] The costs associated with these treatments have not been formally evaluated and are significant.

Chronic urticaria, a heart-sink dermatosis,[62] is challenging for the attending physicians. They are dealing with patients who have a frustrating, unpredictable condition and note that the care of patients with urticaria is time consuming and expensive.[63] The patients have high expectations, severely impaired QoL, and a significant emotional burden.[63] There is significant economic cost and loss to patients and society because of chronic urticaria. There are also intangible costs[64] as a result of the impact of chronic urticaria on the patient's QoL.

ACKNOWLEDGMENTS

Thank you to the Illustrations Department, St John's Institute of Dermatology, London for **Figs. 1** and **2**.

REFERENCES

 1. Czarnetzki BM. Acute and chronic urticaria. In: Czarnetzki BM, editor. Urticaria. Berlin, Heidelberg, New York, Tokyo: Springer-Verlag; 1986. p. 26–46.
 2. Maurer M, Ortonne JP, Zuberbier T. Chronic urticaria: an internet survey of health behaviours, symptom patterns and treatment needs in European adult patients. Br J Dermatol 2009;160(3):633–41.
 3. Greaves MW. Chronic urticaria. N Engl J Med 1995;332:1767–72.
 4. Maurer M, Weller K, Bindslev-Jensen C, et al. Unmet clinical needs in chronic spontaneous urticaria. A GA^2LEN task force report. Allergy 2011;66(3):317–30.
 5. Zuberbier T, Asero R, Bindslev-Jensen C, et al. EAACI/GA(2)LEN/EDF/WAO guideline: definition, classification and diagnosis of urticaria. Allergy 2009; 64(10):1417–26.
 6. Barlow RJ, Warburton F, Watson K, et al. Diagnosis and incidence of delayed pressure urticaria in patients with chronic urticaria. J Am Acad Dermatol 1993;29:954–8.
 7. Gill TM, Feinstein AR. A critical appraisal of the quality of quality-of-life measurements. JAMA 1994;272(8):619–26.
 8. Croog SH, Levine S, Testa MA, et al. The effects of antihypertensive therapy on the quality of life. N Engl J Med 1986;314:1657–64.
 9. Slevin ML, Plant H, Lynch D, et al. Who should measure quality of life, the doctor or the patient? Br J Cancer 1988;57:109–12.
10. Maurer M, Ortonne JP, Zuberbier T. Chronic urticaria: a patient survey on quality-of-life, treatment usage and doctor-patient relation. Allergy 2009;64(4):581–8.
11. Baiardini I, Bousquet PJ, Brzoza Z, et al. Recommendations for assessing patient-reported outcomes and health-related quality of life in clinical trials on allergy: a GA(2)LEN taskforce position paper. Allergy 2010;65(3):290–5.
12. Patrick DL, Burke LB, Powers JH, et al. Patient-reported outcomes to support medical product labeling claims: FDA perspective. Value Health 2007; 10(Suppl 2):S125–37.
13. Worth A, Hammersley VS, Nurmatov U, et al. Systematic literature review and evaluation of patient reported outcome measures (PROMs) for asthma and related allergic diseases. Prim Care Respir J 2012;21(4):455–8.
14. Baiardini I, Braido F, Bindslev-Jensen C, et al. Recommendations for assessing patient-reported outcomes and health-related quality of life in patients with urticaria: a GA(2)LEN taskforce position paper. Allergy 2011;66(7):840–4.
15. Both H, Essink-Bot ML, Busschbach J, et al. Critical review of generic and dermatology-specific health-related quality of life instruments. J Invest Dermatol 2007;127(12):2726–39.
16. Finlay AY, Khan GK. Dermatology Life Quality Index (DLQI)–a simple practical measure for routine clinical use. Clin Exp Dermatol 1994;19(3):210–6.
17. Basra MK, Fenech R, Gatt RM, et al. The Dermatology Life Quality Index 1994-2007: a comprehensive review of validation data and clinical results. Br J Dermatol 2008;159(5):997–1035.
18. Loo WJ, Diba V, Chawla M, et al. Dermatology Life Quality Index: influence of an illustrated version. Br J Dermatol 2003;148(2):279–84.
19. Hongbo Y, Thomas CL, Harrison MA, et al. Translating the science of quality of life into practice: what do dermatology life quality index scores mean? J Invest Dermatol 2005;125(4):659–64.
20. Grob JJ, Gaudy-Marqueste C. Urticaria and quality of life. Clin Rev Allergy Immunol 2006;30(1):47–51.

21. O'Donnell BF, Lawlor F, Simpson J, et al. The impact of chronic urticaria on the quality of life. Br J Dermatol 1997;136(2):197–201.
22. Hunt SM, McKenna SP, McEwen J, et al. A quantitative approach to perceived health status: a validation study. J Epidemiol Community Health 1980;34: 281–6.
23. Hunt SM, McKenna SP, Williams J. Reliability of a population survey tool for measuring perceived health problems: a study of patients with osteoarthrosis. J Epidemiol Community Health 1981;35:297–300.
24. Caine N, Harrison SC, Sharples LD, et al. Prospective study of quality of life before and after coronary artery bypass grafting. Br Med J 1991;302:511–6.
25. Grob JJ, Revuz J, Ortonne JP, et al. Comparative study of the impact of chronic urticaria, psoriasis and atopic dermatitis on the quality of life. Br J Dermatol 2005;152(2):289–95.
26. Baiardini I, Pasquali M, Braido F, et al. A new tool to evaluate the impact of chronic urticaria on quality of life: chronic urticaria quality of life questionnaire (CU-QoL). Allergy 2005;60(8):1073–8.
27. Weller K, Church MK, Kalogeromitros D, et al. Chronic spontaneous urticaria: how to assess quality of life in patients receiving treatment. Arch Dermatol 2011;147(10):1221–3.
28. Finlay AY. Quality of life measurement in dermatology: a practical guide. Br J Dermatol 1997;136(3):305–14.
29. Młynek A, Magerl M, Hanna M, et al. The German version of the Chronic Urticaria Quality-of-Life Questionnaire: factor analysis, validation, and initial clinical findings. Allergy 2009;64(6):927–36.
30. Valero A, Herdman M, Bartra J, et al. Adaptation and validation of the Spanish version of the Chronic Urticaria Quality of Life Questionnaire (CU-Q2oL). J Investig Allergol Clin Immunol 2008;18(6):426–32.
31. Kocatürk E, Weller K, Martus P, et al. Turkish version of the chronic urticaria quality of life questionnaire: cultural adaptation, assessment of reliability and validity. Acta Derm Venereol 2012;92(4):419–25.
32. Brzoza Z, Badura-Brzoza K, Młynek A, et al. Adaptation and initial results of the Polish version of the GA(2)LEN chronic urticaria quality of life questionnaire (CU-Q(2)oL). J Dermatol Sci 2011;62(1):36–41.
33. Dias GA, Pires GV, Valle SO, et al. Cross-cultural adaptation of the Brazilian-Portuguese version of the chronic urticaria quality-of-life questionnaire–CU-Q2oL. Allergy 2011;66(11):1487–93.
34. Greaves MW. Antihistamine treatment: a patient self-assessment method in chronic urticaria. Br Med J 1981;283:1435–6.
35. Młynek A, Zalewska-Janowska A, Martus P, et al. How to assess disease activity in patients with chronic urticaria? Allergy 2008;63(6):777–80.
36. Conrad R, Geiser F, Haidl G, et al. Relationship between anger and pruritus perception in patients with chronic idiopathic urticaria and psoriasis. J Eur Acad Dermatol Venereol 2008;22(9):1062–9.
37. Ferrer M. Epidemiology, healthcare, resources, use and clinical features of different types of urticaria. Alergológica 2005. J Investig Allergol Clin Immunol 2009;19(Suppl 2):21–6.
38. Barbosa F, Freitas J, Barbosa A. Alexithymia in chronic urticaria patients. Psychol Health Med 2011;16(2):215–24.
39. Gupta MA, Gupta AK, Schork NJ, et al. Depression modulates pruritus perception. A study of pruritus in psoriasis, atopic dermatitis and chronic idiopathic urticaria. Psychosom Med 1994;56(1):36–40.

40. Yosipovitch G, Ansari N, Goon A, et al. Clinical characteristics of pruritus in chronic idiopathic urticaria. Br J Dermatol 2002;147(1):32–6.
41. Ozkan M, Oflaz SB, Kocaman N, et al. Psychiatric morbidity and quality of life in patients with chronic idiopathic urticaria. Ann Allergy Asthma Immunol 2007; 99(1):29–33.
42. Ben-Shoshan M, Blinderman I, Raz A. Psychosocial factors and chronic spontaneous urticaria: a systematic review. Allergy 2013;68(2):131–41.
43. Dyke SM, Carey BS, Kaminski ER. Effect of stress on basophil function in chronic idiopathic urticaria. Clin Exp Allergy 2008;38(1):86–92.
44. Brzoza Z, Kasperska-Zajac A, Badura-Brzoza K, et al. Decline in dehydroepiandrosterone sulfate observed in chronic urticaria is associated with psychological distress. Psychosom Med 2008;70(6):723–8.
45. Picardi A, Abeni D, Melchi CF, et al. Psychiatric morbidity in dermatological outpatients: an issue to be recognized. Br J Dermatol 2000;143(5):983–91.
46. Regier DA, Boyd JH, Burke JD Jr, et al. One-month prevalence of mental disorders in the United States. Based on five Epidemiologic Catchment Area sites. Arch Gen Psychiatry 1988;45(11):977–86.
47. Uguz F, Engin B, Yilmaz E. Quality of life in patients with chronic idiopathic urticaria: the impact of Axis I and Axis II psychiatric disorders. Gen Hosp Psychiatry 2008;30(5):453–7.
48. Uguz F, Engin B, Yilmaz E. Axis I and Axis II diagnoses in patients with chronic idiopathic urticaria. J Psychosom Res 2008;64(2):225–9.
49. Staubach P, Dechene M, Metz M, et al. High prevalence of mental disorders and emotional distress in patients with chronic spontaneous urticaria. Acta Derm Venereol 2011;91(5):557–61.
50. Staubach P, Eckhardt-Henn A, Dechene M, et al. Quality of life in patients with chronic urticaria is differentially impaired and determined by psychiatric comorbidity. Br J Dermatol 2006;154(2):294–8.
51. Engin B, Uguz F, Yilmaz E, et al. The levels of depression, anxiety and quality of life in patients with chronic idiopathic urticaria. J Eur Acad Dermatol Venereol 2008;22(1):36–40.
52. Berrino AM, Voltolini S, Fiaschi D, et al. Chronic urticaria: importance of a medical-psychological approach. Eur Ann Allergy Clin Immunol 2006;38(5):149–52.
53. Poon E, Seed PT, Greaves MW, et al. The extent and nature of disability in different urticarial conditions. Br J Dermatol 1999;140(4):667–71.
54. Weller K, Groffik A, Magerl M, et al. Development and construct validation of the angioedema quality of life questionnaire. Allergy 2012;67(10):1289–98.
55. Hergüner S, Kiliç G, Karakoç S, et al. Levels of depression, anxiety and behavioural problems and frequency of psychiatric disorders in children with chronic idiopathic urticaria. Br J Dermatol 2011;164(6):1342–7.
56. Delong LK, Culler SD, Saini SS, et al. Annual direct and indirect health care costs of chronic idiopathic urticaria: a cost analysis of 50 nonimmunosuppressed patients. Arch Dermatol 2008;144(1):35–9.
57. Zazzali JL, Broder MS, Chang E, et al. Cost, utilization, and patterns of medication use associated with chronic idiopathic urticaria. Ann Allergy Asthma Immunol 2012;108(2):98–102.
58. O'Donnell BF, Barr RM, Black AK, et al. Intravenous immunoglobulin in autoimmune chronic urticaria. Br J Dermatol 1998;138(1):101–6.
59. Mitzel-Kaoukhov H, Staubach P, Müller-Brenne T. Effect of high-dose intravenous immunoglobulin treatment in therapy-resistant chronic spontaneous urticaria. Ann Allergy Asthma Immunol 2010;104(3):253–8.

60. Zuberbier T, Asero R, Bindslev-Jensen C, et al. EAACI/GA(2)LEN/EDF/WAO guideline: management of urticaria. Allergy 2009;64(10):1427–43.
61. Grattan CE, Francis DM, Slater NG, et al. Plasmapheresis for severe, unremitting, chronic urticaria. Lancet 1992;339(8801):1078–80.
62. Yosipovitch G, Greaves M. Chronic idiopathic urticaria: a "Cinderella" disease with a negative impact on quality of life and health care costs. Arch Dermatol 2008;144(1):102–3.
63. Weller K, Viehmann K, Bräutigam M. Cost-intensive, time-consuming, problematical? How physicians in private practice experience the care of urticaria patients. J Dtsch Dermatol Ges 2012;10(5):341–7.
64. Bickers DR, Lim HW, Margolis D, et al. The burden of skin diseases: 2004 a joint project of the American Academy of Dermatology Association and the Society for Investigative Dermatology. J Am Acad Dermatol 2006;55(3):490–500.

Treatment of Chronic Urticaria

Riccardo Asero, MD[a],*, Alberto Tedeschi, MD[b],
Massimo Cugno, MD[c]

KEYWORDS

- Chronic urticaria • Therapy • Antihistamines • Corticosteroids • Ciclosporin
- Omalizumab

KEY POINTS

- Second-generation antihistamines are unquestionably the first-line treatment for chronic urticaria and can be used at higher than licensed doses if normal doses fail to control the disease.
- A short course of oral corticosteroids should be considered for patients not responding to antihistamines before trying other immunosuppressive drugs.
- Ciclosporin is effective in most antihistamine-resistant patients who require long-term corticosteroid treatments to control their disease.
- Omalizumab is effective in most subsets of chronic urticaria who do not respond to other treatments but its high cost represents a limitation to its widespread use.

INTRODUCTION

Chronic urticaria (CU) is a skin disorder characterized by the recurrent eruption of short-lived wheals accompanied by redness and itching for at least 6 weeks.[1] CU has an estimated prevalence of 0.5% to 1%, a female predominance (female/male ratio: 2/1),[1,2] and a heavy impact on the quality of life.[3] Recent advances in the knowledge of CU pathophysiology have led to a rethinking of therapeutic strategies. The demonstration of histamine-releasing autoantibodies[4–6] and of increased inflammation and coagulation biomarkers[7,8] has provided the rationale for the use of immunomodulatory and anti-inflammatory drugs in CU.[9] To conjugate the frequent need for long-term treatments aiming to control the disease with the least possible impact in terms of side effects, several therapeutic strategies have been suggested during the last years by scientific panels of experts belonging to national as well as international

[a] Ambulatorio di Allergologia (Allergy Unit), Clinica San Carlo, Via Ospedale 21; 20037, Paderno Dugnano, Milano, Italy; [b] U.O. Allergologia e Immunologia Clinica (Allergy and Clinical Immunology Unit), Fondazione IRCCS Ca' Granda, Ospedale Maggiore Policlinico, Via Pace 9; 20122, Milano, Italy; [c] Internal Medicine, Department of Pathophysiology & Transplantation, Università degli Studi di Milano, IRCCS Fondazione Ca' Granda, Ospedale Maggiore Policlinico, Via Pace 9; 20122, Milano, Italy
* Corresponding author.
E-mail address: r.asero@libero.it

Immunol Allergy Clin N Am 34 (2014) 105–116
http://dx.doi.org/10.1016/j.iac.2013.09.013   immunology.theclinics.com

societies, including the European Academy of Allergy and Clinical Immunology; the American Academy of Allergy, Asthma, and Immunology; and the World Allergy Organization.[10–15] Altogether, except for the fact that some new drugs have been introduced in the therapeutic schemes recently, such documents do not show major conceptual differences and are generally organized as a stepwise treatment to be adapted from one patient to another based on the severity of the disease and on the response to therapy. The pharmacologic treatment of CU is critically reviewed here.

GENERAL MEASURES

Besides pharmacologic treatments, CU patients should follow some general measures aiming at the reduction or minimization of a series of cofactors that might induce an exacerbation of the disease. In general, all the conditions causing vasodilation (eg, alcoholic drinks, excessive ambient temperature, heavy clothing, hot baths or showers, and spicy food) should be avoided because they might trigger a flare of wheals. Overtiredness is another condition that can be associated with the appearance of wheal-and-flare skin reactions in these subjects. Finally, up to 15% of CU patients experience an exacerbation of their disease after taking aspirin or other cycloxygenase-1 (COX-1) inhibitors (eg, diclofenac, propionic acid derivatives, indomethacin, oxicams); thus, the tolerability of COX-1-inhibiting drugs should be ascertained, and in the case of a positive history, patients should be advised to use analgesics or anti-inflammatory drugs exerting little or no activity on COX-1, such as paracetamol, etoricoxib, or tramadol. Oral tolerance tests with the latter drugs should be carried out to ascertain their tolerability.

ANTIHISTAMINES

Second-generation antihistamines (bilastine, cetirizine, desloratadine, ebastine, fexofenadine, levocetirizine, loratadine, mizolastine, rupatadine) are unquestionably the cornerstone of treatment of CU. Their effectiveness in patients with mild or moderate urticaria is shown by several randomized controlled trials.[10–15] The different second-generation antihistamines are not equally effective. Based on studies of inhibition of the wheal induced by histamine or by allergens, as well as on double-blind, placebo-controlled studies, cetirizine and its derivative levocetirizine appear to be the most effective compounds of the group,[16–22] although the recently introduced bilastine showed an efficacy similar to levocetirizine in one study,[23] and in another study, rupatadine was superior to levocetirizine.[24] Studies looking at sedation and psychomotor functions produced variable results with no relevant differences between levocetirizine, cetirizine, and loratadine in some cases,[25] and a greater sedative effect of cetirizine over fexofenadine, or loratadine in other cases.[26]

First-generation antihistamines are effective in patients with CU but their efficacy does not seem superior to second-generation antihistamines,[27–29] although they bear a higher degree of sedation and cognitive impairment.[30] Altogether, in most cases there is no reason to use these drugs as first-line treatment or as an add-on treatment for CU patients who do not respond to second-generation antihistamines.[10–15] However, as studies of the negative effects of first-generation antihistamines have almost exclusively been carried out on healthy subjects, not in patients with severe sleep deprivation due to CU, it cannot be excluded that first-generation antihistamines may be beneficial in some CU patients.

In patients with CU who do not respond adequately to second-generation antihistamines at licensed doses, higher than licensed doses can be given. Such approach is supported by studies carried out in both patients with acquired cold urticaria[31] and spontaneous CU,[32,33] showing a greater therapeutic effect without an increase in side effects. However, the safety of "off-label" dosages of second-generation antihistamines is evidence-based in the short term, but not yet in the long term. Furthermore, increasing the dosage of second-generation antihistamines is not always effective.[34]

Some old studies suggested the efficacy of adding H2-antagonists to H1-antagonists,[35,36] but subsequent investigations yielded conflicting results.[37,38] Thus, in view of the low quality of evidence supporting the use of H2 receptor antagonists in association with H1 antihistamines and of the fact that such association does not seem to produce any real advantage over the use of anti-H1 antihistamines alone, such an approach is presently not recommended. Nonetheless, H2 receptor antagonists may be of value in patients currently or recently treated by oral corticosteroids as well as in patients who have gastric hyperacidity.

CORTICOSTEROIDS

The effectiveness of oral corticosteroids in CU patients not responding to antihistamine therapy is widely recognized. Rather surprisingly, however, controlled studies are lacking; in the largest (retrospective) study carried out so far[39]; prednisone at a dose of about 0.3 to 0.5 mg/kg induced a remission of the disease and subsequent control with antihistamines at licensed doses in about 50% of cases. Most remaining patients responded well also, but relapsed when doses were tapered down, or after the end of the corticosteroid course. In about one-third of temporary responders, a second course of prednisone induced a persistent remission of the disease. Clinical effects were evident as early as the day after the first 25-mg dose. In view of the potentially severe side effects associated with long-term treatment (diabetes, hypertension, osteoporosis, and gastrointestinal bleeding), oral corticosteroids should be used for short periods and at the minimal effective dose.

LEUKOTRIENE RECEPTOR ANTAGONISTS
Montelukast and Zafirlukast

The effectiveness of cysteinyl-leukotriene antagonists as montelukast and zafirlukast in CU is supported by anecdotal reports[40,41] and some placebo-controlled studies.[42–46] Frequently they were used in combination with H1 antihistamines and were particularly effective in CU patients positive for autologous serum skin test (ASST) and with intolerance to aspirin or to food additives.[42,46] However, not all the studies have confirmed the efficacy of leukotriene antagonists, especially when used as monotherapy.[47] In summary, existing evidence of their effectiveness is limited, and the grade of recommendation for their use is low. Nonetheless, these drugs may be tried in patients unresponsive to antihistamines in view of their excellent safety profile.

ANTI-INFLAMMATORY DRUGS

The category of anti-inflammatory drugs includes dapsone, sulfasalazine, and hydroxychloroquine. Evidence for the efficacy of these drugs in the treatment of CU is often limited, but they are cheap and relatively safe, and they could be tried before considering more expensive and/or toxic agents.

Dapsone

Dapsone has been found to be effective in different sorts of CU/angioedema, including spontaneous CU at the dosage of 25 to 50 mg per day.[48,49] In a randomized open study the addition of dapsone to desloratadine did not reduce urticaria activity scores compared with desloratadine alone but was associated with a significantly higher rate of complete remissions.[50] Although generally well tolerated, dapsone may induce dose-related anemia and, infrequently, peripheral neuropathy, skin rash, gastrointestinal complaints, hepatotoxicity, methemoglobinemia, blood dyscrasias, and DRESS (drug reaction with eosinophilia and systemic symptoms) syndrome. Furthermore, it may induce severe hemolysis in G6PD-deficient subjects. Thus, G6PD phenotype should be checked in all patients before starting a treatment with dapsone, and the use of this drug requires a careful follow-up of the patient.

Sulfasalazine

The efficacy of sulfasalazine in CU is supported by some case reports and by a retrospective observational study.[51–54] Effective dose is up to 2 g per day and response occurs within 1 month of therapy. Side effects include nausea, vomiting, dyspepsia and anorexia, and headache, and less frequently, hematologic abnormalities, proteinuria, and hepatotoxicity.

Hydroxychloroquine

Hydroxychloroquine significantly improved the quality of life of CU patients in a randomized, blinded, placebo-controlled study, although urticaria activity scores were only marginally influenced.[55] The most relevant side effect, although very rare, is retinopathy, which is associated with a greater than 5-year use of the drug.

IMMUNOSUPPRESSIVE DRUGS
Calcineurin Inhibitors

The effectiveness of ciclosporin in antihistamine-resistant CU is supported by case reports and case series[56–58] as well as by controlled trials.[59–62] Effective doses range between 3 and 5 mg/kg/d to be given for approximately 3 to 6 months during which period blood pressure, kidney function, and liver function should be regularly monitored. After stopping the drug, complete remission may last up to 9 months in about 50% of patients, whereas other patients show a decreased number of flare-ups and a restored response to antihistamine treatment[60]; a low-dose, long-term maintenance therapy for up to 2 years has been suggested for those who show a marked propensity to relapse after discontinuation.[63]

An observational study found that tacrolimus may be effective in antihistamine-resistant CU.[64]

Other Immunosuppressive Agents

Several other immunosuppressive drugs have been used to treat severe, antihistamine-resistant CU, although most experience relies on uncontrolled studies.[65] Methotrexate at a weekly mean dosage of 15 mg seems effective and safe in most CU patients who are not responsive to conventional therapy.[66,67] Some case reports have shown the efficacy of intravenous and oral cyclophosphamide[68,69] and azathioprine[70] in antihistamine-resistant CU with positive autologous serum skin test. Recently, mycophenolate mofetil, a purine biosynthesis inhibitor, has emerged as a possible therapeutic option for CU patients who do not respond to antihistamines and/or corticosteroids,[71,72] along with another inhibitor of purine biosynthesis, mizoribine.[73]

BIOLOGICALS
Omalizumab

Omalizumab is a recombinant humanized monoclonal IgG antibody that binds free IgE, down-regulates mast cell function. and induces eosinophil apoptosis. It is currently used as add-on therapy for severe allergic asthma and has been demonstrated to be effective in patients with CU. The effectiveness of omalizumab in different subsets of antihistamine-unresponsive CU/angioedema was demonstrated in both autoimmune and nonautoimmune forms by several case reports, case series, and lately by some multicenter double-blind placebo-controlled studies as well.[74–84] A randomized, double-blind placebo-controlled trial involving 323 patients[83] demonstrated the efficacy and tolerability of subcutaneous omalizumab at the dose of 150 or 300 mg in patients aged 12 to 75 years with CU. Over 12 weeks (dosing at 4-week intervals), omalizumab efficacy was found to be dose dependent, with the greatest effects at 300 mg. In another phase III study, 336 patients with H1 antihistamine-resistant CU were randomized to receive 6 subcutaneous injections at 4-week intervals of either 300 mg of omalizumab or placebo, followed by a 16-week observation period. Omalizumab was well tolerated and reduced the signs and symptoms of CU; however, after drug discontinuation, symptoms gradually recurred over a period of about 10 weeks.[84] At the moment, it must be noted that omalizumab is not yet licensed for the treatment of urticaria in Europe or in the United States and its use is limited by the high cost.

Intravenous Immunoglobulin

The possible use of intravenous immunoglobulin has been suggested by some case reports and by an open-label trial[85–89] of CU patients with positive ASST and basophil histamine release assay who did not respond to other therapies. In the trial, 9 of 10 patients responded at a dose of 0.4 g/kg/d for 5 consecutive days and in 3 cases prolonged remission after a 3-year follow-up was observed. However, such favorable results were not observed in another study.[89] Although relatively safe (anaphylactoid reactions, aseptic meningitis, and renal failure are only rarely reported), intravenous immunoglobulins are expensive and should be considered only in patients who do not respond to other treatments.

Rituximab

Rituximab is a chimeric monoclonal antibody against the protein CD20, which is primarily found on the surface of B cells. It destroys B cells and thus reduces the production of antibodies including autoantibodies. Limited experience is available regarding rituximab use in CU; however, it was effective in 2 patients with H1 antihistamine-resistant CU,[90,91] whereas in another patient it failed to control the disease.[92]

ANTICOAGULANTS

CU patients frequently show a marked increase of plasmatic markers of thrombin generation and fibrinolysis during severe exacerbations of the disease[93–95] possibly as a consequence of tissue factor expression by activated eosinophils.[93,96] The activation of coagulation and fibrinolysis decreases until complete normalization during remission.[94,97] Whether this phenomenon (activation of coagulation/fibrinolysis) plays a pivotal role in the disease pathophysiology or acts simply as an amplification system is still to be defined. However, the fact that such an activation parallels the activity of CU may provide the rationale for the evaluation of anticoagulant and antifibrinolytic therapy in patients with CU. The effectiveness of anticoagulant therapy in some patients with refractory CU has been observed as long as a decade ago by the use of both oral anticoagulants and heparin.[98–100] Despite this increasing evidence, anticoagulant therapy cannot yet be recommended as a routine treatment for CU.

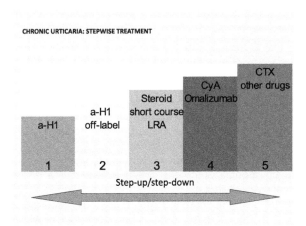

Fig. 1. Suggested stepwise therapeutic approach to CU. a-H1, antihistamine; CTX, cyclophosphamide; CyA, cyclosporin; LRA, leukotriene receptor antagonist.

OTHER TREATMENTS

Plasmapheresis has been suggested as a possible treatment in patients with severe, unremitting, and refractory CU[101]; however, such an approach is not easily available and cannot be recommended for routine use.

TREATMENT STRATEGIES IN CLINICAL PRACTICE

A stepwise treatment strategy should be adopted in patients with CU (Fig. 1), considering that in most cases stepping-up implies an increase in both direct and indirect costs and in the risk of side effects. Omalizumab has been included as a fourth-line treatment, although its high costs and limited availability represent a problem in most settings. In many cases of severe disease a step-down will be possible following a period of treatment with anti-inflammatory/immunosuppressive drugs (eg, systemic corticosteroids or ciclosporin).

REFERENCES

1. Greaves MW, Tan KT. Chronic urticaria: recent advances. Clin Rev Allergy Immunol 2007;33:134–43.
2. Gaig P, Olona M, Munoz Lejarazu D, et al. Epidemiology of urticaria in Spain. J Investig Allergol Clin Immunol 2004;14:214–20.
3. O'Donnell BF, Lawlor F, Simpson J, et al. The impact of chronic urticaria on the quality of life. Br J Dermatol 1997;136:197–201.
4. Grattan CE, Wallington TB, Warin RP, et al. A serological mediator in chronic idiopathic urticaria: a clinical, immunological and histological evaluation. Br J Dermatol 1986;114:583–90.
5. Grattan CE, Francis DM, Hide M, et al. Detection of circulating histamine releasing autoantibodies with functional properties of anti-IgE in chronic urticaria. Clin Exp Allergy 1991;21:695–704.
6. Hide M, Francis DM, Grattan CE, et al. Autoantibodies against the high affinity IgE receptor as a cause of histamine release in chronic urticaria. N Engl J Med 1993;328:1599–604.

7. Tedeschi A, Asero R, Lorini M, et al. Plasma levels of matrix metalloproteinase-9 in chronic urticaria patients correlate with disease severity and C-reactive protein but not with circulating histamine-releasing factors. Clin Exp Allergy 2010; 40:875–81.

8. Asero R, Tedeschi A, Riboldi P, et al. Plasma of patients with chronic urticaria shows signs of thrombin generation, and its intradermal injection causes wheal-and-flare reactions much more frequently than autologous serum. J Allergy Clin Immunol 2006;117:1113–7.

9. Cugno M, Marzano AV, Asero R, et al. Activation of blood coagulation in chronic urticaria: pathophysiological and clinical implications. Intern Emerg Med 2010; 5:97–101.

10. Zuberbier T, Bindslev-Jensen C, Canonica GW, et al. EAACI/GA2LEN guideline: management of urticaria. Allergy 2006;61:321–31.

11. Powell RJ, Du Toit GL, Siddique N, et al, British Society for Allergy and Clinical Immunology (BSACI). BSACI guidelines for the management of chronic urticaria and angio-oedema. Clin Exp Allergy 2007;37:631–50.

12. Tedeschi A, Girolomoni G, Asero R, AAITO Committee for Chronic Urticaria and Pruritus Guidelines. AAITO Position paper. Chronic urticaria: diagnostic workup and treatment. Eur Ann Allergy Clin Immunol 2007;39:225–31.

13. Zuberbier T, Asero R, Bindslev-Jensen C, et al, Dermatology Section of the European Academy of Allergology and Clinical Immunology, Global Allergy and Asthma European Network, European Dermatology Forum, World Allergy Organization. EAACI/GA2LEN/EDF/WAO guideline: management of urticaria. Allergy 2009;64:1427–43.

14. Sánchez-Borges M, Asero R, Ansotegui IJ, et al, WAO Scientific and Clinical Issues Council. Diagnosis and treatment of urticaria and angioedema: a worldwide perspective. World Allergy Organ J 2012;5(11):125–47.

15. Zuberbier T, Aberer W, Asero R, et al. The EAACI/GA2LEN/EDF/AAAAI/WAO/ Guideline for the definition, classification, diagnosis and management of Urticaria. The 2013 revision and update. Allergy, in press.

16. Grant JA, Danielson L, Rihoux JP, et al. A double-blind, single-dose, crossover comparison of cetirizine, ebastine, epinastine, fexofenadine, terfenadine, and loratadine versus placebo: suppression of histamine-induced wheal and flare response for 24 h in healthy male subjects. Allergy 1999;54:700–7.

17. Grant JA, Riethuisen JM, Moulaert B, et al. A double-blind, randomized, single-dose, crossover comparison of levocetirizine with ebastine, fexofenadine, loratadine, mizolastine, and placebo: suppression of histamine-induced wheal-and-flare response during 24 hours in healthy male subjects. Ann Allergy Asthma Immunol 2002;88:190–7.

18. Frossard N, Strolin-Benedetti M, Purohit A, et al. Inhibition of allergen-induced wheal and flare reactions by levocetirizine and desloratadine. Br J Clin Pharmacol 2008;65:172–9.

19. Handa S, Dogra S, Kumar B. Comparative efficacy of cetirizine and fexofenadine in the treatment of chronic idiopathic urticaria. J Dermatolog Treat 2004; 15:55–7.

20. Potter PC, Kapp A, Maurer M, et al. Comparison of the efficacy of levocetirizine 5 mg and desloratadine 5 mg in chronic idiopathic urticaria patients. Allergy 2009;64:596–604.

21. Clough GF, Boutsiouki P, Church MK. Comparison of the effects of levocetirizine and loratadine on histamine-induced wheal, flare, and itch in human skin. Allergy 2001;56:985–8.

22. Popov TA, Dumitrascu D, Bachvarova A, et al. A comparison of levocetirizine and desloratadine in the histamine-induced wheal and flare response in human skin in vivo. Inflamm Res 2006;55:241–4.
23. Zuberbier T, Oanta A, Bogacka E, et al, Bilastine International Working Group. Comparison of the efficacy and safety of bilastine 20 mg vs levocetirizine 5 mg for the treatment of chronic idiopathic urticaria: a multi-centre, double-blind, randomized, placebo-controlled study. Allergy 2010;65:516–28.
24. Maiti R, Jaida J, Raghavendra BN, et al. Rupatadine and levocetirizine in chronic idiopathic urticaria: a comparative study of efficacy and safety. J Drugs Dermatol 2011;10:1444–50.
25. Hindmarch I, Johnson S, Meadows R, et al. The acute and sub-chronic effects of levocetirizine, cetirizine, lotatadine, promethazine and placebo on cognitive function, psychomotor performance, and wheal and flare. Curr Med Res Opin 2001;17:241–55.
26. Curran MP, Scott LJ, Perry CM. Cetirizine: a review of its use in allergic disorders. Drugs 2004;15:55–7.
27. Grant JA, Bernstein DI, Buckley CE, et al. Double-blind comparison of terfenadine, chlorpheniramine, and placebo in the treatment of chronic idiopathic urticaria. J Allergy Clin Immunol 1998;81:574–9.
28. Monroe EW. Relative efficacy and safety of loratadine, hydroxyzine, and placebo in chronic idiopathic urticaria. Clin Ther 1992;14:17–21.
29. Breneman DL. Cetirizine versus hydroxyzine and placebo in chronic idiopathic urticaria. Ann Pharmacother 1996;30:1075–9.
30. Shamsi Z, Hindmarch I. Sedation and antihistamines: a review of inter-drug differences using proportional impairment ratios. Hum Psychopharmacol 2000; 15(S1):S3–30.
31. Siebenhaar F, Degener F, Zuberbier T, et al. High-dose desloratadine decreases wheal volume and improves cold provocation thresholds compared with standard-dose treatment in patients with acquired cold urticaria: a randomized, placebo-controlled, crossover study. J Allergy Clin Immunol 2009; 123:672–9.
32. Kameyoshi Y, Tanaka T, Mihara S, et al. Increasing the dose of cetirizine may lead to better control of chronic idiopathic urticaria: an open study of 21 patients. Br J Dermatol 2007;157:803–4.
33. Staevska M, Popov TA, Kralimarkova T, et al. The effectiveness of levocetirizine and desloratadine in up to 4 times conventional doses in difficult-to-treat urticaria. J Allergy Clin Immunol 2010;125:676–82.
34. Asero R. Chronic unremitting urticaria: is the use of antihistamines above the licensed dose effective? A preliminary study of cetirizine at licensed and above-licensed doses. Clin Exp Dermatol 2007;32:34–8.
35. Monroe EW, Cohen SH, Kalbfleisch J, et al. Combined H1 and H2 antihistamine therapy in chronic urticaria. Arch Dermatol 1981;117:404–7.
36. Bleehen SS, Thomas SE, Greaves MW, et al. Cimetidine and chlorpheniramine in the treatment of chronic idiopathic urticaria: a multi-centre randomized double-blind study. Br J Dermatol 1987;117:81–8.
37. Paul E, Bodeker RH. Treatment of chronic urticaria with terfenadine and ranitidine. A randomized double-blind study in 45 patients. Eur J Clin Pharmacol 1986;31:277–80.
38. Sharpe GR, Shuster R. In dermographic urticaria H2 receptor antagonists have a small but therapeutically irrelevant additional effect compared with H1 antagonists alone. Br J Dermatol 1993;129:575–9.

39. Asero R, Tedeschi A. Usefulness of a short course of oral prednisone in antihistamine-resistant chronic urticaria: a retrospective analysis. J Investig Allergol Clin Immunol 2010;20:386–90.
40. Tedeschi A, Suli C, Lorini M, et al. Successful treatment of chronic urticaria. Allergy 2000;55:1097–8.
41. Asero R, Tedeschi A, Lorini M. Leukotriene receptor antagonists in chronic urticaria. Allergy 2001;56:456–7.
42. Bagenstose SE, Levin L, Bernstein JA. The addition of zafirlukast to cetirizine improves the treatment of chronic urticaria in patients with positive autologous serum skin test results. J Allergy Clin Immunol 2004;113:134–40.
43. Di Lorenzo G, Pacor ML, Mansueto P, et al. Randomized placebo-controlled trial comparing desloratadine and montelukast in monotherapy and desloratadine plus montelukast in combined therapy for chronic idiopathic urticaria. J Allergy Clin Immunol 2004;114:619–25.
44. Nettis E, Colanardi MC, Paradiso MT, et al. Desloratadine in combination with montelukast in the treatment of chronic urticaria: a randomized, double-blind, placebo-controlled study. Clin Exp Allergy 2004;34:1401–7.
45. Erbagci Z. The leukotriene receptor antagonist montelukast in the treatment of chronic idiopathic urticaria: a single-blind, placebo-controlled, crossover clinical study. J Allergy Clin Immunol 2002;110:484–8.
46. Pacor ML, Di Lorenzo G, Corrocher R. Efficacy of leukotriene receptor antagonist in chronic urticaria. A double-blind, placebo-controlled comparison of treatment with montelukast and cetirizine in patients with chronic urticaria with intolerance to food additive and/or acetylsalicylic acid. Clin Exp Allergy 2001; 31:1607–14.
47. Reimers A, Pichler C, Helbling A, et al. Zafirlukast has no beneficial effects in the treatment of chronic urticaria. Clin Exp Allergy 2002;32:1763–8.
48. Boehm I, Bauer R, Bieber T. Urticaria treated with dapsone. Allergy 1999;54: 765–6.
49. Cassano N, D'Argento V, Filotico R, et al. Low-dose dapsone in chronic idiopathic urticaria: preliminary results of an open study. Acta Derm Venereol 2005;85:254–5.
50. Engin B, Ozdemir M. Prospective randomized non-blinded clinical trial on the use of dapsone plus antihistamine vs. antihistamine in patients with chronic idiopathic urticaria. J Eur Acad Dermatol Venereol 2008;22:481–6.
51. Jaffer AM. Sulfasalazine in the treatment of corticosteroid-dependent chronic idiopathic urticaria. J Allergy Clin Immunol 1991;88:964–5.
52. Engler RJ, Squire E, Benson P. Chronic sulfasalazine therapy in the treatment of delayed pressure urticaria and angioedema. Ann Allergy Asthma Immunol 1995;74:155–9.
53. Hartmann K, Hani N, Hinrichs R, et al. Successful sulfasalazine treatment of severe chronic idiopathic urticaria associated with pressure urticaria. Acta Derm Venereol 2001;81:71.
54. McGirt LY, Vasagar K, Gober LM, et al. Successful treatment of recalcitrant chronic idiopathic urticaria with sulfasalazine. Arch Dermatol 2006;142:1337–42.
55. Reeves GE, Boyle MJ, Bonfield J, et al. Impact of hydroxychloroquine therapy on chronic urticaria: chronic autoimmune urticaria study and evaluation. Intern Med J 2004;34:182–6.
56. Fradin MS, Ellis CN, Goldfarb MT, et al. Oral cyclosporine for severe chronic idiopathic urticaria and angioedema. J Am Acad Dermatol 1991;25(6 Pt 1): 1065–7.

57. Toubi E, Blant A, Kessel A, et al. Low-dose cyclosporin A in the treatment of severe chronic idiopathic urticaria. Allergy 1997;52:312–6.
58. Serhat Inaloz H, Ozturk S, Akcali C, et al. Low-dose and short-term cyclosporine treatment in patients with chronic idiopathic urticaria: a clinical and immunological evaluation. J Dermatol 2008;35:276–82.
59. Grattan CE, O'Donnell BF, Francis DM, et al. Randomized double-blind study of cyclosporin in chronic 'idiopathic' urticaria. Br J Dermatol 2000;143: 365–72.
60. Di Gioacchino M, Di Stefano F, Cavallucci E, et al. Treatment of chronic idiopathic urticaria and positive autologous serum skin test with cyclosporine: clinical and immunological evaluation. Allergy Asthma Proc 2003;24:285–90.
61. Baskan EB, Tunali S, Turker T, et al. Comparison of short- and long-term cyclosporine A therapy in chronic idiopathic urticaria. J Dermatolog Treat 2004;15: 164–8.
62. Vena GA, Cassano N, Colombo D, et al, Neo-I-30 Study Group. Cyclosporine in chronic idiopathic urticaria: a double-blind, randomized, placebo-controlled trial. J Am Acad Dermatol 2006;55:705–9.
63. Kessel A, Toubi E. Cyclosporine-A in severe chronic urticaria: the option for long-term therapy. Allergy 2010;65:1478–82.
64. Kessel A, Bamberger E, Toubi E. Tacrolimus in the treatment of severe chronic idiopathic urticaria: an open-label prospective study. J Am Acad Dermatol 2005; 52:145–8.
65. Tedeschi A, Airaghi L, Lorini M, et al. Chronic urticaria: a role for newer immunomodulatory drugs? Am J Clin Dermatol 2003;4:297–305.
66. Perez A, Woods A, Grattan CE. Methotrexate: a useful steroid-sparing agent in recalcitrant chronic urticaria. Br J Dermatol 2010;162:191–4.
67. Sagi L, Solomon M, Baum S, et al. Evidence for methotrexate as a useful treatment for steroid-dependent chronic urticaria. Acta Derm Venereol 2011;91: 303–6.
68. Bernstein JA, Garramone SM, Lower EG. Successful treatment of autoimmune chronic idiopathic urticaria with intravenous cyclophosphamide. Ann Allergy Asthma Immunol 2002;89:212–4.
69. Asero R. Oral cyclophosphamide in a case of cyclosporin and steroid-resistant chronic urticaria showing autoreactivity on autologous serum skin testing. Clin Exp Dermatol 2005;30:582–3.
70. Tedeschi A. Paradoxical exacerbation of chronic urticaria by H1-antihistamines and montelukast. Eur Ann Allergy Clin Immunol 2009;41:187–9.
71. Shahar E, Bergman R, Guttman-Yassky E, et al. Treatment of severe chronic idiopathic urticaria with oral mycophenolate mofetil in patients not responding to antihistamines and/or corticosteroids. Int J Dermatol 2006;45:1224–7.
72. Zimmerman AB, Berger EM, Elmariah SB, et al. The use of mycophenolate mofetil for the treatment of autoimmune and chronic idiopathic urticaria: Experience in 19 patients. J Am Acad Dermatol 2012;66:767–70.
73. Hashimoto T, Kawakami T, Ishii N, et al. Mizoribine treatment for antihistamine-resistant chronic autoimmune urticaria. Dermatol Ther 2012;25:379–81.
74. Boyce JA. Successful treatment of cold-induced urticaria/anaphylaxis with anti-IgE. J Allergy Clin Immunol 2006;117:1415–8.
75. Spector SL, Tan RA. Effect of omalizumab on patients with chronic urticaria. Ann Allergy Asthma Immunol 2007;99:190–3.
76. Kaplan AP, Joseph K, Maykut RJ, et al. Treatment of chronic autoimmune urticaria with omalizumab. J Allergy Clin Immunol 2008;122:569–73.

77. Dreyfus DH. Observations on the mechanism of omalizumab as a steroid-spating agent in autoimmune or chronic idiopathic urticaria and angioedema. Ann Allergy Asthma Immunol 2008;100:624–5.
78. Godse KV. Omalizumab in severe chronic urticaria. Indian J Dermatol Venereol Leprol 2008;74:157–8.
79. Vestergaard C, Deleuran M. Two cases of severe refractory chronic idiopathic urticaria treated with omalizumab. Acta Derm Venereol 2010;90:443–4.
80. Ferrer M, Gamboa P, Sanz ML, et al. Omalizumab is effective in nonautoimmune urticaria. J Allergy Clin Immunol 2011;127:1300–2.
81. Maurer M, Altrichter S, Bieber T, et al. Efficacy and safety of omalizumab in patients with chronic urticaria who exhibit IgE against thyroperoxidase. J Allergy Clin Immunol 2011;128:202–9.
82. Saini S, Rosen KE, Hsieh HJ, et al. A randomized, placebo-controlled, dose-ranging study of single-dose omalizumab in patients with H1-antihistamine-refractory chronic idiopathic urticaria. J Allergy Clin Immunol 2011;128:567–73.
83. Maurer M, Rosén K, Hsieh HJ, et al. Omalizumab for the treatment of chronic idiopathic or spontaneous urticaria. N Engl J Med 2013;368:924–35.
84. Kaplan A, Ledford D, Ashby M, et al. Omalizumab in chronic idiopathic/spontaneous urticaria patients symptomatic despite standard combination therapy. J Allergy Clin Immunol 2013;132:101–9.
85. O'Donnell BF, Barr RM, Kobza Black A, et al. Intravenous immunoglobulin in autoimmune chronic urticaria. Br J Dermatol 1998;138:101–6.
86. Pereira C, Tavares B, Carrapatoso I, et al. Low-dose intravenous gammaglobulin in the treatment of severe autoimmune urticaria. Eur Ann Allergy Clin Immunol 2007;39:237–42.
87. Klote MM, Nelson MR, Engler RJ. Autoimmune urticaria response to high-dose intravenous immunoglobulin. Ann Allergy Asthma Immunol 2005;94:307–8.
88. Wetter DA, Davis MD, Yiannias JA, et al. Effectiveness of intravenous immunoglobulin therapy for skin disease other than toxic epidermal necrolysis: a retrospective review of Mayo Clinic experience. Mayo Clin Proc 2005;80:41–7.
89. Asero R. Are IVIG for chronic unremitting urticaria effective? Allergy 2000;55:1099–100.
90. Arkwright PD. Anti-CD20 or anti-IgE therapy for severe chronic autoimmune urticaria. J Allergy Clin Immunol 2009;123:510–1.
91. Chakravarty SD, Yee AF, Paget SA. Rituximab successfully treats refractory chronic autoimmune urticaria caused by IgE receptor autoantibodies. J Allergy Clin Immunol 2011;128:1354–5.
92. Mallipeddi R, Grattan CE. Lack of response of severe steroid-dependent chronic urticaria to rituximab. Clin Exp Dermatol 2007;32:333–4.
93. Asero R, Tedeschi A, Coppola R, et al. Activation of the tissue factor pathway of blood coagulation in patients with chronic urticaria. J Allergy Clin Immunol 2007;119:705–10.
94. Asero R, Tedeschi A, Riboldi P, et al. Severe chronic urticaria is associated with elevated plasma levels of D-dimer. Allergy 2008;63:176–80.
95. Takeda T, Sakurai Y, Takahagi S, et al. Increase of coagulation potential in chronic spontaneous urticaria. Allergy 2011;66:428–33.
96. Cugno M, Marzano AV, Tedeschi A, et al. Expression of tissue factor by eosinophils in patients with chronic urticaria. Int Arch Allergy Immunol 2009;148:170–4.
97. Khalaf AT, Liu XM, Sheng WX, et al. Efficacy and safety of desloratadine combined with dipyridamole in the treatment of chronic urticaria. J Eur Acad Dermatol Venereol 2008;22:487–92.

98. Parslew R, Pryce D, Ashworth J, et al. Warfarin treatment of chronic idiopathic urticaria and angio-oedema. Clin Exp Allergy 2000;30:1161–5.
99. Chua SL, Gibbs S. Chronic urticaria responding to subcutaneous heparin sodium. Br J Dermatol 2005;153:216–7.
100. Asero R, Tedeschi A, Cugno M. Heparin and tranexamic acid therapy may be effective in treatment-resistant chronic urticaria with elevated D-dimer: a pilot study. Int Arch Allergy Immunol 2010;152:384–9.
101. Grattan CE, Francis DM, Slater NG, et al. Plasmapheresis for severe, unremitting, chronic urticaria. Lancet 1992;339:1078–80.

Pediatric Urticaria

Teresa Tsakok, BM, BCh, MA, MRCP[a], George Du Toit, FRCPCH[b],
Carsten Flohr, BM, BCh, MA, MSc, MRCPCH, PhD[c,d,*]

KEYWORDS

- Urticaria • Pediatric urticaria • Quality of life • Evidence-based approach

KEY POINTS

- Although acute urticaria is common, chronic urticaria is a rare but troubling disorder, for which a stepwise approach is required toward investigations and treatment.
- Unique and varied associations with autoimmune conditions, such as thyroid and celiac disease, are described in a subset of patients, suggesting an underlying autoimmune predisposition.
- Unlike in adults, there is no good evidence that the presence of autoantibodies translates into a more severe and prolonged disease course, but this has been examined in only a few small studies.
- Whatever the cause, families need reassurance that chronic urticaria is a nonallergic condition, with an excellent overall prognosis.
- Symptoms generally respond well to high-dose antihistamine regimens (up to 4 times the standard licensed dose if required), and airway compromise is not a feature, even when angioedema is pronounced.
- More research, including head-to-head drug trials to establish relative efficacy and safety, is needed to gain a deeper understanding of this poorly understood condition in children.

Disclosures: None.
Funding: C. Flohr holds a UK National Institute of Health Research Clinician Scientist Award. The views expressed in this publication are those of the authors and not necessarily those of the National Health Service, the UK National Institute for Health Research, or the UK Department of Health.
[a] Guy's and St Thomas' Hospital NHS Foundation Trust, King's College London, London SE1 7EH, UK; [b] Department of Children's Allergies, Guy's and St Thomas' Hospital NHS Foundation Trust, King's College London, London SE1 7EH, UK; [c] Department of Paediatric Dermatology, St John's Institute of Dermatology, Guy's and St Thomas' Hospitals NHS Foundation Trust, King's College London, London SE1 7EH, UK; [d] Department of Children's Allergies, St John's Institute of Dermatology, Guy's and St Thomas' Hospitals NHS Foundation Trust, King's College London, London SE1 7EH, UK
* Corresponding author. Departments of Paediatric Dermatology and Children's Allergies, St John's Institute of Dermatology, Guy's and St Thomas' Hospitals NHS Foundation Trust, King's College London, London SE1 7EH, UK.
E-mail address: carsten.flohr@kcl.ac.uk

Immunol Allergy Clin N Am 34 (2014) 117–139
http://dx.doi.org/10.1016/j.iac.2013.09.008
0889-8561/14/$ – see front matter © 2014 Elsevier Inc. All rights reserved.
immunology.theclinics.com

INTRODUCTION

Urticaria is a skin condition identified by itchy red wheals that are characteristically transient, with well-defined borders and a central pallor.[1] In up to 50% of cases, sudden swelling of the lower dermis and subcutaneous tissues, known as angioedema, may also occur.[1] Whether urticaria presents with wheals, angioedema, or both, several specific clinical patterns are believed to typify this disease in both children and adults.[2] However, efficient diagnosis and management are hampered by confusion surrounding the numerous classification systems for urticaria, which has resulted in extensive heterogeneity among studies. Furthermore, most data in this field pertain to adults, with a tiny pediatric evidence base that is often of low quality or tends to extrapolate data from studies focusing on older age groups or other clinical conditions, such as allergic rhinitis. Yet, although urticaria is only rarely life-threatening, its impact on quality of life in children should not be overlooked, with 1 study estimating that the negative impact of urticaria is comparable with other chronic diseases of childhood, such as diabetes and epilepsy.[3] A systematic search of online databases, including Medline, was performed to inform this review (search strategy available from the authors on request). This review equips the clinician with an evidence-based approach to all aspects of pediatric urticaria, hinging on an illustrative case and including a summary table of studies (**Table 1**) pertaining to disease management in children.

PATHOGENESIS

Mast cell and basophil degranulation is the fundamental event causing wheal formation. In the classic type 1 immediate hypersensitivity reaction, allergen-specific IgE is produced after initial contact with a particular allergen. On subsequent contact, the allergen, bound to specific IgE, then cross-links high-affinity IgE receptors (FceR1) on the surface of mast cells. This event triggers the mast cells to release histamine and vasoactive mediators, causing vasodilatation, increased blood flow, and enhanced vascular permeability. The resulting erythema, fluid extravasation, and swelling of the superficial dermis together give rise to the urticarial wheal. However, it is also possible for other stimuli such as anti-IgE and anti-FceR1 IgG antibodies to signal via the high-affinity IgE receptors on mast cells[4]; wheals generated in this way are classified as autoimmune urticaria. Nonimmunologic stimuli such as opiates, neuropeptides, and stem cell factor, as well as physical triggers, may also cause wheals by binding to receptors independent of the FceR1 altogether.[5]

CLASSIFICATION

There are numerous overlapping and evolving classification systems for urticaria in both children and adults. Acute urticaria by definition lasts up to 6 weeks; chronic urticaria more than 6 weeks, although the validity of this arbitrary cutoff has been questioned.[6] The term idiopathic was previously widely used in the context of chronic urticaria, until studies indicated that up to half of adult sufferers harbored an autoimmune mechanism. This finding led to reclassification of a large subset of chronic idiopathic urticaria as chronic autoimmune urticaria.[7] More recently, the term chronic spontaneous urticaria has been proposed as a preferable alternative to chronic idiopathic urticaria; this places greater emphasis on clinical course and less on cause, which is often unknown and thus arguably less informative.[2] Nevertheless, when urticaria is triggered by specific stimuli, the term inducible or physical urticaria has been used, comprising a heterogeneous group that includes dermographic, aquagenic,

Table 1
Articles pertaining to urticaria management in children (based on a systematic online literature search)

Reference Country	Article Type	Age (y)	No. of Participants	Focus of Article	Urticaria Type	Key Findings/ Recommendations
Augustin & Ehrle,[77] 2009 Germany	Observational postmarketing surveillance study	2–101	9246	Safety and efficacy of desloratadine in chronic idiopathic urticaria	Chronic idiopathic	Itching, number of wheals, and size of the largest wheal decreased significantly from baseline with desloratadine therapy ($P<.0001$). Improvements in sleep and daily activities were reported by 67% and 71% of patients, respectively ($P<.0001$). In patients who had previously received therapy with cetirizine, loratadine, or fexofenadine alone, patients rated the onset of efficacy of desloratadine as faster in 55.5%, 54.7% and 57.6% of cases, respectively. Incidence of adverse events was low (0.5% of patients), with no serious adverse events

(continued on next page)

Table 1
(continued)

Reference Country	Article Type	Age (y)	No. of Participants	Focus of Article	Urticaria Type	Key Findings/ Recommendations
Beno et al,[78] 2007 United States	Self-administered cross-sectional survey	n/a	1137 physicians (emergency, pediatric emergency, pediatric)	A survey of emergency department management of acute urticaria in children	Acute	First-generation H_1 antagonists alone were the most common therapy used on initial presentation of acute urticaria, followed by corticosteroids, H_2 antagonists, and second-generation H_1 antagonists (used by only 7.8%, despite their recommendation as first-line therapy). Only 14.2% of physicians overall were familiar with guideline recommendations
Bloom et al,[67] 2004 United States	2 parallel RCTs	2–5 6–12	111 120	Safety of desloratadine syrup in children with urticaria or allergic rhinitis	Chronic idiopathic	No serious adverse events; desloratadine syrup is safe for use in children
Boyce,[79] 2006 United States	Case report	12	1	Successful treatment of cold urticaria/anaphylaxis with omalizumab (monoclonal IgE antibody)	Cold	This patient with cold urticaria experienced progressively severe symptoms, resistant to antihistamines and antileukotriene therapy. She was atopic and had moderate persistent asthma. A trial of anti-IgE resulted in complete resolution of her urticaria

Study	Study design	Age	No.	Purpose	Type	Findings
Doshi & Weinberger,[73] 2009 United States	Retrospective case series	9–16	7	Efficacy and safety of cyclosporine in chronic childhood urticaria, unresponsive to conventional therapies	Chronic idiopathic	All had cessation of symptoms. This occurred after 1–4 wk for 6 of the 7 children and after 8 wk for 1. Whereas some experienced relapses, all were eventually off medications and symptom-free. None experienced adverse effects
Frances et al,[80] 2004 Argentina	Case report	Not stated	1	Successful treatment of aquagenic urticaria with hydroxyzine	Aquagenic	Treatment with hydroxyzine (25 mg daily) was successful after a month follow-up in preventing wheals and erythema. However, mild pruritus was still present after contact with water
Giuliodori et al,[81] 2009 Italy	Case report	12	1	Use of cyclosporine in chronic autoimmune urticaria unresponsive to antihistamines, antileukotrienes, and corticosteroids	Chronic autoimmune	Cyclosporine was started at 4 mg/kg/d for 2 mo, decreasing by 0.3 mg/kg/d every 2 mo for 1 y. Renal function was monitored monthly. This treatment induced and maintained remission by the 14th mo of consecutive therapy

(continued on next page)

Table 1
(continued)

Reference Country	Article Type	Age (y)	No. of Participants	Focus of Article	Urticaria Type	Key Findings/ Recommendations
Kaplan et al,[82] 2005 United States	Multicenter randomized placebo-controlled double-blind study	≥12	255	Efficacy and safety of once-daily dosing of fexofenadine hydrochloride (180 mg) on chronic idiopathic urticaria	Chronic	Patients administered with fexofenadine (n = 163) experienced significantly greater improvements in mean number of wheals and pruritus severity scores compared with the placebo group (n = 92) (P<.001 for both). There were no significant differences in the frequency of treatment-emergent adverse events between the 2 treatment groups
McGee et al,[83] 2012 United States	Case report	13	1	Review of current treatments for aquagenic urticaria	Aquagenic	Application of topical petrolatum as a protective barrier against water, resulted in complete remission. Other treatments include antihistamines, anticholinergics, and ultraviolet therapy

Study	Design	Age	N	Objective	Type	Findings
Saini et al,[76] 2011 United States	Phase 2 randomized, placebo-controlled, double-blind, dose-ranging study	12–75	90	Efficacy and safety of omalizumab in patients with chronic idiopathic urticaria who remained symptomatic (urticaria activity score over 7 d >12) despite H_1-antihistamine therapy	Chronic	Both the 300-mg omalizumab group (219.9 vs 26.9, $P<.001$) and the 600-mg omalizumab group (214.6 vs 26.9, $P = .047$) showed greater improvement vs the placebo group in urticaria activity scores. Omalizumab was well tolerated, and the incidence of adverse events was similar across treatment groups
Salmun et al,[84] 2000 United States	Single-dose bioavailability study / Multiple-dose tolerability study (placebo-controlled)	2–5	18 / 121	Pharmacokinetics, electrocardiographic effects, and tolerability of loratadine syrup in children with urticaria or allergic rhinitis	Chronic idiopathic	5 mg loratadine syrup provided exposure similar to that seen in adults with 10 mg. Loratadine was well tolerated in both single and multiple doses. Electrocardiographic parameters were not altered with loratadine compared with placebo
Sanada et al,[74] 2005 Japan	Case series	4–72	25	Effectiveness of montelukast for antihistamine-resistant urticaria	Chronic idiopathic	Urticaria improved in the 1 pediatric patient aged 4 y

(continued on next page)

Table 1
(continued)

Reference Country	Article Type	Age (y)	No. of Participants	Focus of Article	Urticaria Type	Key Findings/ Recommendations
Simons (EPAAC),[64] 2001 Canada	RCT	1–2	817	Effect of long-term treatment with cetirizine in prevention of urticaria in children with eczema	Acute	Acute urticaria occurred in 16.2% of placebo-treated children compared with 5.8% of children treated with cetirizine ($P<.001$). The protective effect of cetirizine disappeared when treatment was stopped. Overall, urticaria episodes were most commonly associated with intercurrent infection or with food ingestion or direct skin contact

Study	Type	Age	N	Aim	Subtype	Results
Simons (EPAAC),[65,66] 2007 Canada	RCT	1–2	510	Effect of long-term treatment with levocetirizine on urticaria in young atopic children		27.5% (70/255) of those taking levocetirizine and 41.6% (106/255) of those taking placebo experienced urticaria ($P<.001$). The mean $\pm$ standard error of the mean number of urticaria episodes was 0.71 ± 0.11 in those receiving levocetirizine and 1.71 ± 0.25 in those receiving placebo ($P<.001$). The mean $\pm$ standard error of the mean duration of urticaria episodes was 4.43 ± 1.57 d in those receiving levocetirizine and 5.36 ± 1.27 d in those receiving placebo ($P<.001$). These results strengthen the evidence base for the use of relatively nonsedating, second-generation H_1-antihistamines in the pediatric population
Visitsunthorn et al,[85] 1995 Thailand	Double-blind crossover study with >5 y follow-up	4–9	6	Comparison of effectiveness of cyproheptadine and ketotifen on clinical symptoms of cold urticaria and ice cube scores	Cold	Efficacy of cyproheptadine and ketotifen was not significantly different ($P>.05$). Both showed good results in the treatment of cold urticaria, with mild side effects. During follow-up, 5 cases showed complete recovery

cold, and cholinergic urticaria. Diseases presenting with urticarial eruptions, such as urticarial vasculitis, and systemic conditions such as autoinflammatory diseases (eg, Schnitzler syndrome) or systemic mastocytosis, are not included in the 2006 European Academy of Allergy and Clinical Immunology (EAACI)/GA^{2}LEN/European Dermatology Forum (EDF)/World Allergy Organization (WAO) classification.[1] However, they should be considered as part of the differential diagnosis on encountering a patient with urticarial symptoms in the clinic.

EPIDEMIOLOGY

Urticaria is common, affecting up to 25% of the population during their lifetime. Most of these episodes are acute, and there is a particular paucity of population-based studies in the pediatric setting. One noninterventional birth cohort study reported that 5.4% of 404 6-year-old children had at least 1 episode of urticaria during the previous year.[8] In line with this finding, Henz and Zuberbier[9] gave a range of 2.1% to 6.7% for all forms of childhood urticaria. Regarding specific urticaria subtypes, Kaplan[7] estimated that 0.1% to 3% of children are diagnosed with chronic urticaria. Another study found that 68% of 66 children with urticaria had presented to the emergency department within the previous year, of whom 18% were described as having chronic urticaria.[10] Although there are fewer data available regarding acute childhood urticaria, 1 notable study[11] reported no difference in the epidemiologic patterns of acute urticaria between northern and southern Europe, despite marked differences in climate and geography.

CLINICAL FEATURES, COURSE, AND PROGNOSIS

As mentioned earlier, the cardinal feature of urticaria is the repeated occurrence of wheals, accompanied by erythema and itching. These wheals can be round or irregular, of varying size, and located at any skin site. However, their defining characteristic is that they are migratory and transient (lasting <24 hours), resolving with no residual skin lesion. When angioedema coexists, it also resolves within 24 hours and is less consistently associated with itching than the skin wheals. Compared with atopic dermatitis (AD), the pattern of itching may seem different. Whereas children with AD often damage the skin by scratching with their nails, children with urticaria more frequently rub firmly with the palm, hence seldom damaging the skin.

There has been some debate about the proportion of children experiencing wheals, angioedema, or both. A prospective study of 94 Thai children with chronic urticaria reported that 51% had wheals with concomitant angioedema,[12] whereas Volonakis and colleagues[13] found that most children (78.4%) had wheals alone, 6.6% had angioedema alone, and only 15% had both. This finding was closer to Liu and colleagues'[14] findings in a large series of 1120 children with an initial episode of acute urticaria, of whom just 8.8% had both. This subset appeared to experience a more severe disease course than those with wheals alone.

The prognosis of childhood urticaria has also been a focus of interest, with most studies focusing on chronic urticaria, because acute urticaria is transient and resolves without sequelae in most cases. In Liu and colleagues' report,[14] only 5.4% of children with acute urticaria continued to experience symptoms after 15 days. The prognosis for chronic urticaria is likewise believed to be favorable, with Sahiner and colleagues[15] reporting complete resolution of symptoms in 50% of children at 5-year follow-up. The suggestion that female gender and age younger than 10 years worsened prognosis was not borne out by multivariate analysis. Du Toit's[16] series of 80 children with chronic urticaria found remission in 36% within 3 years, but was no more successful at identifying predictors of disease course. Khakoo and colleagues'[17] retrospective study of 53 children with physical urticaria may indicate a worse prognosis in this subset of patients compared with those with chronic spontaneous urticaria, with a remission rate of only 38.4% within 5 years. Univariate analysis suggested that a history of other allergies and increased frequency of urticaria episodes were associated with a greater risk of nonremission. Unlike in adults, there does not seem to be a difference between chronic idiopathic and autoimmune urticaria with regard to disease severity, medication requirement, or disease remission in children.[12,18]

CAUSE

Parents are often concerned that allergies, for instance to foods, are to blame for their child's urticaria. However, identifying a cause can prove elusive, and there are widespread inconsistencies in how possible causes are investigated, confirmed, and reported. This situation likely accounts for the wide range (16%–83%) reported in the literature for successful identification of a cause in children with either acute or chronic urticaria.[13,15,19–24]

Infections

Studies of children with both acute and chronic urticaria have indicated that infection is a major cause. In Liu and colleagues'[25] retrospective analysis of 953 children presenting to the emergency department with acute urticaria, infections were the leading cause in infants (56.5%), although prevalence of infections decreased as age increased (51.2% in pre–school-aged children, 42.1% in school-aged children, and 17.1% in adolescents). Another study[26] delved deeper into possible sources of infection, reporting that of 44 children presenting with acute urticaria associated with clinical infection or a febrile illness, 40 had respiratory tract symptoms and only 4 had gastrointestinal symptoms. Viral screens were suggestive of viral cause in 79.5% patients. However, 47.7% patients had received antibiotics before developing the urticaria, making it difficult to attribute symptoms to infection alone. Potential causality was perhaps better addressed in Konstaninou and colleagues'[11] epidemiologic study, showing that seasonal variations in respiratory viral infections coincided with variations in acute urticaria.

Bacterial infections have also been implicated in acute childhood urticaria, with Schuller and Elvey's 1980 study suggesting that β-hemolytic streptococci had a role in 13 of 32 cases.[27] *Mycoplasma pneumoniae* has been reported in both case series[28] and larger observational studies.[26] More recently, Sackesen and colleagues[29] recommended that urinalysis and cultures should be performed on children presenting with urticaria. These investigators detected urinary tract infection in 6 children with acute urticaria, of 54 participating children with various forms of urticaria. Five of the 6 children were asymptomatic from their urinary tract infection, and none was taking antibiotics at the time of diagnosis. Treatment of the infection resulted in clearance of urticaria.

The contribution of infection to chronic childhood urticaria is less clear. Sackesen and colleagues'[29] study reported infection in 6 of 17 (35%) participants suffering from this form of the condition, whereas Kilic and colleagues[18] were unable to identify infection as a cause in any of their 40 children with chronic urticaria. Infectious agents reported to cause chronic childhood urticaria range from viruses (Epstein-Barr) to bacteria (staphylococci, streptococci, *Helicobacter pylori*, *Escherichia coli*) and parasites (*Blastocystis hominis*).[30] Yet again, Sackesen and colleagues[29] highlighted the potential significance of silent infection, documenting *H pylori* in 3 of 17 children, all without gastrointestinal symptoms. One child had urticaria remission after *H pylori* eradication. Meanwhile, Hameed and colleagues[31] reported resolution of urticaria symptoms at 1-year follow-up associated with eradication of *Blastocystis hominis*, and a study in Thai children described urticaria remission in 2 of 5 patients treated for parasitic infections.[12] This report seems to be supported by Du Toit and colleagues'[16] finding that 2.5% children with chronic urticaria had stool samples positive for parasites, compared with 0% children with AD ($P = .005$). However, such reports predominantly hail from geographic areas in which parasitic infection remains common.

Drugs

Drug hypersensitivity is a commonly suspected cause of both acute and chronic urticaria in children, with medication use implicated in up to 29.8% and 17% cases, respectively.[11,22,23,25,29,32] Antibiotics and nonsteroidal antiinflammatory drugs are the usual culprits. However, both these agents are often prescribed during infections, making it difficult to ascertain true causality.[22,25] In line with this finding, Caubet and colleagues[33] were able to reproduce an urticarial reaction in only 6.8% of 88 children presenting to the emergency department within 72 hours of ingesting β-lactams. These investigators suggested that viral infections for which β-lactams may have been prescribed were more likely to play a role. To complicate matters further, identification of true drug hypersensitivity can prove elusive, with 2 studies of more than 40 children with a history of drug allergy showing that more than 90% could tolerate the drug after appropriate workup.[34,35]

Food

Acute urticaria is a cardinal clinical feature of IgE-mediated food hypersensitivity. However, food allergy seems to be an uncommon cause of childhood urticaria, with several studies reporting that it accounts for less than 7% of cases.[11,23,29] The main foods implicated include egg, milk, soy, peanut, and wheat in infants, and fish, seafood, and nuts in older children. A study of 94 Thai children found that 33 had positive skin prick tests, of whom only 39% had a history to suggest clinical food allergy, and only in these cases was elimination of the implicated food beneficial.[12] Meanwhile, Du Toit and colleagues[16] reported that elimination diets did not seem to affect the natural history of disease and described lower rates of food sensitization among children with chronic urticaria than children with AD. A few studies have attempted to use pseudoallergen-free diets in order to elucidate a role for food additives in pediatric urticaria. Ehlers and colleagues[36] recruited 16 German children with chronic urticaria to a 3-week low-pseudoallergen diet, reporting that symptoms in 12 remitted and then reappeared when pseudoallergen-rich foods were reintroduced. Double-blind placebo-controlled food challenges then showed that reactions occurred mainly to coloring agents and preservatives. However, the numbers of children used in such studies are too small for pseudoallergen dietary avoidance to be recommended as a routine part of management.

Autoreactivity

Despite a sea change in the classification of adult urticaria, with the realization that much so-called idiopathic urticaria may be autoimmune, only a few studies have investigated the prevalence of an autoimmune pathogenesis in children. Brunetti and colleagues[37] reported that 40% of 52 children had autoantibodies to either the α-chain of the high-affinity IgE receptor or to IgE itself, as seen in adults. These investigators also estimated that the correct identification of the autoimmune subtype by testing for autoreactivity (autologous serum skin test [ASST] and basophil histamine release assay [BHRA]) would potentially reduce the diagnosis of idiopathic urticaria from 52% to 29%. This finding differed from Du Toit and colleagues'[16] study, which identified autoantibodies to the IgE receptor in 47% of 78 children but could not find a correlation between ASST and either histamine-releasing factors or IgE receptor autoantibodies. Nevertheless, Jirapongsansanuruk and colleagues[12] used a positive ASST result to diagnose chronic autoimmune urticaria in 38% of 94 patients, commenting that there were no differences in medication requirement or disease remission between children with negative versus positive ASST results. As mentioned earlier, this finding contrasts strongly with evidence in adults that a positive ASST identifies a subset of urticaria sufferers with higher disease activity and more severely impaired quality of life.[38]

Physical Triggers

Physical triggers are the most commonly documented cause of chronic urticaria in children, underlying up to 53% of cases[29] and often occurring concomitantly with other forms of urticaria. The physical urticarias are referred to by the precipitating factor, with the main types including dermographic, cholinergic, aquagenic, cold, solar, delayed pressure, vibratory, and exercise-induced. Whereas Sackesen and colleagues[29] found that cholinergic and solar triggers were most common, Khakoo and colleagues[17] performed the largest study of physician-diagnosed physical urticaria in children and reported the 3 main subtypes as dermographic (38%), cholinergic (19%), and mixed (17%). These investigators documented concomitant angioedema in 67% cases. As highlighted earlier, they also found evidence that children with physical urticaria had a longer and more severe disease course than children with other forms of urticaria. That symptom severity should not be underestimated was also highlighted in a study of cold urticaria,[39] in which a third of 30 children experienced anaphylactic reactions. These investigators recommended that adrenaline autoinjectors be dispensed to all children with this urticaria subtype. Likewise, a poor chance of disease remission was observed in a historical cohort study of 87 patients with solar urticaria, in which most were still affected at 5-year and 10-year follow-up.[40]

ASSOCIATIONS

Childhood urticaria has been linked to a higher incidence of autoimmune disease and more rarely to underlying malignancy, but these seem to be associations as opposed to being directly causal.

Autoimmune Diseases

Several autoimmune conditions have been associated with childhood urticaria, including thyroid disease, celiac disease, juvenile rheumatoid arthritis, systemic lupus erythematosus (SLE), and type 1 diabetes.[41] A family history of such disorders may be identified.[41–43] Kilic and colleagues[18] reported a 14.8% prevalence of thyroid autoimmunity in children with chronic urticaria, whereas Levy and colleagues[42] reported a prevalence of 4.3%, and a recent case-control study from Taiwan found antithyroid antibodies in 27% of children with chronic urticaria compared with 0% of controls.[44] Such figures are significantly higher than age-matched healthy children (0.35%–1.6%),[45–47] although they are generally low compared with the prevalence of thyroid autoimmunity in adults with chronic urticaria (14%–33%).[48,49] This finding may perhaps be explained by the fact that autoimmunity develops with age and the evolving immune system. Because most patients with thyroid autoimmunity remain clinically euthyroid, thyroid autoantibodies are likely to represent an underlying autoreactive predisposition rather than being pathogenic in themselves.

Celiac disease has also been linked with childhood urticaria, with Caminiti and colleagues'[50] case-control study diagnosing celiac disease in 5% of children with chronic urticaria compared with just 0.67% of healthy controls. Children experienced complete remission of their urticaria after 5 to 10 weeks of a gluten-free diet, an observation also documented elsewhere.[43,51,52] This finding has been taken as long-awaited evidence of dietary-gastrointestinal-cutaneous interplay, which is likely to be a key driver in the pathogenesis of urticaria. Associations with other autoimmune disorders have not been extensively investigated, although a large Brazilian study found urticaria to be a first manifestation of juvenile SLE in 0.7% of patients,[53] and there are also numerous case reports in the literature, including one in which a 12-year old boy developed both autoimmune thyroid disease and insulin-dependent diabetes in addition to his urticaria.[54]

Malignancy

Several case reports have suggested an association between childhood urticaria and underlying malignancy. Breda and colleagues[55] described a 3-month-old infant presenting with recurrent generalized urticaria, subsequently diagnosed with acute myeloid leukemia. Two weeks of combined chemotherapy led to complete remission of both conditions. In another case, a 12-year-old girl experienced urticaria for 3 months before lip fasciculation was observed and she underwent brain computed tomography. This revealed a grade II astrocytoma, which was treated with radiotherapy, resulting in remission of both urticaria and lip fasciculations.[56] A 17-year-old girl with chronic urticaria was found to have an occult cholangiocarcinoma, with symptoms resolving after a liver transplant.[57] However, there is a lack of evidence from larger studies investigating a true association between urticaria and malignancy in the pediatric setting.

INVESTIGATIONS

Whatever the uncertainties in this field, it is widely accepted that the history and physical examination are the most important steps toward establishing a diagnosis, identifying possible triggers, and determining the need for further investigations. Although acute urticaria rarely warrants a battery of tests, the usefulness of laboratory investigations in chronic urticaria has been evaluated in a large systematic review including 6462 patients of all ages.[58] The investigators commented that a detailed history did seem to be most useful, whereas laboratory tests appeared to be useful only when performed because of the history. Similarly, allergy testing should be conducted only in the light of a detailed history, because results can be difficult to interpret, and there is also a high probability of false-positive results. Thomas and colleagues[59] comment that additional investigations (other than skin prick or specific IgE) in children with chronic urticaria had such a low positive outcome rate (5.2%) that performing them at all may be of questionable value. If autoreactivity is suspected, the ASST or BHRA are sometimes performed, because a positive result suggests an autoimmune component to the disease process (including autoantibodies). However, the uncertainty surrounding the usefulness of ASST and BHRA in children has been outlined above. In addition, the ASST is time consuming and not well tolerated by children. Neither the ASST nor the BHRA is diagnostic of autoimmune urticaria per se, and although used for research purposes, they are not readily available to the practicing clinician. By contrast, if inducible or physical urticaria is suspected, provocation tests such as stroking the skin with a calibrated dermographometer, applying an ice cube, or exercising the patient may prove useful and practical for diagnosing dermographic, cold, and cholinergic urticaria, respectively. A recommended approach has been summarized by the EAACI[1] and the British Society for Allergy and Clinical Immunology (BSACI),[60] stating that laboratory investigations are rarely useful when history and physical examination indicate a diagnosis of chronic urticaria. Allergy testing may be useful if an allergen is implicated by the history and physical examination, and other specific tests may be considered only if clinically relevant, including urinalysis, a full blood count, inflammatory markers, liver function tests, celiac disease screen, thyroid function and thyroid antibody testing, physical provocation tests, elimination diets, antinuclear antibodies, skin biopsy, C3/4 complement and C1 esterase inhibitor assays, serum cryoproteins, and an infectious disease screen.

MANAGEMENT

Episodes of acute urticaria are normally transient, uncomplicated, and easily managed by single-dose antihistamines in the primary-care setting. Urticaria that arises because of an acute allergic reaction typically settles spontaneously within hours and responds favorably to antihistamines. Urticaria of an infective nature often waxes and wanes over a few days, with a sluggish response to antihistamines. However, it is important to distinguish acute urticaria from urticaria associated with anaphylaxis, which may present with urticaria as its first manifestation. In this scenario, an adrenaline autoinjector should be used immediately, and hospitalization is required if the patient shows respiratory distress or other signs of anaphylaxis such as hypotension or hypotonia.[61] However, the management of chronic urticaria is less clear-cut, and is now discussed in further detail.

Education and Counseling

It is helpful to explain to patients what urticaria is, as well as reassure them that in most cases, there is no serious underlying disease causing symptoms. Fatalities are not described, because parents are often concerned that the risks pertaining to conditions such as peanut allergy also apply here, particularly if angioedema is an associated feature. However, this is not the case, and adrenaline is not indicated in the management of chronic urticaria. It is equally important to reiterate that urticaria is as yet poorly understood and not merely caused by allergies, thus extensive allergy testing and lifestyle restrictions are rarely warranted in the absence of a strongly suggestive history. The BSACI recommends asking patients with refractory disease to keep a symptom diary, recording each episode of urticaria and possible precipitant factors.[60] If one is identified, then trigger avoidance is key.

Antihistamines

Symptom control is the mainstay of pharmacologic management of urticaria, and antihistamines continue to be widely used in this setting. However, first-generation antihistamines such as chlorphenamine have been shown to have anticholinergic side effects, cause cognitive impairment, and disrupt sleep patterns in children.[62] These risks have been underlined in the latest GA^2LEN position paper,[63] and the EAACI/GA^2LEN/EDF/WAO now categorically state that nonsedating second-generation antihistamines should be used as first-line therapy, with escalation to up to 4 times the standard dose in refractory cases. However, this recommendation is based on scant high-quality data in the specific context of pediatric urticaria. Simons and colleagues[64–66] have conducted randomized controlled trials (RCTs) looking at the use of the histamine 1 (H_1) receptor antagonists (H1RA) cetirizine and levocetirizine to reduce frequency of urticaria episodes in infants with AD, whereas Bloom and colleagues[67] were able to include children with urticaria in an RCT on desloratadine. However, other RCTs have focused on children with respiratory symptoms and allergic rhinitis.[68,69] As Marrouche and Grattan[2] have commented, it is clear that large-scale head-to-head comparison studies are needed to elucidate the risks and benefits of different second-generation antihistamines in the treatment of childhood urticaria. H2RAs such as ranitidine or cimetidine are occasionally used to treat urticaria, but there is little evidence that they improve symptom control in the adult setting, let alone in children. This finding may be related to reports that although both H_1 and H_2 receptors are involved in the wheal response, H_1 receptors seem primarily responsible for flare and itch.[70] Accordingly, the BSACI does not recommend H2RAs as monotherapy, stating that they can be used as a second-line therapy in combination with H1RAs, although it is usually more effective to increase the H1RA dose first.[60] Meanwhile, the EAACI guideline places H2RAs on the lowest rung of its drug algorithm for chronic urticaria.[71]

Other Therapeutic Options

The recent clinical care pathway published by the Royal College of Pediatrics and Child Health recommends cyclosporine and prednisolone as effective second-line treatments.[72] Cyclosporine was tolerated at a dose of 3 mg/kg/d in 1 retrospective case series of 7 children with chronic urticaria,[73] leading to eventual remission of symptoms in all. However, overall experience with this immunomodulating therapy is limited. Corticosteroids can control urticaria symptoms effectively, but prolonged use may be limited by their well-established side effects. Montelukast is licensed for use in children, but its usefulness in childhood urticaria has not been extensively investigated,[74] although several guidelines recommend their use in conjunction with H_1 antihistamines.[60,71] Anti-IgE antibody treatment represents another therapeutic avenue that is already well established in adolescents and adults[75]; a 2011 phase II RCT of omalizumab, including children as young as 12 years old, reported significant improvements in urticaria activity scores with active treatment.[76] Other systemic treatments, sometimes successfully used in adults, should be considered on an individual basis, including methotrexate and mycophenolate mofetil, intravenous immunoglobulin, and induction of tolerance in some inducible urticaria subtypes. However, there is no published evidence for any of these treatment modalities in children.

Box 1
Illustrative case

An 8-year-old girl was referred to our children's urticaria service with a 3-month history of near-daily urticaria and asymmetrical facial swelling, particularly of the lips and eyelids (**Figs. 1–3**). She also reported symptoms of grass pollen–induced rhinoconjunctivitis, but otherwise enjoyed excellent health. Her urticarial lesions were reported to make her itchy and uncomfortable, and her facial swelling was causing her embarrassment. She had recently missed many days of school. Her symptoms had persisted despite a daily dose of cetirizine 10 mg. She had once been administered a dose of intramuscular adrenaline when assessed in the emergency department for facial angioedema, and she now carried an adrenaline autoinjector. Clinical examination confirmed her good health; there were no skin changes to suggest urticarial vasculitis, nor were there signs or symptoms suggesting an autoimmune condition or other underlying systemic disease.

This case highlights a classic presentation of spontaneous chronic urticaria in childhood. The patient's investigations and management were discussed, after we had outlined the background of this poorly understood condition.

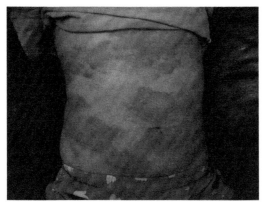

Fig. 1. Wheals on patient's torso.

MANAGEMENT OF ILLUSTRATIVE CASE

With the patient's history and physical examination complete (**Box 1**), we performed several investigations. First, physical stimuli were tested as triggers or exacerbating factors for her urticaria. Standardized techniques for the application of cold, heat, and pressure (using a calibrated dermatographometer) were used, with negative results. The patient's mother had reported that her own irritable bowel syndrome had benefited from a gluten-free diet, so allergy skin prick testing was undertaken to reassure the family that the patient was not food allergic and that wheat (which she tolerated in her diet) was an unlikely cause of her urticaria. Skin prick testing to aeroallergens showed positivity for grass pollen, in keeping with the history of hay fever. However, the patient's urticarial symptoms reportedly came on during the winter pollen-free season, making this an unlikely trigger. Because the child was systemically well, no other investigations were performed.

Based on the skin prick results, the patient's parents were reassured that dietary modification would not be required and that a stepwise approach to treatment was likely to significantly improve symptom control. Her cetirizine dose was increased to

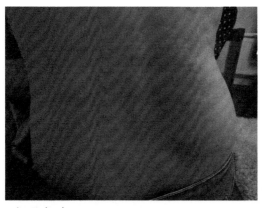

Fig. 2. Wheals on patient's back.

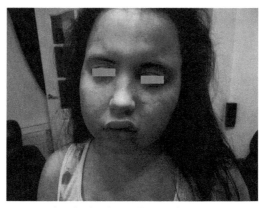

Fig. 3. Angioedema causing facial wheals and lip swelling.

10 mg twice a day (twice the standard dose at this age). It was also explained that chronic urticaria usually remits spontaneously in a matter of years and is unlikely to cause airway compromise, despite frequent and significant facial swelling. The adrenaline autoinjector was therefore withdrawn from her treatment plan.

At 4-week follow-up, the patient's family reported that despite the increased dose of cetirizine, she had not yet achieved an acceptable level of symptom control and was still missing multiple days of school. The decision was then made to use a combined therapy with 2 H1RAs at double the standard dose. Because further improvement was still only moderate at the next clinic visit, montelukast was added, resulting in marginal relief of the spontaneous swelling, but little impact on her wheals.

Frustratingly, after an additional 6 weeks on her new treatment regimen, the patient's symptoms persisted at a level that was unacceptable to both the patient and her family. The use of either oral prednisolone or cyclosporine was then roundly discussed, and the decision made to proceed with cyclosporine, with close monitoring for renal complications. Adequate control was achieved on a daily dose of 3 mg/kg, and the patient remains on this therapy with a plan for gradual weaning once 4 asymptomatic months are achieved.

SUMMARY

This case study of spontaneous chronic urticaria highlights the multiple issues faced by patients, their families, and treating clinicians. Whereas acute urticaria is common, chronic urticaria is a rare but troubling disorder, for which a stepwise approach is required toward investigations and treatment. Unique and varied associations with autoimmune conditions, such as thyroid and celiac disease, are described in a subset of patients, suggesting an underlying autoimmune predisposition. Unlike in adults, there is no good evidence that the presence of autoantibodies translates into a more severe and prolonged disease course, but this has been examined in only a few small studies. Whatever the cause, families need reassurance that chronic urticaria is a nonallergic condition, with an excellent overall prognosis. Symptoms generally respond well to high-dose antihistamine regimens (up to 4 times the standard licensed dose if required), and airway compromise is not a feature, even when angioedema is pronounced. However, this review highlights the paucity of high-quality data pertaining to the presentation, natural history, investigation, and management of urticaria in the pediatric setting. More research, including head-to-head drug trials to establish relative efficacy and safety, is needed to gain a deeper understanding of this poorly understood condition in children.

REFERENCES

1. Zuberbier T, Bindslev-Jensen C, Canonica W, et al. EAACI/GA2LEN/EDF guideline: definition, classification and diagnosis of urticaria. Allergy 2006;61(3): 316–20.
2. Marrouche N, Grattan C. Childhood urticaria. Curr Opin Allergy Clin Immunol 2012;12(5):485–90.
3. Beattie PE, Lewis-Jones MS. A comparative study of impairment of quality of life in children with skin disease and children with other chronic childhood diseases. Br J Dermatol 2006;155(1):145–51.
4. Niimi N, Francis DM, Kermani F, et al. Dermal mast cell activation by autoantibodies against the high affinity IgE receptor in chronic urticaria. J Invest Dermatol 1996;106(5):1001–6.
5. Deacock SJ. An approach to the patient with urticaria. Clin Exp Immunol 2008; 153(2):151–61.
6. Maurer M, Weller K, Bindslev-Jensen C, et al. Unmet clinical needs in chronic spontaneous urticaria. A GA^{2}LEN task force report. Allergy 2011;66(3):317–30.
7. Kaplan AP. Chronic urticaria: pathogenesis and treatment. J Allergy Clin Immunol 2004;114(3):465–74 [quiz: 475].
8. Kjaer HF, Eller E, Høst A, et al. The prevalence of allergic diseases in an unselected group of 6-year-old children. The DARC birth cohort study. Pediatr Allergy Immunol 2008;19(8):737–45.
9. Henz BM, Zuberbier T. Urticaria. New developments and perspectives. Hautarzt 2000;51(5):302–8 [in German].
10. Ibáñez MD, Garde JM. Allergy in patients under fourteen years of age in Alergológica 2005. J Investig Allergol Clin Immunol 2009;19(Suppl 2):61–8.
11. Konstantinou GN, Papadopoulos NG, Tavladaki T, et al. Childhood acute urticaria in northern and southern Europe shows a similar epidemiological pattern and significant meteorological influences. Pediatr Allergy Immunol 2011;22(1 Pt I):36–42.
12. Jirapongsananuruk O, Pongpreuksa S, Sangacharoenkit P, et al. Identification of the etiologies of chronic urticaria in children: a prospective study of 94 patients. Pediatr Allergy Immunol 2010;21(3):508–14.
13. Volonakis M, Katsarou-Katsari A, Stratigos J. Etiologic factors in childhood chronic urticaria. Ann Allergy 1992;69(1):61–5.
14. Liu TH, Lin YR, Yang KC, et al. Significant factors associated with severity and outcome of an initial episode of acute urticaria in children. Pediatr Allergy Immunol 2010;21(7):1043–51.
15. Sahiner UM, Civelek E, Tuncer A, et al. Chronic urticaria: etiology and natural course in children. Int Arch Allergy Immunol 2011;156(2):224–30.
16. Du Toit G, Prescott R, Lawrence P, et al. Autoantibodies to the high-affinity IgE receptor in children with chronic urticaria. Ann Allergy Asthma Immunol 2006; 96(2):341–4.
17. Khakoo G, Sofianou-Katsoulis A, Perkin MR, et al. Clinical features and natural history of physical urticaria in children. Pediatr Allergy Immunol 2008;19(4): 363–6.
18. Kilic G, Guler N, Suleyman A, et al. Chronic urticaria and autoimmunity in children. Pediatr Allergy Immunol 2010;21(5):837–42.

19. Harris A, Twarog FJ, Geha RS. Chronic urticaria in childhood: natural course and etiology. Ann Allergy 1983;51(2 Pt 1):161–5.
20. Kauppinen K, Juntunen K, Lanki H. Urticaria in children. Retrospective evaluation and follow-up. Allergy 1984;39(6):469–72.
21. Ghosh S, Kanwar AJ, Kaur S. Urticaria in children. Pediatr Dermatol 1993;10(2):107–10.
22. Balaban J. Medicaments as the possible cause of urticaria in children. Acta Dermatovenerol Croat 2002;10(3):155–9.
23. Ricci G, Giannetti A, Belotti T, et al. Allergy is not the main trigger of urticaria in children referred to the emergency room. J Eur Acad Dermatol Venereol 2010;24(11):1347–8.
24. Gupta SP, Jindal N, Gupta S, et al. Clinico-etiological study with response to specific treatment in childhood urticaria. Indian Dermatol Online J 2011;2(2):64–6.
25. Liu TH, Lin YR, Yang KC, et al. First attack of acute urticaria in pediatric emergency department. Pediatr Neonatol 2008;49(3):58–64.
26. Bilbao A, García JM, Pocheville I, et al. Round Table: urticaria in relation to infections. Allergol Immunopathol (Madr) 1999;27(2):73–85 [in Spanish].
27. Schuller DE, Elvey SM. Acute urticaria associated with streptococcal infection. Pediatrics 1980;65(3):592–6.
28. Kano Y, Mitsuyama Y, Hirahara K, et al. Mycoplasma pneumoniae infection-induced erythema nodosum, anaphylactoid purpura, and acute urticaria in 3 people in a single family. J Am Acad Dermatol 2007;57(Suppl 2):S33–5.
29. Sackesen C, Sekerel BE, Orhan F, et al. The etiology of different forms of urticaria in childhood. Pediatr Dermatol 2004;21(2):102–8.
30. Wedi B, Raap U, Wieczorek D, et al. Urticaria and infections. Allergy Asthma Clin Immunol 2009;5(1):10.
31. Hameed DM, Hassanin OM, Zuel-Fakkar NM. Association of Blastocystis hominis genetic subtypes with urticaria. Parasitol Res 2011;108(3):553–60.
32. Mortureux P, Léauté-Labrèze C, Legrain-Lifermann V, et al. Acute urticaria in infancy and early childhood: a prospective study. Arch Dermatol 1998;134(3):319–23.
33. Caubet JC, Kaiser L, Lemaître B, et al. The role of penicillin in benign skin rashes in childhood: a prospective study based on drug rechallenge. J Allergy Clin Immunol 2011;127(1):218–22.
34. Rebelo Gomes E, Fonseca J, Araujo L, et al. Drug allergy claims in children: from self-reporting to confirmed diagnosis. Clin Exp Allergy 2008;38(1):191–8.
35. Seitz CS, Bröcker EB, Trautmann A. Diagnosis of drug hypersensitivity in children and adolescents: discrepancy between physician-based assessment and results of testing. Pediatr Allergy Immunol 2011;22(4):405–10.
36. Ehlers I, Niggemann B, Binder C, et al. Role of nonallergic hypersensitivity reactions in children with chronic urticaria. Allergy 1998;53(11):1074–7.
37. Brunetti L, Francavilla R, Miniello VL, et al. High prevalence of autoimmune urticaria in children with chronic urticaria. J Allergy Clin Immunol 2004;114(4):922–7.
38. Metz M, Giménez-Arnau A, Borzova E, et al. Frequency and clinical implications of skin autoreactivity to serum versus plasma in patients with chronic urticaria. J Allergy Clin Immunol 2009;123(3):705–6.
39. Alangari AA, Twarog FJ, Shih MC, et al. Clinical features and anaphylaxis in children with cold urticaria. Pediatrics 2004;113(4):e313–7.
40. Beattie PE, Dawe RS, Ibbotson SH, et al. Characteristics and prognosis of idiopathic solar urticaria: a cohort of 87 cases. Arch Dermatol 2003;139(9):1149–54.

41. Dalal I, Levine A, Somekh E, et al. Chronic urticaria in children: expanding the "autoimmune kaleidoscope". Pediatrics 2000;106(5):1139–41.
42. Levy Y, Segal N, Weintrob N, et al. Chronic urticaria: association with thyroid autoimmunity. Arch Dis Child 2003;88(6):517–9.
43. Levine A, Dalal I, Bujanover Y. Celiac disease associated with familial chronic urticaria and thyroid autoimmunity in a child. Pediatrics 1999;104(2):e25.
44. Wan KS, Wu CS. The essential role of anti-thyroid antibodies in chronic idiopathic urticaria. Endocr Res 2013;38(2):85–8.
45. Rallison ML, Dobyns BM, Meikle AW, et al. Natural history of thyroid abnormalities: prevalence, incidence, and regression of thyroid diseases in adolescents and young adults. Am J Med 1991;91(4):363–70.
46. Jaksić J, Dumić M, Filipović B, et al. Thyroid diseases in a school population with thyromegaly. Arch Dis Child 1994;70(2):103–6.
47. Marwaha RK, Tandon N, Karak AK, et al. Hashimoto's thyroiditis: countrywide screening of goitrous healthy young girls in postiodization phase in India. J Clin Endocrinol Metab 2000;85(10):3798–802.
48. Heymann WR. Chronic urticaria and angioedema associated with thyroid autoimmunity: review and therapeutic implications. J Am Acad Dermatol 1999;40(2 Pt 1):229–32.
49. Zauli D, Deleonardi G, Foderaro S, et al. Thyroid autoimmunity in chronic urticaria. Allergy Asthma Proc 2001;22(2):93–5.
50. Caminiti L, Passalacqua G, Magazzù G, et al. Chronic urticaria and associated coeliac disease in children: a case-control study. Pediatr Allergy Immunol 2005; 16(5):428–32.
51. Meneghetti R, Gerarduzzi T, Barbi E, et al. Chronic urticaria and coeliac disease. Arch Dis Child 2004;89(3):293.
52. Peroni DG, Paiola G, Tenero L, et al. Chronic urticaria and celiac disease: a case report. Pediatr Dermatol 2010;27(1):108–9.
53. Spadoni M, Jacob C, Aikawa N, et al. Chronic autoimmune urticaria as the first manifestation of juvenile systemic lupus erythematosus. Lupus 2011;20(7): 763–6.
54. Hyman SJ, Shreffler WG, Rapaport R. Type 1 diabetes, autoimmune thyroid disease, and chronic urticaria. Pediatr Diabetes 2008;9(5):508–11.
55. Breda L, Di Marzio D, Rollo V, et al. Acute myeloid leukaemia presenting as recurrent generalized urticaria in infancy. Eur J Pediatr 2008;167(6):697–8.
56. Shamsadini S, Varesvazirian M, Shamsadini A. Urticaria and lip fasciculation may be prodromal signs of brain malignancy. Dermatol Online J 2006;12(3):23.
57. Naimeh LG, Muller BA. Chronic urticaria in a 17-year-old patient with a past history of bowel disease. Ann Allergy Asthma Immunol 2001;86(5):511–6.
58. Kozel MM, Bossuyt PM, Mekkes JR, et al. Laboratory tests and identified diagnoses in patients with physical and chronic urticaria and angioedema: a systematic review [Internet]. J Am Acad Dermatol 2003;48(3):409–16. Available at: http://eutils.ncbi.nlm.nih.gov/entrez/eutils/elink.fcgi?dbfrom=pubmed&id= 12637921&retmode=ref&cmd=prlinks.
59. Thomas P, Perkin MR, Rayner N, et al. The investigation of chronic urticaria in childhood: which investigations are being performed and which are recommended? Clin Exp Allergy 2008;38(6):1061–2.
60. Powell RJ, Toit Du GL, Siddique N, et al. BSACI guidelines for the management of chronic urticaria and angio-oedema. Clin Exp Allergy 2007;37(5): 631–50.
61. Huang SW. Acute urticaria in children. Pediatr Neonatol 2009;50(3):85–7.

62. Pampura AN, Papadopoulos NG, Spičák V, et al. Evidence for clinical safety, efficacy, and parent and physician perceptions of levocetirizine for the treatment of children with allergic disease. Int Arch Allergy Immunol 2011;155(4): 367–78.
63. Church MK, Maurer M, Simons FE, et al. Risk of first-generation H(1)-antihistamines: a GA(2)LEN position paper. Allergy 2010;65(4):459–66.
64. Simons FE. Prevention of acute urticaria in young children with atopic dermatitis. J Allergy Clin Immunol 2001;107(4):703–6.
65. Simons FE, Early Prevention of Asthma in Atopic Children (EPAAC) Study Group. Safety of levocetirizine treatment in young atopic children: an 18-month study. Pediatr Allergy Immunol 2007;18(6):535–42.
66. Simons FE, Early Prevention of Asthma in Atopic Children Study Group. H1-antihistamine treatment in young atopic children: effect on urticaria. Ann Allergy Asthma Immunol 2007;99(3):261–6.
67. Bloom M, Staudinger H, Herron J. Safety of desloratadine syrup in children. Curr Med Res Opin 2004;20(12):1959–65.
68. Grimfeld A, Holgate ST, Canonica GW, et al. Prophylactic management of children at risk for recurrent upper respiratory infections: the Preventia I Study. Clin Exp Allergy 2004;34(11):1665–72.
69. Hampel FC, Kittner B, van Bavel JH. Safety and tolerability of fexofenadine hydrochloride, 15 and 30 mg, twice daily in children aged 6 months to 2 years with allergic rhinitis. Ann Allergy Asthma Immunol 2007;99(6):549–54.
70. Greaves MW, Davies MG. Histamine receptors in human skin: indirect evidence. Br J Dermatol 1982;107(Suppl 23):101–5.
71. Zuberbier T, Asero R, Bindslev-Jensen C, et al. EAACI/GA^{2}LEN/EDF/WAO guideline: management of urticaria. Allergy 2009;64(10):1427–43.
72. Leech S, Grattan C, Lloyd K, et al. The RCPCH care pathway for children with urticaria, angio-oedema or mastocytosis: an evidence and consensus based national approach. Arch Dis Child 2011;96:i34–7.
73. Doshi DR, Weinberger MM. Experience with cyclosporine in children with chronic idiopathic urticaria. Pediatr Dermatol 2009;26(4):409–13.
74. Sanada S, Tanaka T, Kameyoshi Y, et al. The effectiveness of montelukast for the treatment of anti-histamine-resistant chronic urticaria. Arch Dermatol Res 2005; 297(3):134–8.
75. Maurer M, Rosén K, Hsieh HJ, et al. Omalizumab for the treatment of chronic idiopathic or spontaneous urticaria. N Engl J Med 2013;368(10):924–35.
76. Saini S, Rosen KE, Hsieh HJ, et al. A randomized, placebo-controlled, dose-ranging study of single-dose omalizumab in patients with H1-antihistamine-refractory chronic idiopathic urticaria. J Allergy Clin Immunol 2011;128(3): 567–73.e1.
77. Augustin M, Ehrle S. Safety and efficacy of desloratadine in chronic idiopathic urticaria in clinical practice: an observational study of 9246 patients. J Eur Acad Dermatol Venereol 2009;23(3):292–9.
78. Beno SM, Nadel FM, Alessandrini EA. A survey of emergency department management of acute urticaria in children. Pediatr Emerg Care 2007;23(12): 862–8.
79. Boyce JA. Successful treatment of cold-induced urticaria/anaphylaxis with anti-IgE. J Allergy Clin Immunol 2006;117(6):1415–8.
80. Frances AM, Fiorenza G, Frances RJ. Aquagenic urticaria: report of a case. Allergy Asthma Proc 2004;25(3):195–7.

81. Giuliodori K, Ganzetti G, Campanati A, et al. A non-responsive chronic auto-immune urticaria in a 12-year-old autistic girl treated with cyclosporin. J Eur Acad Dermatol Venereol 2009;23(5):619–20.
82. Kaplan AP, Spector SL, Meeves S, et al. Once-daily fexofenadine treatment for chronic idiopathic urticaria: a multicenter, randomized, double-blind, placebo-controlled study. Ann Allergy Asthma Immunol 2005;94(6):662–9.
83. McGee JS, Kirkorian AY, Pappert AS, et al. An Adolescent Boy with Urticaria to Water: Review of Current Treatments for Aquagenic Urticaria. Pediatr Dermatol 2012.
84. Salmun LM, Herron JM, Banfield C, et al. The pharmacokinetics, electrocardio-graphic effects, and tolerability of loratadine syrup in children aged 2 to 5 years. Clin Ther 2000;22(5):613–21.
85. Visitsunthorn N, Tuchinda M, Vichyanond P. Cold Urticaria in Thai Children: Comparison between Cyproheptadine and ketotifen in the Treatment. Asian Pacific journal of allergy and immunology/launched by the Allergy and Immunology Society of Thailand 1995;13:29–35.

Urticarial Vasculitis and Schnitzler Syndrome

H.C. Torsten Zuberbier, MD*,
Marcus Maurer, MD

KEYWORDS

- Urticaria • Schnitzler syndrome • Interleukin-1 • Urticarial vasculitis
- Leucocytoclastic vasculitis • Myeloma

KEY POINTS

- Newly defined diagnostic criteria of urticaria vasculitis and Schnitzler syndrome.
- Better understanding of pathophysiology.
- New treatment options described.

INTRODUCTION

Urticarial vasculitis is no longer classified as part of urticaria in the current guidelines for urticaria due to the underlying nature of the disease. It is defined as a leukocytoclastic vasculitis that presents, clinically, with wheals. In contrast to the histamine-induced wheals in urticaria, the wheals in urticarial vasculitis are not fleeting but often stay for more than 24 hours and sometimes leave small patches of a brownish color due to microbleedings.

The disease may be seen as a stage between severe chronic spontaneous urticaria and leucocytoclastic vasculitis in association with autoimmune processes. Minimal histologic signs of vasculitis may also occur in chronic urticaria patients and in a series of 83 patients with chronic urticaria 10 exhibited histologic features of urticarial vasculitis.

The clinical picture of urticarial vasculitis is diverse, and more severely affected patients often exhibit hypocomplementemia. The typical age group consists of young to middle-aged women.[1]

Schnitzler syndrome is related to urticarial vasculitis. It is defined as a disease with a monoclonal mostly immunoglobulin IgM gammopathy, increased markers of systemic inflammation such as C-reactive protein (CRP), and the chronic appearance of wheals, which, on histopathological examination, often show signs of urticarial vasculitis.[2]

Department of Dermatology and Allergy, Allergy Center, Charité-Universitätsmedizin Berlin, Charitéplatz 1, Berlin 10117, Germany
* Corresponding author.
E-mail address: torsten.zuberbier@charite.de

Immunol Allergy Clin N Am 34 (2014) 141–147
http://dx.doi.org/10.1016/j.iac.2013.09.007
0889-8561/14/$ – see front matter © 2014 Elsevier Inc. All rights reserved.
immunology.theclinics.com

CLINICAL ASPECTS
Skin Lesions and Symptoms

Both in urticarial vasculitis and in Schnitzler syndrome wheals are typically generalized in distribution and sometimes faintly red but often, especially in urticarial vasculitis, deeply red or purplish-red in color. Sometimes punctate purpura may be observed within the lesions. The major points of differentiation against wheals in chronic spontaneous urticaria are their duration and resolution. Urticarial vasculitis wheals generally persist for more than 24 hours and up to 72 hours (ie, longer than the wheals in chronic spontaneous urticaria) and they resolve, in many cases, by developing a mild residual hyperpigmentation with small signs of bleeding, which is not seen in chronic spontaneous urticaria unless vigorous rubbing or scratching has caused bruising. Like in urticaria, most patients experience pruritus at the sites of lesions but sometimes also complain of burning sensations.[1]

Extracutaneous Signs and Symptoms

In addition to the wheals, extracutaneous signs and symptoms are often observed in both urticarial vasculitis and Schnitzler syndrome. The variety of clinical and laboratory findings are summarized in **Boxes 1** and **2** and **Tables 1–3**.

Course of Disease and Prognosis

The clinical course of urticarial vasculitis is often benign with resolution of the disease within 1 year in 30% to 40% of patients. In Schnitzler syndrome, the disease is normally lifelong or chronic, although single cases have been reported whereby a permanent resolution of the disease was observed together with the resolution of monoclonal gammopathy.[3,4]

Other related diseases sometimes showing signs of urticarial vasculitis are Muckle-Wells syndrome and autoimmune diseases, such as systemic lupus erythematosus, Still disease, or Sjögren syndrome.

In Schnitzler syndrome one of the key clinical features is recurrent fever, which is seen in more than 90% of patients. Recurrent fever was already described by Dr Schnitzler in her first description of the disease in 1972.[5] Monoclonal gammopathy, a key feature of Schnitzler syndrome, is not necessarily present at disease onset and may occur only after several years. On the other hand, the 10-year risk of developing a lymphoproliferative disorder in patients with Schnitzler syndrome, in most

---

Box 1
Diagnostic signs of urticarial vasculitis

1. Idiopathic chronic urticaria, vessel damage, wheals lasting >24 h

2. Leukocytoclastic vasculitis on histology

3. Purpuric or erythema multiforme-like lesions

4. Clinical signs of multisystem disease (see **Table 1**)

5. ESR, circulating immune complexes, positive direct immunofluorescence, Ø serum complement (see **Table 2**)

6. Resistance to therapy with antihistamines

7. Serologic evidence of connective tissue disease (+double-stranded ANF; +lupus band on immunofluorescence)

Data from Czarnetzki BM. Urticaria. Berlin: Springer; 1986.

Box 2
Schnitzler syndrome: Strasbourg diagnostic criteria

Obligate criteria

• Chronic urticarial rash and

• Monoclonal IgM or IgG

• Minor criteria

• Recurrent fever[a]

• Objective findings of abnormal bone remodeling with or without bone pain[b]

• A neutrophilic dermal infiltrate on skin biopsy[c]

• Leukocytosis and/or elevated CRP[d]

Definite diagnosis if

• Two obligate criteria AND at least 2 minor criteria if paraprotein IgM, and 3 minor criteria if paraprotein IgG

Probable diagnosis if

• Two obligate criteria AND at least 1 minor criterion if IgM, and 2 minor criteria if IgG

    [a] A valid criterion if objectively measured. Must be >38°C and otherwise unexplained. Occurs usually, but not obligatory, together with the skin rash.
    [b] As assessed by bone scintigraphy, MRI, or elevation of bone alkaline phosphatase.
    [c] Corresponds usually to the entity described as "neutrophilic urticarial dermatosis" (Medicine 2009;88:23–31); absence of fibrinoid necrosis and significant dermal edema.
    [d] Neutrophils >10,000/mm^3 and/or CRP >30 mg/L.
    From Simon A, et al. Schnitzler's syndrome: diagnosis, treatment, and follow-up. Allergy 2013;68(5):562–8; with permission.

---

cases Waldenström macroglobulinemia, is estimated to be 15%,[2] although it is unclear which patients are at increased risk.

As for diagnostic criteria for Schnitzler syndrome, there was no internationally accepted consensus for a long time until recently an expert meeting was organized; the results have been published in *Allergy* 2013 (Simon 2013). The publication summarizes the recent literature and the expert consensus suggests that Schnitzler syndrome should be suspected in patients usually older than 40 years with (1) wheals, (2) a monoclonal gammopathy, which defines the syndrome, but a suspicion of Schnitzler syndrome arises when any of the symptoms listed in **Box 2** are present with fever ≥38.5°C with no other apparent cause. On the other hand, as there is no single blood or laboratory test available for the definite diagnosis, it is also important to remember that monoclonal gammopathy of unknown significance is relatively common in elderly patients and co-occurrence can thus be by chance with chronic urticaria. Other diseases that need to be ruled out are adult-onset Still disease and cryopyrin-associated periodic syndromes, especially Muckle-Wells syndrome, which normally occurs at a younger age.

The definite diagnosis is therefore based on estimating the probability according to the so-called Strasbourg diagnostic criteria, as summarized in **Box 2**.

HISTOPATHOLOGY AND LABORATORY FINDINGS

The histologic and laboratory findings characteristic for urticarial vasculitis are summarized in **Box 1** and **Table 2**. Urticarial vasculitis must be confirmed histologically.

Table 1
Clinical symptoms of urticarial vasculitis

Organ	Frequency of Involvement (%)	Clinical Manifestation
Skin	100	Pruritic or burning wheals (lasting >24 h), angioedema, bullae, lesions resembling erythema multiforme, livedo reticularis, Raynaud phenomenon, purpura
Joints	75	Arthralgias, swelling, stiffness, arthritis of single or multiple joints
Kidneys	60	Hematuria, proteinuria, decreased creatinine clearance
Respiratory system	55	Chronic obstructive pulmonary disease, pleuritic chest pain, laryngeal edema
Eyes	35	Uveitis, episcleritis, conjunctivitis, loss of vision
Gastrointestinal tract	30	Nausea, vomiting, diarrhea, abdominal pain
Nervous system	12	Mononeuritis, myositis, seizures, pseudotumor cerebri, increased central nervous system pressure
Cardiovascular and hematological systems	5	Raynaud syndrome, carditis, lymphadenopathy, leukopenia, thrombocytopenia, anemia
General systemic	10	Fever

Data from Czarnetzki BM. Urticaria. Berlin: Springer; 1986.

The most important diagnostic feature of histopathology is the damage of the walls of the small superficial venules evidenced by endothelial swelling, obstruction of the vessel lumen, and extravasation of erythrocytes into the dermis. In addition, fibrinoid material can be detected in most cases around the vessel walls. Leukocytoclasia and neutrophilic as well as eosinophilic infiltration is frequently observed but not mandatory. Histopathology and laboratory findings in Schnitzler syndrome overlap with urticarial vasculitis and are summarized in **Table 3** and **Box 2**.

TREATMENT

In contrast to urticaria, antihistamines are usually ineffective in urticarial vasculitis and Schnitzler syndrome and should therefore no longer be used as monotherapy; however, they may alleviate some symptoms, especially in patients with mild forms of urticarial vasculitis and also in those patients with chronic spontaneous urticaria with an overlap expressing only some features of vasculitis.

In general, in the treatment of urticarial vasculitis nonsteroidal anti-inflammatory drugs, cytostatic drugs, such as azathioprine or cyclophosphamide, and antimalarials have proven to be beneficial.[6]

Almost all patients respond to systemically administered corticosteroids. However, because of their side effects, daily treatment with corticosteroids should not be considered first-line therapy.

Table 2
Laboratory changes in patients with urticarial vasculitis (frequency is shown in parentheses, if known)

Histopathology	Fibrinoid changes in vessel walls (88%)
	Tissue eosinophilia (63%)
	Leukocytoclastic vasculitis (61%)
	Erythrocyte extravasation (58%)
	Neutrophilic infiltration (58%)
	Edema of upper dermis (44%)
Immunopathology (direct IF)	Deposits of (a) IgM, IgG, IgA or (b) CIq, C4, C3 or (c) fibrinogen in vessel walls and at the dermoepidermal junction, 89% of specimens
Changes in peripheral blood	ESR (75%)
	CH50 (35%), CIq, C4, C3 (32%), C5
	Circulating immune complexes, normal or decreased immunoglobulins, rarely positive: ANF, RF cryoglobulins, bacterial or viral antigens; rarely: leukopenia, thrombocytopenia
Autoantibodies against	CIq
	IL-1
	IgE
	FcεRI
	Thyroid microsomal antigens

Abbreviations: ANF, antinuclear factor; ESR, erythrocyte sedimentation rate; IF, immunofluorescence; RF, rheumatoid factor.

Data from Czarnetzki BM. Urticaria. Berlin: Springer, 1986. Chapter 8; and Mehregan DR, Hall MJ, Gibson LE. Urticarial vasculitis: a histopathologic and clinical review of 72 cases. J Am Acad Dermatol 1992;26(3 Pt 2):441–8.

Table 3
Clinical and biological findings in patients with Schnitzler syndrome

Clinical or Biological Finding	Prevalence (%)
Urticarial rash	100
Elevated ESR (≥30)	95
Fever	93
Monoclonal IgM gammopathy	89
Kappa light chain	89
Arthralgia/arthritis	77
Leucocytosis (≥10,000)	76
Bone pain	68
Abnormal bone morphology	62
Palpable lymph nodes	74
Pruritus	45
Liver and/or spleen enlargement	34

From Simon A, et al. Schnitzler's syndrome: diagnosis, treatment, and follow-up. Allergy 2013;68(5):562–8; with permission.

In treatment-resistant urticarial vasculitis, case reports suggest the use of inter-feron-α,[7] mycophenolate mofetil,[8] colchicine,[9,10] or a cyclophosphamide-dexamethasone pulse therapy.[11]

Treatment of Schnitzler syndrome has changed during the recent years. It is impor-tant to define the exact need for treatment together with the patient. It must be noted that the disease severity varies considerably between patients and also in individual patients over the time. Some patients experience daily symptoms, whereas others have flare-ups once or twice a year. Simon and coworkers,[12] during the above-mentioned consensus conference in Strasbourg, devised an algorithm with recom-mendations for treatment. Treatment needs to be adapted based on the results. Apart from the question of significant alterations in quality of life, it is important to measure CRP. If CRP is below 30 mg/L, it is regarded as only a low level of persistent inflam-mation/disease activity.

In these cases an observation and/or treatment choice of colchicine 1 to 2 mg/d, nonsteroidal anti-inflammatory drugs in case of flare-ups, and hydroxychloroquine is recommended. Most important is, however, to follow-up these patients preferably at quarterly intervals per year to ensure that the level of disease remains stable.

In those patients with significant alterations of quality of life or persistent elevation of markers of inflammation (CRP>30 mg/L), the recent awareness of changes in the inter-leukin (IL) -1β as a hallmark of the pathologic abnormality in this disease has led to new possibilities in treatment. Anakinra has become one of the standard drug therapies[13] but also Canakinumab[14,15] as well as Rilonacept[16] have been shown to be effective, safe, and well tolerated.

Although of Schnitzler syndrome is defined as an auto-inflammatory disease of late onset involving IL-1, not all patients respond to anti-IL-1 treatment, showing that other cytokines are involved. In a case study 3 patients who did not respond to anti IL-1 responded well to anti-IL-6 treatment.[14]

Although the role of anti-IL-1 therapy is now widely established in Schnitzler syn-drome, it may also be a treatment option in severe urticarial vasculitis. The results of the first clinical trial in urticarial vasculitis, assessing the effects of the humanized monoclonal anti-IL-1β antibody, demonstrated that a single-dose treatment signifi-cantly reduced disease activity and markers of inflammation.[17]

REFERENCES

1. Czarnetzki BM. Urticaria. Berlin: Springer; 1986.
2. de Koning HD, Bodar EJ, van der Meer JW, et al. Schnitzler syndrome: beyond the case reports: review and follow-up of 94 patients with an emphasis on prog-nosis and treatment. Semin Arthritis Rheum 2007;37(3):137–48.
3. Asli B, Brouet JC, Fermand JP. Spontaneous remission of Schnitzler syndrome. Ann Allergy Asthma Immunol 2011;107(1):87–8.
4. Lipsker D. The Schnitzler syndrome. Orphanet J Rare Dis 2010;5:38.
5. Schnitzler L. Lésion urticariennes chroniques permanents (érythème pètaloide?) case clinique. Journée Dermatologique d'Angers 1972;28(46B).
6. Zuberbier T, Haas N, Henz BM. Urticarial vasculitis. In: Bos JD, editor. The skin immune system (SIS)2. Boca Raton, USA: CRC Press; 1997. p. 489–96.
7. Czarnetzki BM, Algermissen B, Jeep S, et al. Interferon treatment of patients with chronic urticaria and mastocytosis. J Am Acad Dermatol 1994;30(3):500–1.
8. Worm M, Sterry W, Kolde G. Mycophenolate mofetil is effective for maintenance therapy of hypocomplementaemic urticarial vasculitis. Br J Dermatol 2000; 143(6):1324.

9. Werni R, Schwarz T, Gschnait F. Colchicine treatment of urticarial vasculitis. Dermatologica 1986;172(1):36–40.
10. Mehregan DR, Hall MJ, Gibson LE. Urticarial vasculitis: a histopathologic and clinical review of 72 cases. J Am Acad Dermatol 1992;26(3 Pt 2):441–8.
11. Worm M, Muche M, Schulze P, et al. Hypocomplementaemic urticarial vasculitis: successful treatment with cyclophosphamide-dexamethasone pulse therapy. Br J Dermatol 1998;139(4):704–7.
12. Simon A, Asli B, Braun-Falco M, et al. Schnitzler's syndrome: diagnosis, treatment, and follow-up. Allergy 2013;68(5):562–8.
13. Gran JT, Midtvedt O, Haug S, et al. Treatment of Schnitzler's syndrome with anakinra: report of three cases and review of the literature. Scand J Rheumatol 2011; 40(1):74–9.
14. Krause K, Feist E, Fiene M, et al. Complete remission in 3 of 3 anti-IL-6-treated patients with Schnitzler syndrome. J Allergy Clin Immunol 2012;129(3):848–50.
15. Krause K, Feist E, Maurer M, et al. Cryopyrin-assoziierte periodische Syndrome. Kinder- und Jugendmedizin 2011;6:349–57.
16. Krause K, Weller K, Stefaniak R, et al. Efficacy and safety of the interleukin-1 antagonist rilonacept in Schnitzler syndrome: an open-label study. Allergy 2012;67(7):943–50.
17. Krause K, Metz M, Makris M, et al. The role of interleukin-1 in allergy-related disorders. Curr Opin Allergy Clin Immunol 2012;12(5):477–84.

Urticaria and Angioedema in Pregnancy and Lactation

Frances Lawlor, MB.BCh.BAO, DCh, DObst RCOG, MD, FRCP(Irel), FRCP(Lond)[a,b,*]

KEYWORDS

- Urticaria • Ordinary • Physical • Hereditary angioedema • Pregnancy • Labor
- Delivery

KEY POINTS

- Urticaria is part of the management of pregnancy, labor, and delivery.
- Treatment is necessary because urticaria has an impact on quality of life.
- With certain caveats treatment is similar to that of nonpregnant patients.

URTICARIA IN PREGNANCY

Introduction

Urticaria occurs during pregnancy but urticaria is not a pregnancy dermatosis. Although there are specific pregnancy dermatoses and itching (pruritus) is a pregnancy-related problem, there is no specific pregnancy-related urticaria.[1] There are no data relating to the incidence and prevalence of urticaria in pregnancy. Only one type of hereditary angioedema (HAE), type 3, which is rare and considered hormonally influenced, has presented and exacerbated in pregnancy.[2] One eruption said to exacerbate during pregnancy, autoimmune progesterone dermatitis, is reported by some investigators to have a transient urticarial phase.[1,3] This condition might be considered as part of a differential diagnosis. Any discussion about urticaria and pregnancy is usually related to possible effects on fertility, to the behavior and management of specific urticarias coexisting with pregnancy, to information about treatment, and to treatment given to women planning pregnancy and during pregnancy. Any effects on labor, delivery and breastfeeding are also considerations.

It is vital to differentiate urticaria from itch. Urticaria is defined by whealing, which usually itches. When urticaria is present, however, the situation is dynamic and the whealing lesions may be transient, sometimes lasting only hours, so at any one time wheals may not be evident and there may be an erythema, either patchy, linear, or

[a] Department of Cutaneous Allergy, St Thomas' Hospital, Block 7, South Wing, Lambeth Palace Road, London SE17EH, UK; [b] The London Clinic, 120 Harley Street, London W17JG, UK
* The London Clinic, 120 Harley Street, London W17JG, UK.
E-mail address: Frances.Lawlor@gstt.nhs.UK

Immunol Allergy Clin N Am 34 (2014) 149–156
http://dx.doi.org/10.1016/j.iac.2013.09.006   immunology.theclinics.com

annular. Patients should be encouraged to photograph their skin rashes (preferably using dated photographs) to help with diagnosis.

Hormones in Pregnancy

Hormone levels change and increase during pregnancy. During the first few weeks, progesterone, 17- hydroxyprogesterone, estrone, and estradiol levels, produced by the corpus luteum, increase. Human chorionic gonadotropin (hCG) also rises at the beginning of pregnancy, reaching peak levels at 60 to 90 days' gestation, then declines to a plateau until delivery. hCG and the corpus luteum are responsible for several weeks for production of inhibin and relaxin, which stop follicular development and reduce contractility of the uterus. After several weeks, the hormone production is taken over by the placenta and the fetus. The placenta and fetus act as an endocrine system. The placenta is mature by 12 weeks. It connects the fetal and maternal circulation. The fetoplacental unit produces increased amounts of peptides (inhibin, relaxin, and human placental lactogen), neuropeptides (gonadotropin-releasing hormone, corticotropin-releasing hormone, and thyroid-releasing hormone), steroid hormones (progesterone, androgens, estradiol, estrone, and estriol), and peptide growth factors (insulinlike growth factors 1 and 2). All these levels return to normal after a few days of birth.[1]

Hormonal changes have not been studied extensively in urticaria patients and the increases (described previously) seem not to have a deleterious effect on urticaria in pregnancy, although there is a case report of pregnancy-provoked urticaria in two successive pregnancies, resolving after termination, in which the mother whealed 5 minutes after intradermal injection of estradiol benzoate.[4] Some investigators have looked at dehydroepiandrosterone (DHEAS) in nonpregnant urticaria patients and found DHEAS levels significantly lower than in normal controls.[5] It is considered that DHEAS may antagonize the production of T_H2 cytokines.[6] It is not known whether an increase in pregnancy might have a beneficial effect on urticaria in pregnancy but it seems possible.

Concurrent Urticaria and Pregnancy

Acute urticaria is self-limiting and can be one of the manifestations of allergy. It is conventionally defined as lasting up to 6 weeks and there are no data relating either to its incidence or prevalence in pregnancy. In up to approximately 50% of patients, it is related to an ingested food, insect bite, infection, or drug.[7] When it occurs as part of drug-induced anaphylaxis, initial treatment is with subcutaneous or intramuscular adrenaline, followed by supportive treatment, systemic steroid, and antihistamine treatment. There is one report of intravenous adrenaline given safely because of drug-induced anaphylaxis over the course of a labor.[8] Intravenous adrenaline is generally not advisable and joint care with a cardiologist is a suggestion if this were undertaken, because of effects on a patient's heart.

Chronic urticaria is defined as urticaria lasting longer than 6 weeks. It is spontaneous or induced, usually by a physical stimulus (physical urticaria). Chronic spontaneous urticaria may be idiopathic, where no cause is found, or autoimmune due to circulating autoantibodies reactive with the high-affinity IgE receptor expressed on dermal mast cells and basophils or less commonly with IgE itself. Patients considered to be autoimmune usually have a positive basophil histamine release test and often have other organ-specific or non–organ-specific autoantibodies. Chronic spontaneous urticaria may continue during pregnancy and delivery and postpartum.

In cases of a physical urticaria, reproducible whealing occurs in response to a specific physical stimulus or to a rise in core body temperature. Where there is a physical urticaria, a whealing reaction can occur from friction (symptomatic dermographism); sustained pressure (delayed pressure urticaria); vibration (vibratory angioedema); local exposure to heat or cold; sunlight; water; or exercise, heat, cold, and emotion (cholinergic urticaria).[7] Rarer urticarias also occur. These include angioedema with eosinophilia that has been treated in pregnancy (as in nonpregnant patients) with a successful outcome using prednisolone.[9]

Urticaria does not seem to affect fertility. It is not teratogenic and does not affect the fetal development. There are no changes to the onset or progress of labor or delivery. Generally it seems not to worsen during pregnancy and may even improve, although there may be exceptions. It tends not to have an impact on a normal delivery.

Patients with chronic urticaria and the physical urticarias and their health care teams are concerned about how the condition will be treated during pregnancy and if labor and delivery will be more of a problem. Chronic urticaria patients, cholinergic urticaria patients, and symptomatic dermographism patients discuss management during pregnancy and delivery more frequently because these urticarias occur more frequently in younger women. It is possible that delayed pressure urticaria may have some impact postpartum related to various sustained pressure stimuli during delivery, but this has not been documented.

One issue relating to delivery seems to be postpartum development of wheals or swellings that might be considered allergic unless an obstetric team is updated on concurrent skin conditions and the patient fully informed about the situation.

Pregnant women may develop or already suffer from contact urticaria from any substance with which they come in contact, including preservatives and antiseptics in creams and latex. Contact urticaria reactions occur within minutes of contact with the eliciting substance. Reactions are cutaneous or extracutaneous. Cutaneous reactions comprise localized urticaria or dermatitis. Extracutaneous reactions may involve wheezing, runny nose and watery eyes, lip swelling, hoarseness, difficulty swallowing, nausea, vomiting, diarrhea, or cramps. In some reactions, progression to anaphylactic shock occurs. Reactions to latex may be severe. Contact urticaria can be diagnosed and the culprit identified using epicutaneous application, skin prick tests, or scratch tests in selected patients. Caution should be exercised and facilities for resuscitation available due to the (albeit rare) occurrence of anaphylaxis. The eliciting substances must be avoided.[10]

Treatment of Ordinary Urticaria, both Acute and Chronic, and Physical Urticarias in Pregnancy

The treatment of urticaria is with antihistamines. When considering antihistaminic use in pregnancy different views are expressed and, as more work is done and more experience gathered, views will evolve. The US Food and Drug Administration (FDA) has issued pregnancy categories for drug treatment in pregnancy and it is helpful to be aware of these. Pregnancy category A is given if adequate and well-controlled human studies have failed to demonstrate a risk to the fetus in the first trimester of pregnancy (and there is no evidence of risk in later trimesters). Pregnancy category B is given if a drug failed to demonstrate a risk to the fetus in animal reproduction studies and there is a lack of well-controlled studies in pregnant women or if animal studies have shown an adverse effect but adequate and well-controlled studies in pregnant women have failed to demonstrate a risk to the fetus in any trimester. Pregnancy category C is given if animal studies have shown an adverse effect on the fetus and there are no adequate and well-controlled studies in humans but potential benefits may well warrant the use of the drug in pregnant women. Pregnancy category D is applied when there is positive evidence of human fetal risk based on adverse reaction data from investigational or marketing experience or studies in humans, but potential benefits may warrant use of the drug in pregnant women despite potential risks. Pregnancy category X is used when studies in animals or humans have demonstrated fetal abnormalities and/or there is positive evidence of human fetal risk from investigational or marketing experience, and the risks involved in use of the drug in pregnant women clearly outweigh the benefits.[11] The FDA is currently working on modifying this labeling system. Australia and Germany also have pregnancy labeling systems that are not described.

Antihistamines are used in allergy, including drug reactions, allergic rhinitis, conjunctivitis, and insect bites, all of which occur concomitantly in pregnancy. They are also used in the treatment of pruritus and eczema, both atopic and contact. Pruritus is known to be a particularly pregnancy-related affliction. Many antihistamines are available over the counter and their use is not monitored and women may become pregnant while taking these medications. There are no reports of problems in practice from the use of antihistamines in humans and studies have shown no convincing increase in human teratogenicity.[12] An Israeli prospective study on the use of certain antihistamines showed no teratogenicity.[13] Likewise, a prospectively conducted Swedish study in which antihistamines were prescribed for nausea and vomiting showed beneficial effects on delivery outcome,[14] presumably related to control of the nausea and vomiting and no teratogenic effect of the antihistamines studied.

Although each individual's response to antihistamines is idiosyncratic, first-generation antihistamines generally are both sedating and have anticholinergic side effects. For these reasons, minimally sedating (second-generation) antihistamines are the treatment of choice for urticaria in Europe.[15] This group of drugs includes cetirizine, levocetirizine, fexofenadine hydrochloride, loratadine, desloratadine, acrivastine, mizolastine, bilastine, ebastine, and rupatadine.

As the shadow of possible teratogenicity lingers, ordinary urticaria may be undertreated in pregnancy because it is not a life-threatening disorder. It is important to be aware that the FDA gives cetirizine, loratadine, and levocetirizine a category B label and a category C label to fexofenadine and desloratadine. All drugs are given if clinically indicated. Looking at the first-generation antihistamines, the FDA gives chlorpheniramine, cyproheptadine, dexchlorpheniramine, and tripelennamine a B label and gives hydroxyzine and promethazine a C label.[16] All data must be considered against the background of lack of problems with antihistamines in practice and the Chinese saying, "It is easy to stand a pain but difficult to stand an itch."

Allergic rhinitis and its impact on asthma guidelines suggest that first-generation antihistamines should no longer be used.[17] The American College of Obstetricians and Gynecologists have suggested chlorpheniramine and tripenelamine or, if necessary, cetirizine and loratadine, after the first trimester.[18]

Both prospective studies used antihistamines, including minimally sedating antihistamines, during the first trimester with good effect. Because a baby is formed in the first trimester, however, many women try to avoid all drugs during this time.

European urticaria treatment guidelines suggest first-line minimally sedating antihistamines be taken regularly as first-line treatment for urticaria and advise updosing up to 4 times the manufacturer recommended dosages, at approximately 2-week intervals, when needed, to achieve control.[15,19] The author uses either cetirizine or loratadine in adequate dosage to control symptoms in pregnancy, although other doctors practice differently and different views are expressed. With regard to treatment during the first trimester, the author advises women that there have been no problems documented in those who have needed to take medication during the first trimester.

The author advises stopping antihistamines 3 to 7 days before delivery to avoid any adverse effects on neonates whose organs may not be sufficiently developed to metabolize the drug in the maternal blood.

There is no place for the use of maintenance systemic steroids in the treatment of urticaria either during pregnancy or outside of pregnancy. Occasional 2 to 3 day courses during a severe exacerbation are now considered appropriate.[15] Systemic corticosteroids are used to control asthma in pregnancy when necessary[17] and occasional use in urticaria is unlikely to cause gestational diabetes or preeclampsia. The question raised in the past relating to the development of cleft palate seems unconfirmed.[20]

Antihistamines are excreted in breast milk. First-generation antihistamines are not advised when breastfeeding; second-generation antihistamines are preferred. Breast milk levels are lower with cetirizine and loratadine and some investigators recommend these if breastfeeding.[21] Neonates are receiving a drug, however, and it might be more correct not to breastfeed.

Leukotriene antagonists (LTAs) are added to antihistamines as additional treatment of urticaria. These drugs are also used in the treatment of asthma. Those patients responding to LTAs can be continued in pregnancy, apart from zileuton, which should be avoided. No neonatal structural abnormalities or other perinatal problems have been identified.[17] The FDA categorizes LTAs as category B, apart from zileuton, which is category C. These drugs are excreted in breast milk. Ciclosporin has been used when necessary in pregnancy.[22] The FDA has labeled it category C. It has not caused teratogenicity but may be implicated, both in toxemia of pregnancy and in premature labor. Because it is excreted in breast milk, breastfeeding should not be carried out.[23]

Labor or delivery is not documented as unusual or different in those with either ordinary or any physical urticaria.

HEREDITARY ANGIOEDEMA

The management of hereditary angioedema (HAE) as part of ordinary urticaria in HAE is different to the treatment of angioedema as part of ordinary angioedema. Antihistamines, adrenaline, systemic steroids, and other standard second-line and third-line treatments are ineffective either as prophylaxis or treatment.

Classic HAE is an autosomal dominantly inherited disease with mutations on the C1-INH gene on chromosome 11. There are often new mutations so a family history is not always given. There are two types: type 1, where there is a quantitative decrease in the inhibitor of C1 esterase (the first component of complement), C1 esterase inhibitor; and type 2 where, the immunoreactive level of C1 esterase inhibitor is normal but there is a functional defect. Type 1 is most common; 85% of patients suffer from this type, with 15% suffering from type 2. The disease affects approximately 1:50,000 people. It most frequently presents in adolescence but presents occasionally in pregnancy and in the puerperium.[24,25]

Patients develop painless longer-lasting swellings, up to 7 days in duration, without urticaria, which affects both the skin and the subcutaneous tissues. These swellings are frequently peripheral but also affect the upper airways and the abdomen, sometimes with associated nausea and vomiting, simulating an acute surgical emergency, and patients can die of laryngeal edema.[26] If a pregnant woman with HAE attends with abdominal pain, it is reasonable to treat immediately for HAE in addition to informing a surgical colleague. The screening test to perform is a C4 level during an attack and, if this is low, to request a C1-INH level both quantitative and functional.

C4 is usually also low in-between attacks but occasionally is normal. The condition does not seem to become worse during pregnancy and there are many articles documenting safe pregnancy and outcome.[27–29] Usually attacks are treated when there is laryngeal involvement or swelling of the face or neck or of there is abdominal pain or in other body areas if they are severe. Maintenance treatment is given to prevent attacks. This increases the C1-INH levels; 50% of the normal C1-INH level seems to be adequate to avert attacks. Trauma provokes attacks and prophylaxis is given prior to trauma caused by dental or surgical interventions.[26] Although delivery is traumatic, complications during vaginal delivery are rare, but prophylaxis is advised before any intervention, including vacuum extraction, forceps, and caesarean section. The usual maintenance treatment given to these patients, danazol, cannot be used in pregnancy, because it may cause virilization in the female fetus if used after 8 weeks. This virilization is sometimes transient, sometimes is minor, and sometimes requires surgery in childhood.[30]

Other prophylactic treatments such as tranexamic acid and epsilon amino caproic acid are not recommended in pregnancy.

The current recommendation is that plasma-derived C1-INH be given during pregnancy as prophylaxis and treatment.[31] This is given intravenously and those patients with infrequent mild attacks generally attend the hospital. Ideally, when possible, and particularly when onset of attacks is rapid and hospital access difficult, patients should be offered a self-infusion program and trained to cannulate themselves and self-treat, under the guidance of an HAE unit.[32,33] One article describes twice-weekly C1-INH as prophylaxis during pregnancy and use in one patient during labor prior to delivery and 2 days later.[34] C1-INH has no adverse effects on the neonate. It seems prudent to have C1-INH available during delivery and the postpartum period. If a caesarean section is necessary, regional anesthesia is preferable to intubation because of the possible laryngeal trauma induced.[26] C1-INH cover is advised before and during any surgical intervention. If C1-INH is not available in an emergency, fresh frozen plasma may be substituted although it has theoretic disadvantages. The antikallirein inhibitor, ecallantide, and the bradykinin inhibitor, icatibant, are not yet considered as prophylaxis or treatment in pregnancy. In cases of laryngeal involvement, an ear, nose, and throat surgeon should be called immediately in addition to medical treatment being given.

The third type of HAE, type 3, usually occurs in families and in women, and occasionally men, and often exacerbates if an oral contraceptive pill is taken during the second half of the menstrual cycle and during pregnancy, when attacks may first present and may become more frequent and more severe. Estrogen may have some relationship with this disease. The C4 level and the C1-INH levels are normal and normally functioning but the symptomatology is the same as in types 1 and 2. In some families, there is a mutation in the gene encoding for factor 12. Treatment of this HAE is not as straightforward as in types 1 and 2 because although some respond to C1-INH, some do not.[26] To date, icatibant has been effective in some patients in whom it has been used. In an emergency it may be necessary to use this drug, although there are no safety data, because deaths occur in this condition, sometimes due to tongue swelling as well as to laryngeal involvement.

There is an acquired form of HAE associated with B-cell lymphoma and with the formation of antibodies. Tests show a normal C4 and a normal C1-INH but a low C1q level. This condition is unlikely to be present in pregnancy. Treatment is with systemic steroids and in association with a specialized clinic.

Overall, urticaria in pregnancy does not generally cause complications. It does not have an adverse impact on labor or delivery. Treatment of urticaria in pregnancy does not differ radically from treatment of nonpregnant patients.

REFERENCES

1. Black MM, Ambros-Rudolph C, Edwards L, et al, editors. Obstetric and Gynaecologic Dermatology. Mosby; 2008.
2. Warin RP, Cunliffe WJ, Greaves MW, et al. Recurrent Angioedema: familial and oestrogen-induced. Br J Dermatol 1986;115:731.
3. Le K, Wood G. A case of autoimmune progesterone dermatitis diagnosed by progesterone pessary. Australas J Dermatol 2011;52(2):139.
4. Lee AY, Lee KH, Lim YG. Oestrogen urticaria associated with pregnancy. Br J Dermatol 1999;141(4):774.
5. Kasperska-Zajac A, Brzoza Z, Rogala B. Lower serum concentration of dehydroepiandesterone sulphate in patients suffering from chronic idiopathic urticaria. Allergy 2007;61(12):1489.
6. Choi IS, Cui Y, Koh YA. Effects of dehydroepiandosterone on Th2 cytokine production in peripheral blood mononuclear cells from asthmatics. Korean J Intern Med 2008;23(4):176.
7. Lawlor F, Kobza Black A. In: Katsambas AD, Lotti TM, editors. European handbook of dermatological treatments. 3rd edition. Springer, in press.
8. Gei AF, Pacheco LD, Vanhook JW, et al. The use of a continuous infusion of epinephrine for anaphylactic shock during labor. Obstet Gynecol 2003;102(6):1332.
9. Lorraine JK. Successful pregnancy in a woman with cyclic angioedema and eosinophilia. Ann Allergy Asthma Immunol 1996;77(6):497.
10. Amin S, Maibach HI. In: Amin S, Lahti A, Maibach HI, editors. Contact urticaria syndrome. CRC press; 1997.
11. University of Washington Drug Formulary.
12. Gilboa SM, Strickland MJ, Olshan AF. Use of antihistamine medications during early pregnancy and isolated major malformations. Birth Defects Res A Clin Mol Terato 2009;85(2):137.
13. Diav-Citrin O, Shechtman S, Aharonovich A, et al. Pregnancy outcome after gestational exposure to loratadine or antihistamines: a prospective controlled cohort study. J Allergy Clin Immunol 2003;111(6):1239.
14. Kallen B. Use of antihistamine drugs in early pregnancy and delivery outcome. J Matern Fetal Neonatal Med 2002;11(3):146.
15. Zuberbier T. A summary of the new international EAACI/GA2EN/EDF/WAO guidelines in urticaria. World Allergy Organ J 2012;5(1):1.
16. Kar S, Krishnan A, Preetha K, et al. A review of antihistamines used during pregnancy. J Pharmacol Pharmacother 2012;3(2):105.
17. Bousquet J, Van Cauwenberge P, Khaltaev N. Aria workshop group, WHO, Allergic rhinitis and its impact on asthma. J Allergy Clin Immunol 2001;108(5):147.
18. Dombrowski MP, Huff R, Lipkowitz M. The use of newer asthma and allergy medications during pregnancy. Ann Allergy Asthma Immunol 2000;84:475.
19. Zuberbier T. Pharmacological rationale for the treatment of chronic urticaria with second generation non-sedating antihistamines at higher-than-standard doses. J Eur Acad Dermatol Venereol 2012;26:9.
20. Fraser FC, Sajoo A. Teratogenic potential of corticosteroids in humans. Teratology 1997;51:45.
21. Powell RJ, Du Toit GL, Siddique N, et al. BSACI guidelines for the management of chronic urticarial and angio-edema. Clin Exp Allergy 2007;37:631.
22. Wright S, Glover M, Baker H. Psoriasis ciclosporin and pregnancy. Arch Dermatol 1991;127(3):426.

23. American college of rheumatology. Available at: www.rheumatology.org.
24. Greaves MW. Hereditary angioedema. In: Lebwohl M, Heymann WR, Berth-Jones J, et al, editors. Treatment of skin disease. Saunders Elsevier; 2010. p. 292.
25. Cunningham DS, Jensen JT. Hereditary angioedema in the puerperium. J Reprod Med 1991;36(4):312.
26. Anon JB. Hereditary angioedema; a clinical review for the otolaryngologist. Ear Nose Throat J 2011;90:32.
27. Goring HD, Bork K, Spath PJ, et al. Hereditary angioedema in the German-speaking region. Hautarzt 1998;49:114 [in German].
28. Winnewisser J, Rossi M, Spath P, et al. Type 1 hereditary angioedema. Variability of clinical presentation and course within two large kindreds. J Intern Med 1997; 1:39.
29. Cox M, Holdcroft A. Hereditary angioedema; current management in pregnancy. Anaesthesia 1995;50(6):547.
30. Brunskill PJ. The effects of fetal exposure to danazol. Br J Obstet Gynaecol 1992; 99(3):212.
31. Caballero T, Farkas H, Bouillet L, et al. International consensus and practical guidelinws on the gynecologic and obstetric management of female patients with hereditary angioedema caused by C1 inhibitor deficiency. J Allergy Clin Immunol 2013;129(2):308.
32. Levi M, Choi G, Picavet C, et al. Self administration of C!-inhibitor concentrate in patients with hereditary or acquired angioedema caused by C1-inhibitor deficiency. J Allergy Clin Immunol 2006;117(4):904.
33. Longhurst HJ, Carr S, Khair K. C1-inhibitor concentrate home therapy for hereditary angioedema: a viable, effective, treatment option. Clin Exp Immunol 2007; 147(1):11.
34. Baker J, Sheffer A, Christiansen J, et al. Cinryze replacement therapy in hereditary angioedema and pregnancy [abstract]. J Allergy Clin Immunol 2009;123(2): S106.

Immunologic Contact Urticaria

John McFadden, DM, FRCP

KEYWORDS

• Contact urticaria • Atopic • Food • Cosmetics

KEY POINTS

- The wheal and flare reaction from direct contact with a chemical or protein agent is known as *contact urticaria*.
- Contact urticaria can be either nonimmunologic (no sensitization required) or immunologic (sensitization required).
- There are a wide variety of agents that can cause immunologic contact urticaria, and they can be either low-molecular-weight chemicals (haptens) or proteins.
- Immunologic contact urticaria can be easily missed clinically, particularly if the presentation is an apparent worsening of a preexisting dermatitis or urticaria.
- Management requires avoidance of the implicated agent.

NONIMMUNOLOGIC CONTACT URTICARIA

Nonimmunologic contact urticaria (NICU) is caused by a wide variety of agents. NICU reactions tend to be of less severity than immunologic contact urticaria (ICU) reactions. H-1 antihistamines do not seem to protect against NICU reactions from contact with agents such as benzoic acid or cinnamal (Lahti 1980). NICU reactions can be, however, inhibited by either oral or topical nonsteroidal antiinflammatory drugs.[1] Prostaglandin D2 is released during NICU reactions to agents such as benzoic acid and sorbic acid.[1]

Lahti and Basketter (1980) classified NICU agents into the following subheadings: animals (eg, arthropods, caterpillars, corals); foods (pepper mustard thyme); fragrances and flavorings (eg, balsam of Peru, cinnamic acid, cinnamic aldehyde); medicaments (eg, benzocaine, camphor, witch hazel); metals (cobalt); plants (nettles seaweed); and preservatives and disinfectants (eg, benzoic acid, formaldehyde).[2]

Skin testing for NICU can be performed using either an open or closed patch test reading at 20, 40, and 60 minutes.

Conflicts of interest: none.
Department of Cutaneous Allergy, St John's Institute of Dermatology, King's College, St Thomas' Hospital, Lambeth Palace Road, London SE1 7EH, UK
E-mail address: john.mcfadden@kcl.ac.uk

ICU

ICU involves a type 1 hypersensitivity mediated by allergen-specific immunoglobulin E (IgE) and, therefore, requires a sensitization phase. ICU can spread beyond the localized contact point. A staging system reflects the level of spread (**Box 1**).[3]

Broadly, 2 types of agents can cause ICU (Wang and colleagues 2013)[3]: proteins, such as natural rubber latex (NRL), with a high molecular weight that is often more than 10 000 kDA, and hapten chemicals, which conjugate with carrier proteins (eg, albumen), and the hapten-carrier protein can cause sensitization. Atopic individuals are more predisposed to developing ICU.

Diagnostic testing can be performed several ways; but the open test, which consists of gently rubbing the agent onto an open area of clinically normal skin and observing the site for 60 minutes, is most commonly used. Edema and erythema development denotes a positive test. Prick testing (or scratch testing) is also commonly used. As a rough guide, test reactions caused by ICU usually appear within 15 to 20 minutes, whereas reactions caused by NICU usually appear within 45 to 60 minutes.[4] In vitro radioallergosorbent test (RAST) tests for allergen-specific IgE are also used when available.[3]

NRL ALLERGY

Fourteen different allergenic proteins have been identified within NRL.[5] Hev b1 and Hev b 3 are the major protein allergens involved in patients with spina bifida. Hev b 5 is the main allergen in different risk groups and is recognized by 92% of health care workers and 56% of patients with spina bifida. Hev b 5 shows homology with kiwi acid protein. Hev b 6 is a major allergen, more important in health care workers than patients with spina bifida. Its sequence shows more than a 50% identity with chitinases from fruits, such as banana, avocado, and chestnut, giving rise to the latex-fruit syndrome.

Contact urticaria from latex gloves is the most frequent form of presentation of latex allergy and is more common than pruritus alone.[5]

Although rare, latex is the second cause of intraoperative anaphylaxis (after muscle relaxants).[5] Reactions to latex usually occur during the maintenance phase of operation, whereas when anaphylaxis is caused by opiates or muscle relaxants, it is usually during the induction phase.[5] The association between latex and fruit allergy varies, with the reported prevalence ranging between 21% and 58% of cases. The severity can also vary between mild itching and anaphylaxis. The most common foods implicated are banana, avocado, chestnut, and kiwi. Less commonly reported are papaya, lychee, fig, peach, potato, chickpea, spinach, and the leafy green vegetable phukwaan-ban.[4]

Latex allergy may not always be suspected from the history. Prick testing has a sensitivity of 93% and specificity of 100%.[5] The sensitivity of serum RAST for

| Box 1 |
Staging system
Stage 1: Localized urticaria
Stage 2: Generalized urticaria
Stage 3: Urticaria plus extracutaneous manifestations (rhinitis, conjunctivitis, asthma, gastrointestinal symptoms, angioedema)
Stage 4: Systemic anaphylaxis shock

allergen-specific IgE to latex is also high. Prick testing is considered generally safe, but isolated cases of anaphylaxis have been reported.[6]

People with a latex allergy should be aware of products besides gloves that contain latex both in the hospital and home setting. These products include (in the hospital) catheter stoppers, elastic bandages, tourniquets tubes, and masks. In the domestic setting, these include balloons, condoms, mats, bottles, and baby bottle nipples. Alternatives for latex are available and include nitrile, neoprene, and polyvinyl chloride. Nitrile gives similar protection against infection as that offered by latex; synthetic polymers, such as neoprene, can be used as an alternative for surgical procedures.[5]

Occasionally, health care workers can develop contact urticaria to agents other than latex, such as handling the drug **donepezil** (used for Alzheimer), or disinfecting compounds, such as **dodecyl dimethyl ammonium chloride**.[3]

FOOD

Virtually any food is capable of eliciting an ICU response.[7] ICU within the food industry is a major occupational problem. Food handlers can develop ICU from agents such as **apple, potato, carrot,** and **tomato**.[3] Shellfish and seafood are also common sources of ICU. **Prawn** and **lobster** as sources of ICU were recently highlighted.[8] Cooks who have ICU to raw seafood can usually tolerate eating cooked seafood provided the seafood is protein denatured by cooking.[9] Wang and Maibach[3] (2013) highlight the recent problems of **wheat** allergens among bakers. A new group of wheat allergens capable of causing type I hypersensitivity (asthma and contact urticaria) have been identified.[10]

Certain foods are repeatedly reported as causing problems.

Seafood

Hjorth[11] (1975) reported on housewives with atopic dermatitis who develop contact urticaria to **haddock** and **herring**. He also reported a similar case of contact urticaria to **prawns** in a sandwich maker.[12] A 12-year-old atopic boy acquired contact urticaria to codfish.[13] A 19-year-old man developed generalized urticaria, angioedema of the face and lips, and a dry cough 20 minutes after his cousin, a fisherman, had greeted him with an embrace.[14] Open tests with raw **cod** and **sardine** gave large wheal-and-flare responses at both sites after 10 minutes. After 20 minutes, he complained of generalized pruritus and nasal irritation and was tachycardic, necessitating treatment with epinephrine. His RAST test was positive to **codfish, eel,** and **carp**.

Fruit

Konstantinou and Grattan[15] (2008) reviewed the cross-reactivity between pollens and fruit (**Table 1**). Clinically, this usually manifests as a mucosal ICU. They term this *food*

Table 1	
Common cross-reactions between pollen/plant allergens and fruit	
Pollen/Plant Allergen	**Common Fruit Cross-reaction**
Birch	Apple, pear, carrot, celery, tomato, cherry
Mugwort	Carrot, celery, aniseed, peach
Ragweed	Melon
Goosefoot	Banana melon, peach
Latex	Avocado, banana, chestnut, kiwi, mango, melon, fig, papaya, tomato

contact hypersensitivity syndrome (also known as *oral allergy syndrome*). There are oropharyngeal sensations of pruritus, tingling and burning, which are accompanied by angioedema of the lips, oral mucosa, soft palate or tongue, shortly after eating raw (uncooked) foods. Patients may also experience exacerbation of hay fever symptoms. Handling the fruit can also cause contact urticaria. Gastrointestinal symptoms, such as diarrhea and stomachache, are uncommon. Rarely, life-threatening reactions with angioedema or shock have been reported. Denaturing the protein by cooking usually stops any reaction, with the exception of **nuts** and sometimes **celery**.

Immediate hypersensitivity to **apples** is perhaps the most common fruit allergy. In a study of 262 patients who exhibited fresh fruit and vegetable allergic reactions, 139 (53.1%) were allergic to apples.[16] The major allergen in apples is Mal d 1, a protein structure homologous with the birch pollen major protein Bet v 1.[17] In Spain, 70 patients with a **peach** allergy were diagnosed through clinical history, skin prick test, and open oral challenge and rub test.[18] Oral allergy syndrome (86%) was the most common symptom, followed by contact urticaria (61%) and systemic symptoms (26%). Sixty-seven percent were allergic to peach pulp, and 36% reported symptoms to canned peach. Eighty-one percent of the patients with a peach allergy also had a pollen allergy, and 73% had asthma. The nonpollen allergic patients were more prone to systemic symptoms. A patient diagnosed with contact urticaria to **lychee** had positive skin prick tests to both lychee and **mango**, demonstrating the close botanic affinity between these two fruits.[19]

Vegetables

With testing for immediate hypersensitivity on symptomatic gardeners and greenhouse workers, 2 were positive to **lettuce** and 2 to the **tomato** plant.[20] Sensitivity to **potatoes** can be so severe that merely rubbing the intact skin with a raw potato may cause a wheal to form.[13] Contact urticaria to raw potato is not uncommon in chefs and domestic cooks, and the reactions can be severe. A 4-year-old boy who bit a raw potato developed urticaria, angioedema, respiratory distress, vomiting, and diarrhea.[21] A skin prick test was markedly positive. Of 27 patients diagnosed with **asparagus** allergy, 10 had IgE-mediated contact urticaria after handling asparagus.[22] A minority developed systemic symptoms after oral ingestion. An 84-year-old man presented with a 2-year history of swelling of the face, neck, and dorsum of the hands and arms.[23] The eruption would always arise a few minutes after tending **runner bean plants** in his garden. A prick test to runner beans demonstrated a 5-mm wheal. This case was only the second case reported of runner bean ICU. Case reports, often occupational, have also been reported from **carrot, garlic, paprika, and mustard**.[24–27]

Meat

Contact urticaria has been reported with **chicken, lamb, turkey, calf's liver, beef, sausage, and venison**, particularly in patients with preexisting hand dermatitis.[13,28] A 60-year-old woman complained that her hand dermatitis worsened when preparing beef burgers, and her lips would swell when eating beef burgers.[29] A prick test to beef was positive but negative to chicken and pork. A 21-year-old hunter had contact with game most of his life, since he hunted as a boy.[28] Red deer and roe deer were stored around his farm until being sold. Over 2 years, he had noticed localized urticaria after contact with raw meat and the hair of the roe deer. Prick tests and rub tests confirmed immediate hypersensitivity to roe deer meat and hair. A minority of children with meat allergy can experience oral mucosal ICU.[30]

Milk and Egg

Oranje and colleagues[31] report on 40 children presenting with immediate contact urticaria rash around the mouth after consuming egg or milk, and 34 patients out of 40 also suffered from atopic dermatitis. A 25-year-old man developed urticaria when embracing his lactating wife and when in contact with the milky vomitus of his newborn child.[32] A prick test to cow's milk was negative but positive to his wife's milk. Contact urticaria to cow's milk in an 8-month-old girl was reported.[13] After heating the milk to 80°C there was no further problem.

COSMETICS
Fragrances

Fragrances can cause immediate and delayed hypersensitivity reactions. A multicenter study in Hungary found that 6.1% of patients with a contact allergy to fragrance chemicals also had immediate contact urticaria reactions.[33] They found that contact urticaria was provoked by the fragrance chemicals (in order of most frequent) **cinnamic aldehyde, cinnamic alcohol,** and **evernia prunastri**. Cinnamic chemicals may be in some foods, and evernia prunastri is found naturally as oak moss. Some of the reactions from the cinnamic agents may have been nonimmunologic. Yamamoto and colleagues[34] (2002) describe a case of allergic contact dermatitis to **geraniol**.

Ammonium Persulfate

Ammonium persulfate is used in hair bleaching but has been reported to cause contact urticaria. A hairdresser developed contact urticaria and angioedema after airborne exposure.[35] NICU can also occur with ammonium persulfate exposure.

Contact urticaria can occur from exposure to **hydrolyzed wheat protein** in cosmetic creams and shampoos.[36] Three patients reported reactions to a hair conditioner containing hydrolyzed wheat protein, one on the hands and 2 acute urticaria on the head and neck. All were atopic patients.

HAIR DYES

Temesvari[37] (1984) reported a case of contact urticaria from aromatic amine hair dye; since then, there have been a small number of cases continuing to be reported but some of an apparently serious nature.[37] However, before attributing a case of severe contact urticaria from hair dye to the aromatic amine contained in the hair dye, such as **p-phenylenediamine**, 3 points should be considered. Firstly, other agents within the product (such as hydrolyzed protein) may be the culprit. Secondly, other dyes, such as **basic blue 99, henna, and reactive dyes,** may be implicated.[38] Thirdly, a severe allergic contact dermatitis to aromatic amine hair dye with severe facial swelling may mimic angioedema even to the point of difficulty in breathing, which is caused by the edema constricting the airways.[39]

TOPICAL MEDICAMENTS

ICU may occur from the active agent or from the preservative, base, or additives. A wide range of antibiotics (**bacitracin, cephalosporin, chloramphenicol, gentamicin, neomycin, penicillin, rifampicin, and streptomycin**) have been reported as causing contact urticaria and most also have the ability to cause (rarely) anaphylaxis.[13] Topical **local anesthetics** also have the ability to cause ICU. Ryan and colleagues[40] (1980) reported on mucosal contact urticaria to **benzocaine,** whereas Waton and colleagues[41]

(2004) reported on contact urticaria to **lidocaine** from the use of a local anesthetic cream used for venesection. It is claimed that most cases of contact urticaria to local anesthetic agents are nonimmunologic.[42]

A 36-year-old woman and a 16-year-old boy developed contact urticaria to **nitrogen mustard** used for treating mycoses fungoides.[43] Both individuals had urticaria and anaphylactoid reactions, and both had previous exposure to nitrogen mustard.

Sunscreens have been an occasional source of contact urticaria. Landers and colleagues[44] (2003) reported a patient with both immediate and delayed type hypersensitivity to **oxybenzone**.

Additives to topical medicaments can also cause problems. A severe urticarial reaction with systemic involvement resembling an anaphylactic reaction occurred after the use of a topical steroid.[45] It was found that this reaction was caused by **hexylene glycol**, an excipient in the formulation. Glycols are widely used in cosmetics, foods, and drugs, particularly topical medications. A 42-year-old woman presented with a clear history of pruritus and redness within 30 minutes of applying certain topical preparations, including emollients and corticosteroid creams.[46] There were marked urticarial reactions to the preservative **p-chloro-m-cresol** and to the steroid creams and emollient, which contained p-chloro-m-cresol. Codreanu and colleagues[47] (2006) emphasized the importance of possible allergic reactions to food proteins in topical medicaments and cosmetic products.

ANIMAL HANDLERS

Animal handlers can develop ICU to animal hair and secretions.[3] In Finland, cows are kept indoors most of the year so dander exposure is increased. ICU to **cow dander** is one of the most common occupational diseases in Finland.[3] **Dog and rat saliva, animal hair, cow placenta, rat tails, and guinea pigs** can all be causes of ICU on handling animals.[13] Agrup and Sjostedt[48] (1985) investigated 101 laboratory technicians for a possible allergy to laboratory animals. Fourteen cases of contact urticaria caused by rats were found. Other animals causing contact urticaria were mouse (7), guinea pig (4), and cat (2).[48]

PLANT HANDLERS

Exposure to several plants can cause contact urticaria, so it is not surprising that occupational contact urticaria is seen. Some examples are **Compositae and ivy**.[3] Other common causes of ICU to plants in gardeners include **yucca, spathe flower, and Chinese rose**.[3] Paulsen colleagues'[20] report (1998) on gardeners and greenhouse workers implicated **Christmas cactus, Barberton daisy,** and **Madagascar jasmine** as the most common causes of occupational plant ICU. An IgE-binding protein known as profilin is present in several plant species and has been suggested as a common causative agent for ICU.[49]

ENZYMES

After 1 year in his job, a 27-year-old atopic process man in a chemical enzyme factory developed whealing lasting 1 to 2 hours after contact with **detergent protease** enzymes.[50] Prick testing to a *Bacillus subtilis*-derived protease enzyme was strongly positive as was a RAST assay. Other enzymes reported as causing ICU include **amylase** (especially in baker's),[13,51] **cellulose enzymes**,[52] **xylene** (an aromatic hydrocarbon rather than an enzyme) in laboratory workers,[53] and **papain** (wide pharmacologic, domestic, and industrial use).[54]

RECENT CASE REPORTS

A 3-year-old atopic boy was referred after developing urticaria and angioedema immediately after he had applied his mother's moisturizing cream onto her skin.[55] A prick test to the moisturizing cream was positive as was prick tests to **macadamia nuts and hydrolyzed wheat protein**, both contained in the moisturizing cream. Because this was the first time the boy handled the cream sensitization must have been through previous proxy exposure to the cream on the mother's skin. The authors note that complete avoidance of hydrolyzed wheat exposure is hard to achieve through its common use in cosmetics and processed foods.

A 33-year-old man had worked for the last 5 years in a company processing meals containing seafood, mostly **squid**.[56] His professional duties included managing a crusher machine and cleaning these machines after use. After 1 year, he developed asthma, rhinitis, conjunctivitis, and contact urticaria. He had further symptoms 3 years later when cleaning the crusher machines with pressurized water. On prick testing to squid, there was a positive reaction with 12×30 mm wheal reaction after 15 minutes, and then 3 more wheals developed. Occupational allergy to squid has rarely been reported before.

A 19-year-old woman with bleeding gums was advised to use oral prophylaxis and was prescribed **chlorhexidine** mouthwash to be used twice daily for 3 weeks.[57] The next day, she presented with urticaria on her forehead and face, the front of her elbows and forearms, the side and upper back region of the neck, and on the lower abdomen. On questioning, she had used the mouthwash for 1 minute. Prick testing to chlorhexidine confirmed type 1 hypersensitivity. In a previous study, 6 patients were reported to develop urticaria, dyspnea and anaphylactic shock caused by topical application of chlorhexidine, with testing confirming type 1 hypersensitivity.[58] Chlorhexidine can also be a rare contact allergen, usually from its use in the health care setting, the resulting dermatitis marked by the severity of the reaction.[59]

ICU to another antiseptic agent has also recently been highlighted. A 44-year-old nonatopic woman presented with a 5-year history of pruritic reddish wheals on her skin/mucosa immediately after contact with some soaps and topical products.[60] Recently, the use of a certain toothpaste had caused immediate swelling of her lips and tongue, leading to breathing difficulties. Kissing her husband, who was using the same toothpaste, caused swelling of her lips within minutes. The suspected products that she reacted to, namely, a toothpaste, moisturizer, metronidazole cream, and antibacterial liquid soap, all contained **triclosan** at concentrations of 0.2% to 0.5%. Early reading of patch tests showed severe urticarial reactions to the metronidazole cream and triclosan (2.0% pet.) within 10 to 15 minutes. No reactions were observed with other ingredients that could potentially cause ICU. Delayed type reactions to triclosan were negative. Triclosan is a broad-spectrum antiseptic used in a variety of household and personal care products, such as deodorants, toothpastes, hand soaps, dish soaps, facial cleansers, bath oils, emollients, and topical medicaments. It is also used as an antiseptic in hospitals. The researchers concluded that the diagnosis was ICU rather than NICU because the reaction did not stay localized, with angioedema leading to breathing difficulties. Also, the immediate skin test appeared within 15 minutes, favoring ICU, whereas NICU reactions often occur within 45 to 60 minutes.

A 27-year-old woman applied 0.5% **levofloxacin** eyedrops.[61] Immediately, she developed conjunctival hyperemia, nasal discharge, and sneezing. Subsequently, facial edema, pruritic rash on the trunk and extremities, and mild dyspnea developed. Prick testing to 0.5% levofloxacin hydrate solution was positive. The researchers noted that levofloxacin is the most widely used antibiotic eyedrop in Japan. Although contact urticaria syndrome to these eyedrops is rare, 2 cases of anaphylaxis had been reported directly to the pharmaceutical company.

A 26-year-old woman experienced several episodes of fish allergy since she was 2 years old, developing respiratory distress and widespread wheals within 15 minutes after eating fish.[62] She subsequently strictly avoided eating fish. She also had a history of asthma, atopic dermatitis, allergic rhinitis, and egg allergy. When she was 24 years old, she developed an urticarial eruption on the site where she had applied a cosmetic cream containing **codfish-derived elastin**. The RAST test was positive for codfish, tuna, salmon, mackerel, flatfish, sardine, and salmon. Immunoblot analysis confirmed the presence of IgE antibodies to codfish elastin. Elastin, which is commonly used in cosmetic topical formulations, is traditionally isolated from bovine tendon. Because of the perceived risk of bovine spongiform encephalopathy, there has been a trend to use elastin extracted from fish, particularly the aortic arch of codfish, bonito, yellowtail, and tuna.

A woman (age undisclosed) ingested **sesame**-coated sticks.[63] She suffered intense swelling of the oral mucosa after 15 minutes. She had previously been asymptomatic when ingesting sesame, and personal medical history was unremarkable except for Graves disease. Dermatologic examination revealed edema and erythema on the buccal mucosa, the hard palate, and tongue. The reaction faded within 6 hours after the use of antihistamine and local corticosteroid administration. Prick testing revealed a positive reaction of a 5-mm wheal to sesame. An oral provocation test 1 month later replicated the patient's symptoms. Sesame allergy has increased in the last few years because of the ubiquitous use of oil-rich sesame seeds in cooked and processed food, such as buns, bread, cakes, cereals, salad dressings, and humus.[64] Sesame may also be present in oriental and Middle Eastern foods. Sesame allergy may either coexist or cross-react with peanut allergy. An atopic background is noted with most patients with a sesame allergy. Despite the high population exposure to sesame, there is a paucity of case reports involving sesame allergy.

A 29-year-old woman was referred with recurrent urticarial wheals on the forearms.[65] She was employed as a forensic technician and had regular exposure to *Cannabis* plants at work for the last 2 years. More recently, she noticed this rash developing within a few minutes of contact with the plant, particularly the *Cannabis* flowers. Prick testing with dried extract of *Cannabis* produced a 4-mm wheal; but a 13-mm wheal and flare was observed with an extract of immature flowering plant, and a 15-mm wheal and flare was observed with an extract of flowering material, implicating the flowering version as more allergenic. The researchers note that 4 people in the same workplace reported similar symptoms, so ICU to *Cannabis* may be more common than reported.

REFERENCES

1. Lahti A. Non-immunologic contact urticaria. Acta Derm Venereol 1980;60:1–49.
2. Lahti A, Basketter DA. Immediate contact reactions. Chapter 5. In: Rycroft R, editor. Contact dermatitis. 3rd edition. Berlin: Springer-Verlag; 2001. p. 111–32.
3. Wang CY, Maibach HI. Immunologic contact urticaria- the human touch. Cutan Ocul Toxicol 2013;32(2):154–60.
4. Amin S, Lahti A, Maibach HI. Contact urticaria and contact urticaria syndrome (immediate contact reactions). In: Zhai H, Wilhelm KP, Maibach HI, editors. Marzulli and Maibach's dermatotoxicology. 7th edition. Boca Raton (FL): CRC Press; 2008. p. 525–36.

5. Cabanes N, Igea JM, de la Hoz B, et al. Latex allergy: position paper. J Investig Allergol Clin Immunol 2012;22(5):313–30.
6. Nicolau N, Johnston GA. Anaphylaxis following prick testing with natural rubber latex. Contact Dermatitis 2002;47(2):251–2.
7. Brancacio RR, Alvarez MS. Contact allergy to food. Dermatol Ther 2004;17: 302–13.
8. Teo S, Teik-Jin Goon A, Siang LH, et al. Occupational dermatoses in restaurant, catering, and fast-food outlets in Singapore. Occup Med 2009;59:466–71.
9. Onesimo R, Giorgio G, Pill S, et al. Isolated contact urticaria caused by immunoglobulin E-mediated fish allergy. Isr Med Assoc J 2012;14:11–3.
10. Cirla AM. Asthma and baker's allergy: experience with health programs. G Ital Med Lav Ergon 2011;7:152–5.
11. Hjorth N, Reed-Petersen J. Berufsekzeme durch proteine. Z Hautkr 1975;50: 85–7.
12. Hjorth N, Weissmann K. Occupational dermatitis in chefs and sandwich makers. Contact Dermatitis Newsletters 1972;11:300.
13. Rietschel RL, Fowler JS. Contact urticaria. Chapter 34. In: Rietschel RL, Fowler FS, editors. From fisher's contact dermatitis. Baltimore (MD): Wilkins and Wilkins; 1995. p. 778–807.
14. Kalogeromitros D, Armenaka M, Katsarou A. Contact urticaria and systemic anaphylaxis from codfish. Contact Dermatitis 1999;41:170–1.
15. Konstantinou GN, Grattan CEH. Food contact hypersensitivity syndrome: the mucosal contact urticaria paradigm. Clin Exp Dermatol 2008;33:383–9.
16. Ortolani C, Ispano M, Pastorello E, et al. The oral allergy syndrome. Ann Allergy 1988;61:47–52.
17. Holm J, Baerentzen G, Gajhede M, et al. Molecular basis of allergic cross-reactivity between group 1 major allergens from birch and apple. J Chromatogr B Biomed Sci Appl 2001;756:307–13.
18. Cuesta-Herranz J, Lazaro M, de las Heras M, et al. Peach allergy pattern: experience in 70 patients. Allergy 1998;53:78–82.
19. Giannattasio M, Serafini M, Guarrera P, et al. Contact urticaria from litchi fruit (Litchi chinensis Sonn). Contact Dermatitis 1995;33:67.
20. Paulsen E, Stahl Skov P, Andersen KE. Immediate skin and mucosal symptoms from pot plants and vegetables in gardeners and greenhouse workers. Contact Dermatitis 1998;39:166–70.
21. Beausoleil J, Spergel JM, Pawlowski NA. Anaphylaxis to raw potato. Ann Allergy Asthma Immunol 2001;86:68–70.
22. Tabar AL, Alvarez-Puebla MJ, Gomez B, et al. Diversity of asparagus allergy: clinical and immunological features. Clin Exp Allergy 2004;34:131–6.
23. Narayan S, Sansom JE. Contact urticaria from runner bean. Contact Dermatitis 2002;47:243–4.
24. Moreno-Ancillo A, Gil-Adrados AC, Dominiquez-Noche C, et al. Occupational asthma due to carrot in a cook. Allergol Immunopathol 2005;33(5):288–90.
25. Jappe U, Bonnekoh B, Hausen BM, et al. Garlic-related dermatoses: case report and review of the literature. Am J Contact Dermatitis 1999;10:37–9.
26. Foti C, Carino M, Cassano N, et al. Occupational contact urticaria from paprika. Contact Dermatitis 1997;37:135.
27. Valsecchi R, Leghissa P, Cortinovis R, et al. Contact urticaria syndrome from mustard in anchovy fillet sauce. Contact Dermatitis 2000;42:114.
28. Geyer E, Kranke B, Derhaschnig J, et al. Contact urticaria from roe deer meat and hair. Contact Dermatitis 1998;39:34.

29. Fisher AA. Allergic contact urticaria to raw beef: histopathology of the two specific wheal and flare reaction at the scratch test site. Contact Dermatitis 1982; 8(6):425.

30. Theler B, Brockow K, Dutta M, et al. Clinical presentation and diagnosis of meat allergy in Switzerland and Southern Germany. Swiss Med Wkly 2009; 139(17–18):264–70.

31. Oranje AP, Aarsen RS, Mulder PG, et al. Immediate contact reaction's to cow's milk and egg in atopic children. Acta Derm Venereol 1991;71(3):263–6.

32. Makinen-Kiljunen S, Plosila M. A father's IgE-mediated contact urticaria from mother's milk. J Allergy Clin Immunol 2004;113:353–4.

33. Temesvari E, Nemeth I, Balo-Banga M, et al. Multicentre study of fragrance allergy in Hungary. Contact Dermatitis 2002;46:325–30.

34. Yamamoto A, Morita A, Tsuji T, et al. Contact urticaria from geraniol. Contact Dermatitis 2002;46(1):52.

35. Poltronieri A, Patrini L, Pigatto P, et al. Occupational allergic 'march'. Med Lav 2010;101:403–8.

36. Niinimaka A, Niinimaka M, Makinen-Kiijunen S, et al. Contact urticaria from protein hydrolysates in hair conditioners. Allergy 1998;53:1078–82.

37. Temesvari E. Contact urticaria from paraphenylenediamine. Contact Dermatitis 1984;11(2):125.

38. Davari P, Maibach HI. Contact urticaria to cosmetic and industrial dyes. Clin Exp Dermatol 2010;36:1–5.

39. Tukenmez Demerci G, Kivanic Altunay I, Atis G, et al. Allergic contact dermatitis mimicking angioedema due to paraphenylenediamine hypersensitivity: a case report. Cutan Ocul Toxicol 2012;31(3):250–2.

40. Ryan ME, Davis BM, Marks JG. Contact urticaria and allergic contact dermatitis to benzocaine gel. J Am Acad Dermatol 1980;2:221–2.

41. Waton J, Boulanger A, Trechot PH, et al. Contact urticaria from EMLA cream. Contact Dermatitis 2004;51:284–7.

42. Phillips JF, Yates AB, Deshazo RD. Approach to patients with suspected hypersensitivity to local anaesthetics. Am J Med Sci 2007;334(3):190–6.

43. Grunnet E. Contact urticaria and anaphylactoid reaction induced by topical application of nitrogen mustard. Br J Dermatol 1976;94:101–3.

44. Landers M, Laws S, Storrs FJ. Contact urticaria, allergic contact dermatitis, and photoallergic contact dermatitis from oxybenzone. Am J Contact Dermatitis 2003;14:33–4.

45. Spoerl D, Schere K, Bircher AJ. Contact urticaria with systemic symptoms due to hexylene glycol in a topical corticosteroid: case report and review of hypersensitivity to glycols. Dermatology 2010;220(3):238–42.

46. Walker SM, Chalmers RJ, Beck MH. Contact urticaria due to p-chloro-m-cresol. Br J Dermatol 2004;151:936–7.

47. Codreanu F, Morisset M, Cordebar V, et al. Risk of allergy to food proteins in topical medicinal agents and cosmetics. Eur Ann Allergy Clin Immunol 2006; 38(4):126–30.

48. Agrup G, Sjostedt L. Contact urticaria in laboratory technicians working with animals. Acta Derm Venereol 1985;65(2):111–5.

49. Amaro C, Goosens AN. Immunological occupational contact urticaria and contact dermatitis from proteins: a review. Contact Dermatitis 2008;58: 67–75.

50. Kanerva L, Vanhanen M. Occupational allergic contact urticaria and rhinoconjunctivitis from a detergent protease. Contact Dermatitis 2001;45:49–51.

51. Kanerva L, VAnhanen M, Tupasela O. Occupational allergic contact dermatitis from fungal but not bacterial alpha-amylase. Contact Dermatitis 1997;36(3): 306–7.
52. Kanerva L, Vanhanen M, Tupasela O. Occupational contact urticaria from cellulase enzyme. Contact Dermatitis 1998;38:176–7.
53. Weiss RR, Mowad C. Contact urticaria from xylene. Am J Contact Dermatitis 1998;9(2):125–7.
54. Quinones D, Alonso S, Lopez R, et al. Contact urticaria, rhinoconjunctivitis and bronchial asthma from occupational use of papain. Allergol Immunopathol 1998; 27:273–5.
55. Leheron C, Bourrier T, Albertini M, et al. Immediate contact urticaria caused by hydrolysed wheat proteins in a child via maternal skin contact sensitisation. Contact Dermatitis 2013;68:376–83.
56. Wiszniewska M, Tymoszuk D, Pas-Wyroslak A, et al. Occupational allergy to squid *(Loligo valgaris)*. Occup Med 2013;63:298–300.
57. Chopra V, Chopra H, Sharma A. Allergic urticaria: a case report of rare skin allergy with a common mouthwash. Indian J Dermatol 2013;58(1):298–301.
58. Okano M, Nomura M, Hata S, et al. Anaphylactic symptoms due to chlorhexidine gluconate. Arch Dermatol 1989;125:50–2.
59. Goon AT, White IR, Rycroft RJ, et al. Allergic contact dermatitis from chlorhexidine. Dermatitis 2004;15(1):45–7.
60. Ozkaya E, Bozkurt PK. An unusual case of triclosan-induced immunological contact urticaria. Contact Dermatitis 2013;68:117–28.
61. Saito M, Nakada T. Contact urticaria syndrome from eye drops: levofloxacin hydrate ophthalmic solution. J Dermatol 2013;40(2):130–1.
62. Nishida K, Tateishi C, Tsurata D, et al. Contact urticaria caused by a fish-derived elastin-containing cosmetic cream. Contact Dermatitis 2012;67:171–7.
63. Erkek E, Sahin S, Ince U, et al. Mucosal contact urticaria to sesame seeds. J Eur Acad Dermatol Venereol 2012;26:790–1.
64. Perkins MS. Raising awareness of sesame allergy. Pharm J 2001;267:757–8.
65. Williams C, Thompstone J, Wilkinson M. Work-related contact urticaria to Cannabis sativa. Contact Dermatitis 2008;58:62–3.

Hereditary Disorders Presenting with Urticaria

Nobuo Kanazawa, MD, PhD

KEYWORDS

- KIT • C1-inhibitor • Bradykinin • NLRP3 inflammasome • IL-1β • NLRP12 • PLCγ2
- Autoinflammatory syndrome

KEY POINTS

- Hereditary disorders presenting with urticaria are not common and may not be encountered by most physicians.
- Hereditary disorders presenting with urticaria can be easily missed or misdiagnosed without correct knowledge.
- With proper diagnosis and understanding of the genetic cause and consequent pathogenesis, disease-specific essential therapeutic regimens can be offered.
- Recent discovery of the genetic origins for rare cases with distinct hereditary cold urticaria encourages examination of more cases.
- With rapid progress in genetic analysis, further insights into undefined hereditary urticaria will emerge in the near future.
- The knowledge obtained is promising for the development of novel therapeutics.

INTRODUCTION

Hereditary diseases listed in the latest clinical guideline for urticaria include *KIT* mutations–induced urticaria pigmentosa (mastocytosis), *C1NH* mutations–induced hereditary angioedema (HAE), and *NLRP3* mutations–induced cryopyrin-associated periodic syndromes (CAPS).[1] Although acquired somatic mutations in the *KIT* gene have a central role in the pathogenesis of mastocytosis, some germline *KIT* mutations have been reported in rare familial cases of pediatric mastocytosis.[2] HAE is a potentially life-threatening disease, and a precise diagnosis is required for replacement therapy of complement component 1 inhibitor (C1-INH).[3] CAPS are the most studied hereditary autoinflammatory disorders with dysregulated inflammasome signaling,

Funding Sources: Japan Society for the Promotion of Science, Ministry of Health, Labor and Welfare.
Conflict of Interest: None.
Department of Dermatology, Wakayama Medical University, 811-1 Kimiidera, Wakayama 641-0012, Japan
E-mail address: nkanazaw@wakayama-med.ac.jp

Immunol Allergy Clin N Am 34 (2014) 169–179
http://dx.doi.org/10.1016/j.iac.2013.08.001
0889-8561/14/$ – see front matter © 2014 Elsevier Inc. All rights reserved.

immunology.theclinics.com

for which a precise diagnosis is also critical for early intervention with anti-interleukin (IL)-1β therapy.[4]

In recent years, distinct syndromes with urticarial skin lesions, termed familial cold-induced autoinflammatory syndrome 2 (FCAS2) and FCAS3, have been designated as NLRP12-associated periodic syndromes (NAPS12) and PLCG2-associated antibody deficiency and immune dysregulation (PLAID), respectively, by identification of their genetic origins.[5–7] Moreover, there still remain more than a few cases with genetically undefined hereditary urticaria. The diseases discussed in this article are summarized in **Table 1**.

MASTOCYTOSIS

Mastocytosis (also known as mast cell disease, OMIM #154800) is divided into cutaneous mastocytosis (CM) and systemic mastocytosis (SM).[2] CM includes urticaria pigmentosa (UP), mastocytoma of the skin, and diffuse CM. In contrast to CM confined to the skin, SM is defined by mast cell infiltration in at least one extracutaneous lesion with or without cutaneous involvement (**Table 2**). CM is more commonly observed in children, especially before 6 months of age, but also affects adults mainly in the third to fourth decade.[8] Whereas pediatric CM spontaneously regresses before puberty in most cases, UP in adults has a significant risk of progression to SM.[9] UP is the most common variant of CM, and is characterized by disseminated brown macules or papules.[10] Consistent with the histologic feature showing massive mast cell infiltration in the papillary dermis with epidermal hypermelanosis, scratching the lesions induces mast cell degranulation and causes local flare and wheal reaction. This phenomenon, called Darier's sign, is useful for the diagnosis of UP. Similarly, cutaneous symptoms such as urticarial rashes, edema, and pruritus can be triggered by mechanical and thermal stimuli. Mastocytoma of the skin usually presents a few brown or orange plaques or

Table 1
Hereditary diseases with urticaria

Designation		OMIM Number	Responsible Gene
Mastocytosis		#154800	*KIT*
Hereditary angioedema (HAE)	Types I and II	#106100	*CINH*
	Type III	#610618	*F12*
Cryopyrin-associated periodic syndrome (CAPS)	Familial cold-induced autoinflammatory syndrome (FCAS)	#120100	*NLRP3*
	Muckle-Wells syndrome (MWS)	#191900	
	Chronic infantile neurologic cutaneous articular (CINCA) syndrome	#607115	
NLRP12-associated periodic syndrome (NAPS12)		#611762	*NLRP12*
PLCG2-associated antibody deficiency and immune dysregulation (PLAID)		#614468	*PLCG2*
Aquagenic urticaria		191850	Unknown
Familial localized heat urticaria		191950	Unknown
Dermodistortive urticaria		125630	Unknown
Familial dermographism		125635	Unknown

Table 2		
Classification of mastocytosis		
Variant	**Subvariant**	**Prognosis (Expected Median Survival)**
Cutaneous mastocytosis (CM)	Urticaria pigmentosa (UP)	Good
	Mastocytoma of the skin	
	Diffuse CM	
Systemic mastocytosis (SM)	Indolent SM	Good (>16 y)
	SM with an associated clonal hematologic non–mast cell lineage disease (SM-AHNMD)	Poor (2 y)
	Aggressive SM	Poor (3.5 y)
	Mast cell leukemia	Very poor (2 mo)
	Mast cell sarcoma	Very poor
	Extracutaneous mastocytoma	Good

nodules, larger than 1 cm in diameter.[11] Diffuse CM is an extremely rare variant of CM, in which the skin undergoes generalized infiltration and may even cause erythroderma. Because of the dense infiltration of mast cells, bullous lesions can appear after stimuli or even spontaneously, more commonly in the latter 2 variants of CM.[12] Although evidence of systemic involvement (eg, bone marrow infiltration) is common, systemic symptoms are rare (indolent systemic mastocytosis).[13] Rarely, florid systemic symptoms (diarrhea, wheezing, syncope, and even anaphylaxis) may occur (aggressive systemic mastocytosis) after extensive release of mast cell mediators.

Functional mutations in the *KIT* gene have been detected from mast cells in the lesional skin, and rarely in the blood or bone marrow, indicating the somatic occurrence of these mutations.[14] KIT (CD117) is a receptor for stem cell factor (SCF), the essential growth factor for mast cells and melanocytes, and functions as a receptor tyrosine kinase. The most common activating *KIT* mutation, D816V, can be identified in mast cells from more than 90% of SM cases in adults. By contrast, the same mutation has been found in mast cells from only about one-third of pediatric CM patients.[15] The remaining 5% of adult SM cases and more than half of pediatric CM cases predictably show other *KIT* mutations.[16,17] It should be noted that the presence of the mutation in D816V does not alone induce malignant transformation of mast cells, and pediatric CM cases with this mutation reportedly fail to segregate with progressive or persistent disease.[18,19] Most strikingly, as predicted by an early report of an occurrence of mastocytosis in familial traits and monogenic twins, germline *KIT* mutations have been identified in some familial cases, indicating that mastocytosis can be a hereditary disease with a KIT mutation.[20,21]

HAE

HAE (OMIM #106100) is a rare autosomal dominant disorder with recurrent attacks of nonpitting tissue edema, as a result of increased vascular leakage in subcutaneous or submucosal tissue.[3] Although a description of this disease originates from the late nineteenth century, the underlying deficiency of C1-INH was identified in the 1960s.[22,23] The tissue edema is self-limited, with a longer duration than the wheals of chronic spontaneous urticaria. However, swelling of the extremities, face, and genitals often interferes with daily life, and laryngeal and upper airway swelling is potentially life-threatening and needs emergency control. Abdominal pain with nausea, vomiting, and diarrhea caused by intestinal edema may be misdiagnosed as acute abdomen and treated surgically. Moreover, facial edema, especially affecting the eyelids or lips, can damage the patient's body image and impair the quality of life of patients and their families.[24]

HAE is classified into 3 types depending on the level and activity of C1-INH (**Table 3**). Type I, with low level and activity of CI-INH, accounts for approximately 85% of HAE cases. Type II, with normal or elevated CI-INH level and impaired functional activity, affects the remaining 15% or so. Both types are caused by heterozygous mutations in the *C1NH* (also called *SERPING1*) gene, possibly leading to haploinsufficiency of the C1-INH activity. More than 200 disease-related mutations, deletions, or insertions causing reduced production of the C1-INH protein are associated with type I HAE, whereas point mutations in the protease-binding region of the C1-INH protein are linked to type II HAE.[25] By contrast, type III HAE (OMIM #610618), with normal level and activity of C1-INH, is rare but restricted to females.[26] In 2006, a unique heterozygous missense mutation in the *F12* gene was identified in 4 families with a founder effect.[27,28] This gain-of-function mutation has been shown to increase the activity of factor XII (also called Hageman factor), which is involved in the generation of kinins and is regulated by estrogens.

C1-INH is a plasma protein belonging to a family of serine protease inhibitors (serpins) and plays a regulatory role in multiple steps of the complement, contact, and coagulation systems (**Fig. 1**). The effect of C1-INH deficiency in the complement system has a diagnostic value, because a low serum C4 level is highly suggestive of C1-INH deficiency. By contrast, the role of C1-INH in the contact system is more important for the pathogenesis of HAE. In the case of C1-INH deficiency, activation of this system is exaggerated by hyperactivation of factor XII and prekallikrein, leading to overproduction of bradykinin, a potent vasodilator and inducer of vasopermeability. In fact an increased plasma bradykinin level has been revealed in HAE patients, especially during attacks.[29]

Appropriate management of HAE requires urgent therapy, and short-term and long-term prophylaxis.[30] For acute attacks neither corticosteroid nor epinephrine is effective, and plasma-derived pasteurized C1-INH is most widely administered. Fresh frozen plasma is still used in cases of emergency, but should be used carefully because of a risk of worsening the attack. Recently, a kallikrein inhibitor (ecallantide) and a selective bradykinin B2 receptor antagonist (icatibant) have been approved in Europe and the United States for the treatment of acute attacks. For short-term prophylaxis before dental manipulation or surgery, danazol has been used and, recently, nanofiltered C1-INH has been used for adult and adolescent cases. The same regimens have been used for long-term prophylaxis.

CAPS

Familial cold urticaria (FCU), showing recurrent attacks of urticarial rashes after general exposure to the cold, was first described in 1940.[31] Arthralgia, myalgia, chills, and fever accompanied attacks. A related hereditary disease with recurrent episodes of urticarial

Table 3 Classification of HAE			
	C4 Level	**C1-INH Level**	**C1-INH Activity**
Type I	Low	Low	Low
Type II	Low	Normal or elevated	Low
Type III	Normal	Normal	Normal

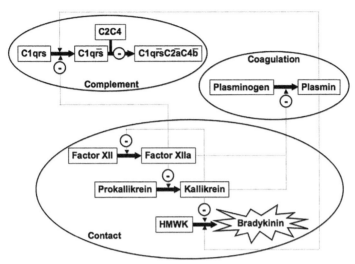

Fig. 1. The regulatory role of C1-INH in the complement, contact, and coagulation systems. Action points of CI-INH are indicated by dashes within circles. HMWK, high molecular weight kininogen.

rash with accompanying symptoms without cold exposure was first described in 1962.[32] Development of late-onset sensorineural deafness and renal amyloidosis was possible, and the disease was called urticaria-deafness-amyloidosis or Muckle-Wells syndrome (MWS; OMIM #191900). In 2001, a new gene in chromosome 1q44 was identified as being responsible for both diseases.[33] The identified gene product has been designated as cryopyrin, which means "cold-induced fever," because of its similarity to pyrin, the *MEFV* gene product responsible for familial Mediterranean fever.[34] Moreover, based on the genetic and clinical similarities to hereditary periodic fever syndromes, the name of the disease has been changed from FCU to familial cold-induced autoinflammatory syndrome (FCAS; OMIM #120100). In 2002, mutations in the same gene were further detected in more severe hereditary disorder, chronic infantile neurologic cutaneous and articular (CINCA) syndrome (OMIM #607115), characterized by a neonatal-onset triad of rash, chronic meningitis, and joint inflammation with recurrent fever.[35,36] Thus these 3 disorders sharing the same genetic origin are defined as forming a sequential spectrum of CAPS.[37] Although CAPS patients may show absence for *NLRP3* mutations, especially in the case of the severe variant, somatic mosaicism of the *NLRP3* mutation has globally been identified in some of these cases.[38]

Cryopyrin is composed of the N-terminal pyrin domain (PYD), central nucleotide oligomerization domain (NOD), and C-terminal leucine-rich repeats (LRR). This molecule is one of the most characterized NOD-like receptor (NLR) family molecules, and has formally been designated as NLRP3.[39] When stimulated with various danger signals, NLRP3 forms a pentamer and associates with procaspase-1 containing the caspase-recruitment domain (CARD), through an adaptor molecule, "apoptosis-associated speck-like protein with a CARD (ASC)," consisting of both PYD and CARD. This NLRP3–ASC–procaspase-1 complex, formed through homophilic interaction of each domain (PYD-PYD and CARD-CARD), has been designated as the NLRP3 inflammasome.[40] This complex works as a cytoplasmic platform activating caspases-1–mediated IL-1β/IL-18 secretion. In the case of CAPS, missense mutations in NLRP3 cause constitutive formation of the inflammasome complex and subsequent IL-1β secretion

(**Fig. 2**). NLRP3 activation in monocytes results in elevated serum IL-1β level, while its activation and IL-1β secretion by dermal mast cells are associated with vascular leakage and neutrophil recruitment in the urticarial rash.[41]

Anti–IL-1 therapies, including recombinant IL-1 receptor antagonist (IL-1Ra) known as anakinra, rilonacept, composed of extracellular IL-1RI and accessory protein (AcP), and anti–IL-1β antibodies such as canakinumab, dramatically improve almost all symptoms of CAPS, indicating the critical role played by IL-1β in the development of CAPS.[42–44]

NAPS12

Two unrelated families with an autosomal dominantly inherited periodic fever syndrome were reported from Guadeloupe in 2008.[5] In one family, twin sons and their father were affected. The sons showed episodic fever, arthralgia, and myalgia induced by generalized cold exposure since the first days of life. Urticaria was also observed twice in each patient. Headache and lower limb pain occurred during and between episodes, and both patients had bilateral sensorineural hearing loss. Their father had also experienced occasional attacks during childhood and still showed episodes of fever and urticaria triggered by physical activities, without hearing loss. An affected daughter in the second family developed cold-induced episodic fever with abdominal pain, vomiting, arthralgia, buccal aphthous ulcers, and lymphadenopathy since the

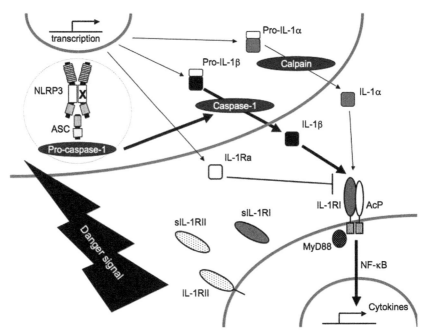

Fig. 2. Molecular pathogenesis of CAPS. In CAPS, a heterozygous *NLRP3* mutation (indicated by X in dimerized molecules) causes constitutive activation of the inflammasome complex (surrounded by a broken-lined circle), leading to cleavage of preformed pro-IL-1β with activated caspase-1 and secretion of mature IL-1β to cause sustained inflammation. On danger, only one signal to induce transcription of pro-IL-1β mRNA is enough for secretion of mature IL-1β. The decoy receptor IL-1RII, soluble (s) IL-1RI and sIL-1RII, as well as IL-1Ra, are all negative regulators of IL-1 signaling.

first year of life. Her affected father also had attacks with fever and abdominal pain between the ages of 5 and 12 years.

Because of the similarity of their symptoms to CAPS, their disease was designated as FCAS2 (OMIM #611762). Through an extensive search for mutations in NLR family molecules, heterozygous nonsense or insertion mutations in the *NLRP12* gene have been identified in each family.[5] A base-pair insertion within the donor splice site of intron 3 activates a cryptic donor splice site, resulting in a frame shift and a premature termination. As NLRP12 has been shown to be a negative regulator of nuclear factor (NF)-κB signaling and such an inhibitory effect was actually impaired by these mutations, their heterozygosity seems to cause haploinsufficiency in patients.[45]

PLAID

Three unrelated families with autosomal dominantly inherited atypical cold urticaria were first reported in 2009.[46] As a characteristic feature, water evaporation seems to be the most effective stimulus, which is occasionally induced by tears flowing down the cheeks or warm water on the skin exposed to room temperature. Accordingly, the patients show a negative cold-stimulation test using ice cubes, whereas urticarial rashes appear after direct contact of ice to the skin followed by rewarming to room temperature. Outdoor cold air also induces urticarial rash over unprotected areas. All patients experienced pruritus and erythema, whereas angioedema was experienced by less than half of the cases. Reactions are local rather than generalized, are not accompanied by systemic complications, and usually resolve within 30 minutes. Of note, ingestion of cold foods or beverages caused oropharyngeal swelling in some cases. Most patients develop the symptoms before 6 months of age and sustain them for life, although their severity usually improves after 30 years of age. The disease has been designated as familial atypical cold urticaria (FACU) or FCAS3 (OMIM #614468), which is clearly distinguished from FCAS by the absence of systemic involvement.

In 2012, immunologic abnormalities were added to their clinical features. These abnormalities include recurrent infections associated with low immunoglobulin (Ig)A and IgM, and high IgE levels in the serum, decreased circulating B cells and natural killer (NK) cells, and development of autoantibodies or autoimmune diseases and granulomatous skin lesions.[6] Through linkage analysis, 3 different heterozygous deletions in the *PLCG2* gene have been identified as responsible, and the disease has been designated as PLAID. Phospholipase C (PLC) family enzymes hydrolyze membranous phospholipids and generate diacylglycerols and inositol triphosphate to activate calcium influx. Among them, PLCγ2 is expressed in B, NK, and mast cells, and involves signaling through various receptor tyrosine kinases. All 3 deletions are included in the C-terminal Src-homology-2 (SH2) domain with an autoinhibitory role, and lack of this domain has been shown to increase the phospholipase activity of PLCγ2. The downstream functions of the immune cells, however, were mostly decreased, probably as a result of chronic signaling. By contrast, mast cells with mutant *PLCG2* showed spontaneous degranulation at 20°C, probably responsible for cold urticaria.[6]

Almost simultaneously, familial cases showing recurrent blistering skin lesions with inflammatory lesions of the joints, eyes, and gastrointestinal tract were reported.[7] Their skin lesions resembled epidermolysis bullosa in infancy, but progressed to erythematous plaques with vesiculopustules, which worsened with heat and sun exposure. These patients also showed mild deficiency of humoral immunity causing recurrent sinopulmonary infections, without circulating autoantibodies. Through whole exome sequencing, a heterozygous gain-of-function missense mutation in the *PLCG2*

Table 4			
Hereditary diseases with cold-induced urticaria			
		Episodic Symptoms	Sustained/Progressive Symptoms
CAPS	FCAS	Urticarial rash, arthralgia, myalgia, chills, fever, swelling of the extremities	Renal amyloidosis
	MWS	Urticarial rash, arthralgia, chills, fever	Sensorineural deafness, renal amyloidosis
	CINCA	Fever	Rash, arthritis, chronic meningitis, visual defect, deafness, growth retardation, renal amyloidosis
NAPS12 (FCAS2)		Fever, arthralgia, myalgia, urticaria, abdominal pain, aphthous ulcers, lymphadenopathy	Sensorineural deafness
PLAID (FCAS3)		Urticaria induced by evaporative cooling, sinopulmonary infections	Serum low immunoglobulin (Ig)M and IgA levels, high IgE levels, decreased B and NK cells, granulomata, antinuclear antibodies

gene has been identified as being responsible.[7] Despite some distinctive clinical and genetic features, the diseases in this family and the families with PLAID possibly form a distinct type of hereditary autoinflammatory syndrome with immunodeficiency. The clinical features of hereditary diseases with cold-induced urticaria are summarized in **Table 4**.

OTHER GENETICALLY UNDEFINED HEREDITARY URTICARIA

On searching the OMIM database, several disorders with distinct OMIM numbers remain to be genetically defined. Aquagenic urticaria (OMIM 191850) is characterized by urticaria induced by contact with water but not by heat or cold, and its familial occurrence was reported in 1979.[47] Familial cases with delayed heat urticaria were reported as familial localized heat urticaria (OMIM 191950),[48] in which the lesions were limited to the areas of contact with heat and were completely inhibited by local lidocaine pretreatment. Another 2 forms of familial physical urticaria, dermodistortive urticaria (OMIM 125630) and familial dermographism (OMIM 125635), are also registered.[49,50] The former is induced by repetitive vibratory or stretching stimulation, whereas the latter is defined by wheal formation on the skin after a single stroke with moderate pressure.

SUMMARY

Hereditary disorders presenting with urticaria are not common and may not be encountered by most physicians. However, without the correct knowledge they can be easily missed or misdiagnosed. With proper diagnosis and understanding of the genetic cause and consequent pathogenesis, disease-specific essential therapeutic regimens can be offered. Recent discovery of the genetic origins of rare cases with distinct hereditary cold urticaria encourages the examination of more cases. As technology in genetic analysis progresses rapidly, further insights into undefined hereditary urticaria will emerge in the near future. The knowledge obtained promises to lead to the development of novel therapeutics.

REFERENCES

1. Hide M, Hiragun T. Japanese guidelines for diagnosis and treatment of urticaria in comparison with other countries. Allergol Int 2012;61:517–27.
2. Fuller SJ. New insights into the pathogenesis, diagnosis, and management of mastocytosis. Hematol Oncol Clin North Am 2012;26:1143–68.
3. Cicardi M, Johnston DT. Hereditary and acquired complement component 1 esterase inhibitor deficiency: a review for the hematologist. Acta Haematol 2012;127:208–20.
4. Yu JR, Leslie KS. Cryopyrin-associated periodic syndrome: an update on diagnosis and treatment response. Curr Allergy Asthma Rep 2011;22:12–20.
5. Jeru I, Duquesnoy P, Fernandes-Alnemri T, et al. Mutations in NALP12 cause hereditary periodic fever syndromes. Proc Natl Acad Sci U S A 2008;105:1614–9.
6. Ombrello MJ, Remmers EF, Sun G, et al. Cold urticaria, immunodeficiency, and autoimmunity related to PLCG2 deletions. N Engl J Med 2012;366:330–8.
7. Zhou Q, Lee GS, Brady J, et al. A hypermorphic missense mutation in PLCG2, encoding phospholipase Cγ2, causes a dominantly inherited autoinflammatory disease with immunodeficiency. Am J Hum Genet 2012;91:713–20.
8. Kettelhut BV, Metcalfe DD. Pediatric mastocytosis. J Invest Dermatol 1991;96:15S–8S.
9. Middelkamp Hup MA, Heide R, Tank B, et al. Comparison of mastocytosis with onset in children and adults. J Eur Acad Dermatol Venereol 2002;16:115–20.
10. Topar G, Staudacher C, Geisen F, et al. Urticaria pigmentosa: a clinical, hematopathologic, and serologic study of 30 adults. Am J Clin Pathol 1998;109:279–85.
11. Wolff K, Komr M, Petzelbauer P. Clinical and histopathological aspects of cutaneous mastocytosis. Leuk Res 2001;25:519–28.
12. Golitz LE, Weston WL, Lane AT. Bullous mastocytosis: diffuse cutaneous mastocytosis with extensive blisters mimicking scalded skin syndrome or erythema multiforme. Pediatr Dermatol 1984;1:288–94.
13. Horny HP, Parwaresch MR, Lennert K. Bone marrow findings in systemic mastocytosis. Hum Pathol 1985;16:808–14.
14. Longley BJ, Metcalfe DD, Tharp M, et al. Activating and dominant inactivating c-KIT catalytic domain mutations in distinct clinical forms of human mastocytosis. Proc Natl Acad Sci U S A 1999;96:1609–14.
15. Bodemer C, Hermine O, Palmerini F, et al. Pediatric mastocytosis is a clonal disease associated with D816V and other activating c-KIT mutations. J Invest Dermatol 2010;130:804–15.
16. Garcia-Montero AC, Jara-Acevedo M, Teodosio C, et al. KIT mutation in mast cells and other bone marrow hematopoietic cell lineages in systemic mast cell disorders: a prospective study of the Spanish Network on Mastocytosis (REMA) in a series of 113 patients. Blood 2006;108:2366–72.
17. Fett NM, Teng J, Longley BJ. Familial urticarial pigmentosa: report of a family and review of the role of KIT mutations. Am J Dermatopathol 2013;35:113–6.
18. Gleixner KV, Mayerhofer M, Ceyny-Reiterer S, et al. KIT-D816V-independent oncogenic signaling in neoplastic cells in systemic mastocytosis: role of Lyn and Btk activation and disruption by dasatinib and bosutinib. Blood 2011;118:1885–98.
19. Yanagihori H, Oyama N, Nakamura K, et al. c-KIT Mutations in patients with childhood-onset mastocytosis and genotype-phenotype correlation. J Mol Diagn 2005;7:252–7.

20. Shaw JM. Genetic aspects of urticaria pigmentosa. Arch Dermatol 1968;97: 137–8.
21. Wasag B, Niedoszytko M, Piskorz A, et al. Novel, activating KIT-N822I mutation in familial cutaneous mastocytosis. Exp Hematol 2011;39:859–65.
22. Quincke HI. Uber akutes umschriebenes Hautoderm. Monatsh Prakt Derm 1882;1:129–31.
23. Donaldson VH, Evans RR. A biochemical abnormality in hereditary angioneurotic edema: absence of serum inhibitor of C′1-esterase. Am J Med 1963;35:37–44.
24. Lumry WR, Castaldo AJ, Vernon MK, et al. The humanistic burden of hereditary angioedema: impact on health-related quality of life, productivity, and depression. Allergy Asthma Proc 2010;31:407–14.
25. Nzeako UC, Frigas E, Tremaine WJ. Hereditary angioedema: a broad review for clinicians. Arch Intern Med 2001;161:2417–29.
26. Bork K, Barnstedt SE, Koch P, et al. Hereditary angioedema with normal C1-inhibitor activity in woman. Lancet 2000;356:213–7.
27. Dewald G, Bork K. Missense mutations in the coagulation factor XII (Hageman factor) gene in hereditary angioedema with normal C1 inhibitor. Biochem Biophys Res Commun 2006;343:1286–9.
28. Cichon S, Martin L, Hennies HC, et al. Increased activity of coagulation factor XII (Hageman factor) causes hereditary angioedema type III. Am J Hum Genet 2006;79:1098–104.
29. Nussberger J, Cugno M, Amstutz C, et al. Plasma bradykinin in angio-oedema. Lancet 1998;351:1693–7.
30. Bowen T, Cicardi M, Farkas H, et al. 2010 international consensus algorithm for the diagnosis, therapy and management of hereditary angioedema. Allergy Asthma Clin Immunol 2010;6:24.
31. Kile RL, Rusk HA. A case of cold urticaria with unusual family history. JAMA 1940;114:1067–8.
32. Muckle TJ, Wells M. Urticaria, deafness and amyloidosis: a new heredo-familial syndrome. Q J Med 1962;31:235–48.
33. Hoffman HM, Mueller JL, Broide DH, et al. Mutation of a new gene encoding a putative pyrin-like protein causes familial cold autoinflammatory syndrome and Muckle-Wells syndrome. Nat Genet 2001;29:301–5.
34. Kastner DL, O'Shea JJ. A fever gene comes in from the cold. Nat Genet 2001; 29:241–2.
35. Feldmann J, Prieur AM, Quartier P, et al. Chronic infantile neurological cutaneous and articular syndrome is caused by mutations in *CIAS1*, a gene highly expressed in polymorphonuclear cells and chondrocytes. Am J Hum Genet 2002;71:198–203.
36. Aksentijevich I, Nowak M, Mallah M, et al. De novo CIAS1 mutations, cytokine activation, and evidence for genetic heterogeneity in patients with neonatal-onset multisystem inflammatory disease (NOMID): a new member of the expanding family of pyrin-associated autoinflammatory diseases. Arthritis Rheum 2002;46:3340–8.
37. Arostegui JI, Aldea A, Modesto C, et al. Clinical and genetic heterogeneity among Spanish patients with recurrent autoinflammatory syndromes associated with the CIAS1/PYPAF1/NALP3 gene. Arthritis Rheum 2004;50:4045–50.
38. Tanaka N, Izawa K, Saito MK, et al. High incidence of NLRP3 somatic mosaicism in patients with chronic infantile neurologic, cutaneous, articular syndrome: results of an international multicenter collaborative study. Arthritis Rheum 2011; 63:3625–32.

39. Kersse K, Bertrand MJ, Lamkanfi M, et al. NOD-like receptors and the innate immune system: coping with danger, damage and death. Cytokine Growth Factor Rev 2011;22:257–76.
40. McDermott MF, Tschopp J. From inflammasomes to fevers, crystals and hypertension: how basic research explains inflammatory diseases. Trends Mol Med 2007;13:381–8.
41. Nakamura Y, Kambe N, Saito M, et al. Mast cells mediate neutrophil recruitment and vascular leakage through the NLRP3 inflammasome in histamine-independent urticaria. J Exp Med 2009;206:1037–46.
42. Hoffman HM, Rosengren S, Boyle DL, et al. Prevention of cold-associated acute inflammation in familial cold autoinflammatory syndrome by interleukin-1 receptor antagonist. Lancet 2004;364:1779–85.
43. Hoffman HM, Throne ML, Amar NJ, et al. Efficacy and safety of rilonacept (interleukin-1 Trap) in patients with cryopyrin-associated periodic syndromes: results from two sequential placebo-controlled studies. Arthritis Rheum 2008;58:2443–52.
44. Lachmann HJ, Kone-Paut I, Kuemmerle-Deschner JB, et al, Canakinumab in CAPS Study Group. Use of canakinumab in the cryopyrin-associated periodic syndrome. N Engl J Med 2009;360:2416–25.
45. Lich JD, Ting JP. Monarch-1/pypaf7 and other CATERPILLER (CLR, NOD, NLR) proteins with negative regulatory functions. Microbes Infect 2007;9:672–6.
46. Gandhi C, Healy C, Wanderer AA, et al. Familial atypical cold urticaria: description of a new hereditary disease. J Allergy Clin Immunol 2009;124:1245–50.
47. Bonnetblanc JM, Andrieu-Pfahl F, Meraud JP, et al. Familial aquagenic urticaria. Dermatologica 1979;158:468–70.
48. Michaelsson G, Ros AM. Familial localized heat urticaria of delayed type. Acta Derm Venereol 1971;51:279–83.
49. Epstein PA, Kidd KK. Dermo-distortive urticaria: an autosomal dominant dermatologic disorder. Am J Med Genet 1981;9:307–15.
50. Jedele KB, Michels VV. Familial dermographism. Am J Med Genet 1991;39:201–3.

Mastocytosis

Melody C. Carter, MD, Dean D. Metcalfe, MD,
Hirsh D. Komarow, MD*

KEYWORDS

• Mast cell • Mastocytosis • KIT • Bone marrow • Skin • Urticaria

KEY POINTS

• The pathologic proliferation of mast cells is a defining feature of mastocytosis.
• Cutaneous manifestations may occur alone or in association with systemic disease at any age.
• The most commonly affected site is the skin.
• Mastocytosis in children is usually limited to the skin and resolves by adulthood.
• Patients with systemic disease often have a somatic activating mutation in the KIT oncogene, which may direct the diagnosis and treatment.
• Treatment is primarily symptomatic for nonaggressive variants of mastocytosis.
• Patients with aggressive disease may benefit from cytoreductive therapies.

INTRODUCTION

Mastocytosis is a disorder of increased mast cell proliferation, with both cutaneous and systemic manifestations. Clinical features of mastocytosis include flushing, pruritus, abdominal pain, diarrhea, hypotension, syncope, and musculoskeletal pain. These features are primarily the result of mast cell mediator release and infiltration into skin, gastrointestinal (GI) tract, liver, spleen, lymph nodes, and bone marrow. The skin is the most common site of involvement. Cutaneous disease manifestations include urticaria pigmentosa, diffuse cutaneous mastocytosis (DCM), mastocytoma, and telangiectasia macularis eruptiva perstans. Mastocytosis occurs in both children and adults, although children tend to primarily manifest cutaneous lesions. Most cases seem to be spontaneous. Inherited patterns of mastocytosis are unusual.

This work was supported by the Division of Intramural Research, National Institute of Allergy and Infectious Disease, NIH.
Conflict of Interest: None.
Laboratory of Allergic Diseases, National Institute of Allergy and Infectious Diseases, National Institutes of Health, 10 Center Drive, Bethesda, MD 20892, USA
* Corresponding author. Laboratory of Allergic Diseases, National Institute of Allergy and Infectious Diseases, National Institutes of Health, Building 10, Room 1C129A1, 10 Center Drive, Bethesda, MD 20892-1960.
E-mail address: komarowh@niaid.nih.gov

Immunol Allergy Clin N Am 34 (2014) 181–196
http://dx.doi.org/10.1016/j.iac.2013.09.001
0889-8561/14/$ – see front matter Published by Elsevier Inc.

immunology.theclinics.com

Mastocytosis has been classified into disease variants, which are listed in **Box 1** according to a World Health Organization (WHO) consensus.[1] Children with cutaneous mastocytosis (CM) generally have resolution of symptoms by adulthood. In adults, cutaneous disease is usually accompanied by evidence of mastocytosis in other organ systems. Indolent systemic mastocytosis (ISM) (**Fig. 1**) is the least severe systemic variant, and patients with ISM or isolated CM are generally managed long-term with symptomatic therapies. Other forms with more severe manifestations carry a poorer prognosis and include systemic mastocytosis with an associated clonal, hematologic non–mast-cell lineage disease (SM-AHNMD), aggressive systemic mastocytosis (ASM), mast cell leukemia (MCL) and mast cell sarcoma. Of these forms, MCL, although rare, is the most aggressive and may be characterized by the presence of immature mast cells in peripheral blood.

CAUSES AND PATHOGENESIS
Mast Cell Origin, Growth, and Development

Human mast cells develop from $CD34^+$ pluripotent progenitor cells.[2-5] Committed bone marrow– derived mast cell progenitors enter the bloodstream, then migrate to peripheral tissue, where they mature and become terminally differentiated. Mature mast cells tend to reside in tissue close to blood vessels, nerves, and glandular structures. They are particularly numerous in the skin, GI tract, respiratory tract, and lymphoid tissue. Mast cells have cytoplasmic granules that contain histamine and a multitude of other inflammatory mediators. Mature mast cells are long lived and tend to have a limited ability to differentiate.[6] Mast cell survival is particularly dependent on the presence of stem cell factor (SCF) in the surrounding milieu.

Mast cells, as well as melanocytes, express KIT, a transmembrane tyrosine kinase receptor for SCF. The interaction between KIT and SCF seems to play an essential role in the development of mastocytosis.[7] Activating somatic mutations in *c-kit*, which encodes for KIT, have been detected in the bone marrow as well as skin and peripheral blood cells in patients with mastocytosis. The most common somatic mutation,

---

Box 1
World Health Organization classification of mastocytosis

CM

　Urticaria pigmentosa = maculopapular CM

　DCM

　Mastocytoma of skin

ISM

　Smoldering systemic mastocytosis

　Isolated bone marrow mastocytosis

Systemic mastocytosis with associated clonal, hematologic non–mast-cell lineage disease

Aggressive systemic mastocytosis

Mast cell leukemia

Mast cell sarcoma

Extracutaneous mastocytoma

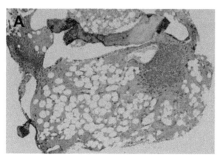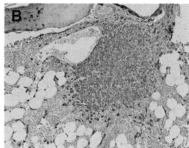

Fig. 1. Bone marrow histopathology in an adult with ISM. Mast cell aggregates shown by staining with tryptase in (*A*) (×40) and (*B*) highlights the mast cell component of the aggregate and the prominent abnormal spindle-shaped mast cells (×100).

Asp816Val (D816V), is located in catalytic domain of KIT and results in augmented mast cell proliferation and survival.[8,9] The D816V mutation is less common in children, especially in those with CM. Other c-kit mutations including V560G, D816Y, D816F, D816H, and E839K have been identified in mast cell lines, MCL, and pediatric mastocytosis.[10,11] Whether these are activating mutations or contribute to ligand-independent activation and suppression of apoptosis has not been fully elucidated. A subgroup of patients who present with hypereosinophilic syndrome have the FIP1L1/PDGRFA fusion tyrosine kinase, which can be found in multiple cell lineages, including mast cells and eosinophils. This genetic abnormality is associated with increased mast cells in the bone marrow, an increased tryptase level, and peripheral eosinophilia, thus highlighting a role for non-KIT–dependent pathways in the pathogenesis of mast cell proliferation.[12]

Pathologic Effects of Mast Cell Mediators

After activation and degranulation, mast cells secrete and generate a host of mediators that contribute to allergic inflammation. The disease manifestations shown in mastocytosis are a consequence of increased mast cells present in tissue and the degree of release of mast cell mediators. **Table 1** summarizes the clinical features associated with mast cell mediators. Mast cell mediator release causes both local tissue and distal inflammation as they are released in to the bloodstream. Clinically, the most significant mediator is histamine. Histamine acts through 4 different receptors, H_1 to H_4, to mediate vasopermeability, vasodilation, GI and bronchial smooth muscle contraction, gastric acid production and pruritus.[13] H_1 receptors modulate bronchial and GI smooth muscle contraction and may be blocked by antihistamines such as diphenhydramine (Benadryl) and cetirizine (Zyrtec). Stimulation of gastric acid secretion by parietal cells is regulated by H_2 receptors and is inhibited by H_2 antagonists like ranitidine (Zantac). Mast cells have abundant secretary granule proteases, which make up most of the proteins present in mast cells, and the major protease is tryptase. Total tryptase comprises mature tryptase stored in granules and released only on activation and immature (pro) tryptase, which is constitutively secreted by the mast cell. Patients with mastocytosis generally have increased serum tryptase and histamine levels.[14,15] Other clinically relevant mediators are prostaglandin D_2 and leukotriene C_4, which cause similar effects. Growth factor and inflammatory cytokines also produced by mast cells include interleukin 3 (IL-3), IL-16, and tumor necrosis factor α.[16]

Table 1
Clinical manifestations and related mast cell mediators

Skin	
Pruritus	Histamine, PAF
Flushing	PGD_2
Urticaria	Histamine, PAF, LTC_4
Blistering	IL-6, tryptase, PGD_2, PAF
Constitutional	
Fatigue, weight loss, cachexia	Tumor necrosis factor α, IL-1β, IL-6
Systemic	
Hypotension and swelling	Histamine, PAF, PGD_2, LTC_4, LTD_4, LTE_4, endothelin
Eosinophilia	IL-5
Mast cell proliferation	SCF, IL-3, IL-6, chymase
Fibrosis	Transforming growth factor β
Inhibition of localized clotting	Heparin
Lymphadenopathy	IL-16, lymphotaxin
Gastrointestinal	
Increased gastric acid	Histamine
Intestinal cramping	Histamine, PAF, LTC_4
Skeletal system	
Osteoporosis	Heparin, tryptase
Lungs	
Bronchoconstriction	Histamine, PGD_2, PAF, LTC_4, LTD_4, endothelin
Mucus and edema	Histamine, PGD_2, PAF, LTC_4, proteases

Abbreviations: IL, interleukin; LT, leukotriene; PAF, platelet-activating factor; PG, prostaglandin; SCF, stem cell factor.

CLINICAL FEATURES
Cutaneous Patterns of Mastocytosis

All variants of mastocytosis share clinical features, but skin is the most common organ site of involvement and is often the first sign of the disease. In children, the skin may be the only manifestation of the disease.[17] In 2007, a proposed additional diagnostic category to the WHO nomenclature, termed mastocytosis of the skin (MIS), was introduced.[18] MIS proposes to assess disease status based on cutaneous findings, before performing a bone marrow biopsy. The diagnosis of MIS is based on the findings of a typical mastocytosis exanthema, comprising the major criterion, and 1 of 2 minor criteria as determined from a lesional skin biopsy showing either abnormal mast cells in clusters (>15) or more than 20 scattered per high-power field or detection of a dermal KIT mutation at codon 816. In terms of standard nomenclature, the term CM is reserved for cutaneous disease only and subdivided into maculopapular CM or urticaria pigmentosa (UP), DCM, mastocytoma, and telangiectasia macularis eruptiva perstans (TMEP).

The most common skin manifestation in both adults (**Fig. 2**) and children (**Fig. 3**) is UP, but the size and number are more variable in children with CM and they are more uniform in adults.[19] The typical appearance of UP are yellow-tan to reddish-brown macules or slightly raised papules scattered mainly on the trunk and legs, with generally less involvement of the sun-exposed areas. The palms, soles, face, and scalp are generally spared, especially in adults. Dermatologic symptoms include pruritus, flushing, and

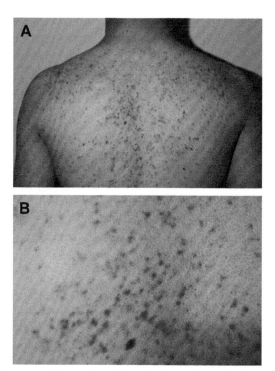

Fig. 2. Urticaria pigmentosa in an adult. (*A*) Typical maculopapular lesions of uniform size, generally less than 0.5 mm and (*B*) a closeup with color variation from red to brown.

blistering, with blistering almost uniquely seen in children. Darier sign is the local wheal-ing of a lesion induced by friction but is inconsistently elicited. UP lesions are seen in greater than 90% of patients with ISM and less than 50% in patients with SM-AHNMD or ASM and may fade over time. Regression of the lesions may not indicate disease improvement. Studies in adults have reported lesional regression to be occa-sionally associated with increased serum tryptase levels and worsening disease.[19–21]

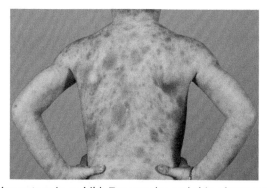

Fig. 3. Urticaria pigmentosa in a child. Tan papules and thin plaques on this child's back reflect the larger size of lesions that may be seen in children compared with those in adults. Lesions on sun-exposed areas such as the extremities tend to appear less active, as in this case.

DCM and mastocytomas have an onset almost exclusively in children. Although DCM may persist into adulthood, mastocytomas usually regress spontaneously. DCM is characterized by thickened skin and may show a peau d'orange appearance, with a reddish-brown discoloration without characteristic lesions of UP (**Fig. 4**A), but may also have scattered nodules similar in appearance to mastocytomas. The skin may be dermatographic, and the formation of hemorrhagic blisters is common. Bullous formation is limited to pediatric-onset cutaneous disease and is usually associated with lesional skin. Bullae may erupt spontaneously or in association with physical stimuli, infection, and immunization (see **Fig. 4**B). This feature is mostly limited to the first few years of life and may need to be distinguished from other bullous diseases of childhood. Solitary mastocytomas are red-brown or yellow-orange nodules, which when traumatized may cause systemic symptoms, such as flushing and hypotension (**Fig. 5**). Solitary mastocytomas generally appear before age 6 months, and it is unusual to develop subsequent skin lesions more than 2 months after the presentation of the initial lesion.[17] UP and DCM are associated with pruritus of varied intensity, which may be exacerbated by changes in climatic temperature, skin friction, and ingestion of hot beverages, spicy foods, alcohol, or certain drugs.

TMEP is the least common CM variant and is almost exclusively seen in adults. It appears as red-brown telangiectatic macules with irregular borders.

GI Symptoms

GI symptoms in patients with mastocytosis are highly prevalent, often severe, and associated with decreased quality of life.[22–25] In a recent study of 83 patients with mastocytosis, the most common symptoms were diarrhea and bloating, followed by nausea and abdominal pain, all of which were significantly more frequent than in healthy age-matched individuals.[23] This recent study is consistent with an earlier report that abdominal pain and diarrhea are present in 80% of patients.[22] However, vomiting was less common and noted in less than 10% of patients. The risk of gastroduodenal ulcers was also found to be greater in these patients and was likely caused by increased gastric acid secretion that resulted from higher histamine production, consistent with other reports.[22,23] The frequency of GI symptoms did not seem to correlate with the presence of the D816V mutation or the level of serum tryptase nor the age of onset of mastocytosis.[23,26] Also, no correlation was found between histologic findings of mast cell infiltration in GI biopsies and GI symptoms. These symptoms

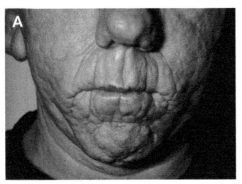
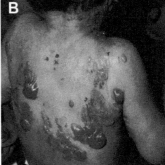

Fig. 4. DCM. (*A*) Diffuse dermal thickening, pachydermic flesh-colored lesions, and (*B*) bullous eruption in a child.

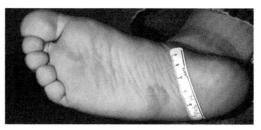

Fig. 5. Solitary mastocytoma on the foot sole of a child. A flat red-to-tan nodule with clearly defined border.

were similar to those in patients with inflammatory bowel disease. In an earlier prospective study,[22] most abdominal pain was dyspeptic, because it responded to H_2 antagonists, and most of these patients had increased gastric acid secretion. In addition to peptic ulcer disease, abdominal pain has been associated with edema of the GI tract, or motility dysfunction.[27,28]

In 1 study,[22] increased bowel movements and fecal output were reported in half of the patients, and in the patients in whom diarrhea was greater than 200 g stool/d, there was increased gastric acid secretion. Plasma histamine levels were also increased and correlated with basal acid output but not directly with abdominal pain or diarrhea. Gastric emptying and transit time did not differ between patients and control subjects with diarrhea and abdominal symptoms, and thus, transit time does not seem to be a major factor in GI symptoms.

Based on small studies and case reports, several GI peptides have been implicated in the pathogenesis of diarrhea and abdominal pain in patients with mastocytosis and include vasoactive intestinal peptide, neurotensin, substance P or motilin, and gastrin.[22,29] Although local secretion may play a role in GI signs and symptoms, it does not seem that systemic levels of these peptides are of major pathologic significance.

Musculoskeletal Involvement

Patients with systemic mastocytosis may have associated osteopenia or osteoporosis. Several patients with SM show roentgenographic findings of diffuse osteolysis and osteosclerosis, primarily affecting the axial skeleton and ends of the long bone.[30] Pathologic fractures or osteoporosis may be the presenting manifestation of mastocytosis. Musculoskeletal pain is a common presenting symptom. In a case series of 362 patients with mastocytosis,[31] 54% reported such pain and 18% felt it caused intolerable disability.

Bone Marrow Pathology

Systemic mastocytosis is usually diagnosed by bone marrow histopathology outlined by a WHO consensus panel (**Box 2**).[11] ISM, the most common variant of systemic disease, is diagnosed when criteria for mastocytosis are met and there is no evidence of an associated clonal hematologic disorder or severe liver disease, hypersplenism, or significant lymphadenopathy. Isolated bone marrow mastocytosis is a subvariant of ISM with a low bone marrow burden of mast cells, a lower tryptase value, and the absence of skin lesions. Several clinical conditions should heighten suspicion of this variant, such as idiopathic anaphylaxis, venom anaphylaxis, unexplained osteoporosis, or chronic diarrhea.[32–35]

Box 2
Diagnostic criteria for cutaneous and systemic mastocytosis

CM

Clinical findings consistent with urticaria pigmentosa, maculopapular CM, DCM, or solitary mastocytoma and typical mast cell infiltrates in a multifocal or diffuse pattern on skin biopsy

Systemic Mastocytosis (SM)

Major and 1 minor, or 3 minor, criteria are required for the diagnosis of SM

Major Criteria

- Multifocal dense infiltrates of mast cells (≥15 mast cell in an aggregate) detected in bone marrow or other extracutaneous organs, and confirmed by tryptase immunohistochemistry (or other special stains)

Minor Criteria

- In biopsy sections of bone marrow or other extracutaneous organs, more than 25% of the mast cells in the infiltrates are spindle-shaped or have atypical morphology; or, of all mast cells in the bone marrow aspirate smears, more than 25% are immature or atypical mast cells
- Detection of Kit point mutation at codon 816 in bone marrow, blood, or other extracutaneous organs
- Mast cells in bone marrow, blood, or other extracutaneous organs that coexpress CD117 with CD2 or CD25
- Baseline serum tryptase persistently greater than 20 ng/mL (if there is an associated clonal myeloid disorder, this parameter is invalid)

Hepatic and Splenic Findings

The liver, spleen, and lymph nodes are common organs affected in systemic mastocytosis, especially in patients with aggressive diseases. Specifically, the paratrabecular compartment of the spleen and paracortex of lymph nodes are more common sites of mast cell infiltration.[36] Other compartments may also be involved, with morphologic findings that pose challenges to identifying the source of the infiltration and may resemble other disease entities such as follicular and T-cell lymphoma, B-cell hyperplasia and lymphoma, Langerhans cell granulomatosis, and Kaposi sarcoma. Liver involvement is also common, but extreme liver disease is present only in those with aggressive disease. In a study of 41 patients with mastocytosis, 61% had indications of liver disease. Twenty-four percent had hepatomegaly, with most having increased liver enzyme levels. Increase in alkaline phosphatase levels correlated with hepatosplenomegaly, liver fibrosis, and increase in γ-glutamyl transpeptidase.[37] Other liver findings in patients with severe disease may include portal hypertension and ascites, but cirrhosis is not generally observed.

Diagnosis

Mastocytosis is diagnosed by history, clinical manifestations, histopathology, and laboratory evaluation. It is then classified as a variant based on WHO criteria (see **Boxes 1** and **2**).[11] The presenting constellation of mast cell mediator symptoms mentioned in the previous sections may be observed in patients with any variant of mastocytosis, both in adults and children.

The diagnosis of CM based on macroscopic appearance is confirmed with a lesional skin biopsy, showing characteristic skin histopathology (**Fig. 6**). Blind skin

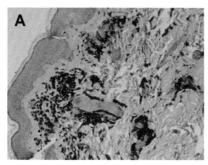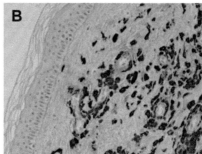

Fig. 6. Histopathology of urticaria pigmentosa from a 7-year-old. Clustering of normal and spindle-shaped mast cells in papillary dermis and extending into the reticular dermis. The tryptase stain highlights perivascular cuffing and interstitial presence of the mast cells. (*A*) Giemsa stain ×40. (*B*) Tryptase stain ×100.

biopsies are not recommended because other skin conditions, including eczema, may be associated with a 2-fold to 4-fold increase in dermal mast cells.[38] In addition, mast cells may also be increased in the skin in conditions such as scleroderma[39] and chronic urticaria,[40] and at sites of prolonged antigenic contact.[41] CM must also be distinguished from other diseases with similar characteristics, as presented in **Box 3**. UP lesions have mast cells in increased numbers in the dermal papillae beneath macules and papules, particularly near blood vessels in the upper dermis.[38] A bandlike infiltrate of mast cells may be seen in the papillary dermis. Mast cells also may appear as nodular infiltrates within the papillary dermis and subcutaneous tissues. Typically, there is a 15-fold to 20-fold increase in mast cells beneath UP lesions. Mast cells may also be found in increased numbers in the normal-appearing skin between lesions of UP.[38] The differences in the histologic pattern in cutaneous disease are generally based on the density of the mast cell infiltrate. In patients with DCM, mast cells are observed around blood vessels and throughout the dermis. These bandlike infiltrates may be indistinguishable from some lesions of UP or from biopsies obtained from mastocytomas. Cutaneous mast cell hyperplasia in patients with TMEP is present around the capillary venules of the superficial plexus. The biopsy of these lesions shows increased numbers of perivascular mast cells.

The diagnosis of mastocytosis should also be considered when a patient, primarily in the adult population, presents with 1 or more of the following: unexplained ulcer disease or malabsorption, radiographic or technetium-99 bone scan abnormalities, hepatomegaly, splenomegaly, lymphadenopathy, peripheral blood abnormalities, venom anaphylaxis, or unexplained flushing or hypotension.[19,42–44] In such patients, the diagnosis of systemic mastocytosis should be considered even in the absence of classic skin lesions.

The current approach to the workup of a patient for systemic mastocytosis consists of a medical evaluation, including a bone marrow biopsy and aspirate, a serum tryptase level, and an analysis for an activating mutation in KIT, preferably on bone marrow mononuclear cells. The diagnosis of systemic disease requires fulfilling the major criterion, consisting of multifocal dense mast cell aggregates, and 1 minor criterion; or 3 minor criteria (see **Box 2**). A bone marrow biopsy in those with pediatric-onset disease is not recommended unless there is evidence of systemic disease, as shown by hepatosplenomegaly, lymphadenopathy or unexplained peripheral blood abnormalities. The most useful stain for mast cells uses a monoclonal antibody to tryptase. In

---

Box 3
Differential diagnosis of cutaneous mast cell manifestations

No apparent lesions

  Idiopathic flushing

  Anaphylaxis with identifiable cause

  Idiopathic anaphylaxis

Diffuse or localized hyperpigmented macules or papules

  Café au lait spots

  Neurofibromatosis

  Albright syndrome

  Postinflammatory hyperpigmentation

  Secondary syphilis

  Chronic urticaria

  Atopic dermatitis

  Addison disease

  Lentigo

Bullous eruptions

  Chronic bullous disease of childhood

  Linear IgA dermatosis

  Staphylococcus infection

  Drug eruption

  Incontinentia pigmenti

  Bullous pemphigoid

  Bullous impetigo of infancy

Solitary or multiple nodules

  Congenital nevus

  Juvenile xanthogranuloma

  Leukemia

  Lymphoma

  Neuroblastoma

---

addition, immunohistochemistry to identify CD25+ mast cells is of value, because CD25 has been shown to be expressed on most clonal mast cells in mastocytosis.[45]

Other tissue specimens, such as those from lymph nodes, spleen, liver, and GI mucosa, may help determine the extent of mast cell involvement, but are not typically necessary. GI biopsies are thus usually obtained only if a GI workup is indicated, and lymph nodes are biopsied only if lymphoma is considered. When biopsies have been obtained of involved tissue, the histopathologic pattern of mast cell aggregates is similar to that seen in the bone marrow and infiltrates are often CD25+.[22,23,46]

In patients suspected of having mastocytosis, the diagnosis of a carcinoid tumor or pheochromocytoma should be ruled out. Patients with mastocytosis do not excrete increased amounts of 5-hydroxyindoleacetic acid in the urine. Patients with carcinoid tumor or pheochromocytoma also do not have histologic evidence of significant mast cell proliferation and should have normal serum tryptase levels.[47]

TREATMENT
Mast Cell–Mediated Therapies

The approach to treatment of patients with mastocytosis begins with management of mast cell–mediated symptoms such as pruritus, flushing, and GI cramping.[48] Specific triggers that cause mast cell mediator release should be avoided. These triggers may include physical and environmental stimuli, emotional stress, infections, medications, vaccinations, and anesthesia. Pruritus and flushing are often treated with an H_1 receptor antagonist such as hydroxyzine or nonsedating antihistamines such as cetirizine or fexofenadine. For additional relief, an H_2 antihistamine may be added such as ranitidine or famotidine. Some patients also benefit from the addition of a leukotriene inhibitor or disodium cromoglycate (cromolyn sodium), which may provide relief for GI symptoms.[49] Despite these medications, patients often continue to report headaches, flushing, GI symptoms, and musculoskeletal pain. This situation is likely caused by the inability of these agents to completely block histamine and other mast cell mediators.

Prompt administration of epinephrine is indicated for treatment of hypotensive episodes, which may be spontaneous or observed after insect stings and injection of contrast media.[50] Patients should be trained in self-administration of injectable epinephrine. Patients with recurrent episodes of hypotension may also benefit from prophylactic administration of H_1 and H_2 antihistamines. Psoralen taken orally in combination with ultraviolet light type A (PUVA) has been used to treat CM and relieve pruritus and flushing in adults.[51,52] In responsive patients, therapeutic effects are usually reached within 2 months, diminish with reduction in therapy, and return to baseline after discontinuation of therapy. Cutaneous mast cell lesions may also be effectively treated with topical corticosteroids under occlusive dressing, which leads to a reduction in the number of dermal mast cells at the treatment site.[53,54] Effects are transient.

GI Manifestations

GI disease is treated with agents that inhibit gastric acid hypersecretion. In general, H_2 antagonists such as ranitidine and proton pump inhibitors like omeprazole are effective. Cromolyn sodium may reduce GI cramping.[14] Severe hepatosplenomegaly and ascites may respond to systemic corticosteroids.[55]

Osteoporosis and Fractures

Patients with systemic disease may suffer from osteoporosis, and in some cases, a presenting feature may be a spontaneous bone fracture. A DEXA scan is used to evaluate bony involvement, including osteoporosis.[56] Treatment options are standard for mild osteoporosis and include calcium supplementation, bisphosphonate therapy, and estrogen replacement in postmenopausal woman. For aggressive disease, consider interferon α-2b and 2-chlorodeoxyadenosine (cladribine/2-CdA), a nucleoside analogue.[57] Potential toxicities of 2-CdA are noteworthy and include myelosuppression and immunosuppression.[58]

Hematologic Involvement

Patients with aggressive forms of systemic mastocytosis may be treated with interferon α-2b,[59] and then 2-CdA. With regard to interferon α-2b, several studies have shown varied responses, with some patients experiencing resolution of symptoms and others a partial or no response.[60] In addition, the side effects, which include fever, nausea, malaise, and a risk for anaphylaxis, should be considered before the initiation of interferon α-2b. In a study of 10 patients with severe systemic disease, 2CdA was shown to decrease symptoms and levels of mast cell mediators in most of the patients.[61]

For targeted therapies, it is important to determine if the D816V mutation is present. Imatinib (Gleevac), a tyrosine kinase inhibitor, has been shown to have a cytotoxic effect in vitro on mast cells that are wild type for KIT, but this effect is less in cells bearing the D816V mutation in KIT. This finding is consistent with the beneficial therapeutic effect of imatinib primarily on patients who do not carry the D816V mutation.[62–64]

Imatinib has been shown to be effective in a group of patients who present with increased mast cells in the bone marrow, increased tryptase levels and peripheral eosinophilia and have the FIP1L1/PDGRFA fusion mutation.[65] Other tyrosine kinase inhibitors, including PKC412 (midostaurin) and masitinib, are being evaluated for efficacy in clinical studies.[66–68] Hematopoietic stem cell transplant was performed in 3 patients, and all encountered disease progression.[69] In patients with severe mast cell disease, splenectomy may improve survival.[70]

Prognosis

In general, children have a more favorable prognosis.[17,21,71,72] Children with CM often experience total or major disease regression by late adolescence.[18,21,73] The resolution of cutaneous disease in adults may correlate with the reduction in clinical skin symptoms but may not indicate disease regression. With adults experiencing a significant reduction in skin lesions, the bone marrow typically continues to show mast cell involvement and a diagnosis of systemic disease by WHO criteria is maintained or confirmed.[18,20] The life expectancy in adult patients with CM and ISM parallels that of the general population.

Patients with SM-AHNMD have a disease course determined by the response of the associated hematologic disorder to therapy. Although there are some cases reports of SM-AHNMD in children,[74–77] this variant is more often seen in adults. ASM and MCL are rare variants, with less favorable outcomes. ASM has a better survival with aggressive cytoreductive therapy, but no therapeutic intervention has reliably extended the life expectancy of patients with MCL.

REFERENCES

1. Horny HP, Metcalfe DD, Bennett JM, et al. Mastocytosis. In: Swerdlow S, Campo E, Harris NL, et al, editors. World Health Organization (WHO) classification of tumours. Pathology & genetics: tumours of haematopoietic and lymphoid tissues. Lyon (France): IARC Press; 2008. p. 54–63.
2. Kirshenbaum AS, Kessler SW, Goff JP, et al. Demonstration of the origin of human mast cells from CD34+ bone marrow progenitor cells. J Immunol 1991; 146(5):1410–5.
3. Kirshenbaum AS, Goff JP, Semere T, et al. Demonstration that human mast cells arise from a progenitor cell population that is CD34(+), c-kit(+), and expresses aminopeptidase N (CD13). Blood 1999;94(7):2333–42.
4. Rottem M, Kirshenbaum AS, Metcalfe DD. Early development of mast cells. Int Arch Allergy Appl Immunol 1991;94(1–4):104–9.
5. Rottem M, Okada T, Goff JP, et al. Mast cells cultured from the peripheral blood of normal donors and patients with mastocytosis originate from a CD34+/Fc epsilon RI- cell population. Blood 1994;84(8):2489–96.
6. Metcalfe DD, Mekori JA, Rottem M. Mast cell ontogeny and apoptosis. Exp Dermatol 1995;4(4 Pt 2):227–30.

7. Longley BJ Jr, Metcalfe DD, Tharp M, et al. Activating and dominant inactivating c-KIT catalytic domain mutations in distinct clinical forms of human mastocytosis. Proc Natl Acad Sci U S A 1999;96(4):1609–14.
8. Horny HP, Sotlar K, Valent P. Mastocytosis: state of the art. Pathobiology 2007; 74(2):121–32.
9. Wilson TM, Maric I, Simakova O, et al. Clonal analysis of NRAS activating mutations in KIT-D816V systemic mastocytosis. Haematologica 2011;96(3): 459–63.
10. Sundstrom M, Vliagoftis H, Karlberg P, et al. Functional and phenotypic studies of two variants of a human mast cell line with a distinct set of mutations in the c-kit proto-oncogene. Immunology 2003;108(1):89–97.
11. Valent P. Diagnostic evaluation and classification of mastocytosis. Immunol Allergy Clin North Am 2006;26(3):515–34.
12. Maric I, Robyn J, Metcalfe DD, et al. KIT D816V-associated systemic mastocytosis with eosinophilia and FIP1L1/PDGFRA-associated chronic eosinophilic leukemia are distinct entities. J Allergy Clin Immunol 2007;120(3):680–7.
13. Akdis CA, Jutel M, Akdis M. Regulatory effects of histamine and histamine receptor expression in human allergic immune responses. Chem Immunol Allergy 2008;94:67–82.
14. Castells M, Metcalfe DD, Escribano L. Diagnosis and treatment of cutaneous mastocytosis in children: practical recommendations. Am J Clin Dermatol 2011;12(4):259–70.
15. Tefferi A, Pardanani A. Systemic mastocytosis: current concepts and treatment advances. Curr Hematol Rep 2004;3(3):197–202.
16. Escribano L, Akin C, Castells M, et al. Current options in the treatment of mast cell mediator-related symptoms in mastocytosis. Inflamm Allergy Drug Targets 2006;5(1):61–77.
17. Caplan RM. The natural course of urticaria pigmentosa. Analysis and follow-up of 112 cases. Arch Dermatol 1963;87:146–57.
18. Valent P, Akin C, Escribano L, et al. Standards and standardization in mastocytosis: consensus statements on diagnostics, treatment recommendations and response criteria. Eur J Clin Invest 2007;37(6):435–53.
19. Brockow K, Akin C, Huber M, et al. Assessment of the extent of cutaneous involvement in children and adults with mastocytosis: relationship to symptomatology, tryptase levels, and bone marrow pathology. J Am Acad Dermatol 2003;48(4):508–16.
20. Brockow K, Scott LM, Worobec AS, et al. Regression of urticaria pigmentosa in adult patients with systemic mastocytosis: correlation with clinical patterns of disease. Arch Dermatol 2002;138(6):785–90.
21. Wolff K, Komar M, Petzelbauer P. Clinical and histopathological aspects of cutaneous mastocytosis. Leuk Res 2001;25(7):519–28.
22. Cherner JA, Jensen RT, Dubois A, et al. Gastrointestinal dysfunction in systemic mastocytosis. A prospective study. Gastroenterology 1988;95(3):657–67.
23. Sokol H, Georgin-Lavialle S, Canioni D, et al. Gastrointestinal manifestations in mastocytosis: a study of 83 patients. J Allergy Clin Immunol 2013;132(4): 866–873.e3.
24. Horan RF, Austen KF. Systemic mastocytosis: retrospective review of a decade's clinical experience at the Brigham and Women's Hospital. J Invest Dermatol 1991;96(3):5S–13S [discussion: 13S–4S].
25. Jensen RT. Gastrointestinal abnormalities and involvement in systemic mastocytosis. Hematol Oncol Clin North Am 2000;14(3):579–623.

26. Gupta R, Bain BJ, Knight CL. Cytogenetic and molecular genetic abnormalities in systemic mastocytosis. Acta Haematol 2002;107(2):123–8.

27. Ammann RW, Vetter D, Deyhle P, et al. Gastrointestinal involvement in systemic mastocytosis. Gut 1976;17(2):107–12.

28. Clemett AR, Fishbone G, Levine RJ, et al. Gastrointestinal lesions in mastocytosis. Am J Roentgenol Radium Ther Nucl Med 1968;103(2):405–12.

29. Wesley JR, Vinik AI, O'Dorisio TM, et al. A new syndrome of symptomatic cutaneous mastocytoma producing vasoactive intestinal polypeptide. Gastroenterology 1982;82(5 Pt 1):963–7.

30. Delsignore JL, Dvoretsky PM, Hicks DG, et al. Mastocytosis presenting as a skeletal disorder. Iowa Orthop J 1996;16:126–34.

31. Hermine O, Lortholary O, Leventhal PS, et al. Case-control cohort study of patients' perceptions of disability in mastocytosis. PLoS One 2008;3(5): e2266.

32. Bonadonna P, Perbellini O, Passalacqua G, et al. Clonal mast cell disorders in patients with systemic reactions to *Hymenoptera* stings and increased serum tryptase levels. J Allergy Clin Immunol 2009;123(3):680–6.

33. Floman Y, Margulies JY, Nyska M, et al. Effect of major axial skeleton trauma on preexisting lumbosacral spondylolisthesis. J Spinal Disord 1991;4(3):353–8.

34. Lidor C, Frisch B, Gazit D, et al. Osteoporosis as the sole presentation of bone marrow mastocytosis. J Bone Miner Res 1990;5(8):871–6.

35. Rueff F, Przybilla B, Bilo MB, et al. Predictors of severe systemic anaphylactic reactions in patients with *Hymenoptera* venom allergy: importance of baseline serum tryptase–a study of the European Academy of Allergology and Clinical Immunology Interest Group on Insect Venom Hypersensitivity. J Allergy Clin Immunol 2009;124(5):1047–54.

36. Travis WD, Li CY. Pathology of the lymph node and spleen in systemic mast cell disease. Mod Pathol 1988;1(1):4–14.

37. Mican JM, Di Bisceglie AM, Fong TL, et al. Hepatic involvement in mastocytosis: clinicopathologic correlations in 41 cases. Hepatology 1995;22(4 Pt 1):1163–70.

38. Garriga MM, Friedman MM, Metcalfe DD. A survey of the number and distribution of mast cells in the skin of patients with mast cell disorders. J Allergy Clin Immunol 1988;82(3 Pt 1):425–32.

39. Nishioka K, Kobayashi Y, Katayama I, et al. Mast cell numbers in diffuse scleroderma. Arch Dermatol 1987;123(2):205–8.

40. Elias J, Boss E, Kaplan AP. Studies of the cellular infiltrate of chronic idiopathic urticaria: prominence of T-lymphocytes, monocytes, and mast cells. J Allergy Clin Immunol 1986;78(5 Pt 1):914–8.

41. Mitchell EB, Crow J, Williams G, et al. Increase in skin mast cells following chronic house dust mite exposure. Br J Dermatol 1986;114(1):65–73.

42. Amon U, Hartmann K, Horny HP, et al. Mastocytosis–an update. J Dtsch Dermatol Ges 2010;8(9):695–711 [quiz: 712].

43. Florian S, Krauth MT, Simonitsch-Klupp I, et al. Indolent systemic mastocytosis with elevated serum tryptase, absence of skin lesions, and recurrent severe anaphylactoid episodes. Int Arch Allergy Immunol 2005;136(3):273–80.

44. Brockow K, Jofer C, Behrendt H, et al. Anaphylaxis in patients with mastocytosis: a study on history, clinical features and risk factors in 120 patients. Allergy 2008;63(2):226–32.

45. Morgado JM, Sanchez-Munoz L, Teodosio CG, et al. Immunophenotyping in systemic mastocytosis diagnosis: 'CD25 positive' alone is more informative than the 'CD25 and/or CD2' WHO criterion. Mod Pathol 2012;25(4):516–21.

46. Hahn HP, Hornick JL. Immunoreactivity for CD25 in gastrointestinal mucosal mast cells is specific for systemic mastocytosis. Am J Surg Pathol 2007; 31(11):1669–76.
47. Schwartz LB, Sakai K, Bradford TR, et al. The alpha form of human tryptase is the predominant type present in blood at baseline in normal subjects and is elevated in those with systemic mastocytosis. J Clin Invest 1995;96(6):2702–10.
48. Worobec AS. Treatment of systemic mast cell disorders. Hematol Oncol Clin North Am 2000;14(3):659–87, vii.
49. Horan RF, Sheffer AL, Austen KF. Cromolyn sodium in the management of systemic mastocytosis. J Allergy Clin Immunol 1990;85(5):852–5.
50. Turk J, Oates JA, Roberts LJ 2nd. Intervention with epinephrine in hypotension associated with mastocytosis. J Allergy Clin Immunol 1983;71(2):189–92.
51. Godt O, Proksch E, Streit V, et al. Short- and long-term effectiveness of oral and bath PUVA therapy in urticaria pigmentosa and systemic mastocytosis. Dermatology 1997;195(1):35–9.
52. Czarnetzki BM, Rosenbach T, Kolde G, et al. Phototherapy of urticaria pigmentosa: clinical response and changes of cutaneous reactivity, histamine and chemotactic leukotrienes. Arch Dermatol Res 1985;277(2):105–13.
53. Guzzo C, Lavker R, Roberts LJ 2nd, et al. Urticaria pigmentosa. Systemic evaluation and successful treatment with topical steroids. Arch Dermatol 1991; 127(2):191–6.
54. Barton J, Lavker RM, Schechter NM, et al. Treatment of urticaria pigmentosa with corticosteroids. Arch Dermatol 1985;121(12):1516–23.
55. Reisberg IR, Oyakawa S. Mastocytosis with malabsorption, myelofibrosis, and massive ascites. Am J Gastroenterol 1987;82(1):54–60.
56. Chen CC, Andrich MP, Mican JM, et al. A retrospective analysis of bone scan abnormalities in mastocytosis: correlation with disease category and prognosis. J Nucl Med 1994;35(9):1471–5.
57. Laroche M, Livideanu C, Paul C, et al. Interferon alpha and pamidronate in osteoporosis with fracture secondary to mastocytosis. Am J Med 2011;124(8): 776–8.
58. Pardanani A. Systemic mastocytosis in adults: 2013 update on diagnosis, risk stratification, and management. Am J Hematol 2013;88(7):612–24.
59. Kluin-Nelemans HC, Jansen JH, Breukelman H, et al. Response to interferon alfa-2b in a patient with systemic mastocytosis. N Engl J Med 1992;326(9): 619–23.
60. Butterfield JH. Response of severe systemic mastocytosis to interferon alpha. Br J Dermatol 1998;138(3):489–95.
61. Kluin-Nelemans HC, Oldhoff JM, Van Doormaal JJ, et al. Cladribine therapy for systemic mastocytosis. Blood 2003;102(13):4270–6.
62. Lim KH, Pardanani A, Butterfield JH, et al. Cytoreductive therapy in 108 adults with systemic mastocytosis: outcome analysis and response prediction during treatment with interferon-alpha, hydroxyurea, imatinib mesylate or 2-chlorodeoxyadenosine. Am J Hematol 2009;84(12):790–4.
63. Vega-Ruiz A, Cortes JE, Sever M, et al. Phase II study of imatinib mesylate as therapy for patients with systemic mastocytosis. Leuk Res 2009;33(11):1481–4.
64. Shah NP, Lee FY, Luo R, et al. Dasatinib (BMS-354825) inhibits KITD816V, an imatinib-resistant activating mutation that triggers neoplastic growth in most patients with systemic mastocytosis. Blood 2006;108(1):286–91.
65. Pardanani A, Ketterling RP, Brockman SR, et al. CHIC2 deletion, a surrogate for FIP1L1-PDGFRA fusion, occurs in systemic mastocytosis associated with

eosinophilia and predicts response to imatinib mesylate therapy. Blood 2003;
102(9):3093–6.

66. Gotlib J, Berube C, Growney JD, et al. Activity of the tyrosine kinase inhibitor
PKC412 in a patient with mast cell leukemia with the D816V KIT mutation. Blood
2005;106(8):2865–70.

67. Paul C, Sans B, Suarez F, et al. Masitinib for the treatment of systemic and cutaneous mastocytosis with handicap: a phase 2a study. Am J Hematol 2010;
85(12):921–5.

68. Aichberger KJ, Sperr WR, Gleixner KV, et al. Treatment responses to cladribine
and dasatinib in rapidly progressing aggressive mastocytosis. Eur J Clin Invest
2008;38(11):869–73.

69. Nakamura R, Chakrabarti S, Akin C, et al. A pilot study of nonmyeloablative allo-
geneic hematopoietic stem cell transplant for advanced systemic mastocytosis.
Bone Marrow Transplant 2006;37(4):353–8.

70. Friedman B, Darling G, Norton J, et al. Splenectomy in the management of systemic mast cell disease. Surgery 1990;107(1):94–100.

71. Kiszewski AE, Duran-Mckinster C, Orozco-Covarrubias L, et al. Cutaneous mastocytosis in children: a clinical analysis of 71 cases. J Eur Acad Dermatol Venereol 2004;18(3):285–90.

72. Lanternier F, Cohen-Akenine A, Palmerini F, et al. Phenotypic and genotypic
characteristics of mastocytosis according to the age of onset. PLoS One
2008;3(4):e1906.

73. Ben-Amitai D, Metzker A, Cohen HA. Pediatric cutaneous mastocytosis: a review of 180 patients. Isr Med Assoc J 2005;7(5):320–2.

74. Gadage VS, Kadam Amare PS, Galani KS, et al. Systemic mastocytosis with
associated acute myeloid leukemia with t (8; 21) (q22; q22). Indian J Pathol Mi-
crobiol 2012;55(3):409–12.

75. Intzes S, Wiersma S, Meyerson HJ. Myelomastocytic leukemia with t(8;21) in a
3-year-old child. J Pediatr Hematol Oncol 2011;33(8):e372–5.

76. Lee JW, Yang WS, Chung SY, et al. Aggressive systemic mastocytosis after
germ cell tumor of the ovary: C-KIT mutation documentation in both disease
states. J Pediatr Hematol Oncol 2007;29(6):412–5.

77. Mahadeo KM, Wolgast L, McMahon C, et al. Systemic mastocytosis in a child
with t(8;21) acute myeloid leukemia. Pediatr Blood Cancer 2011;57(4):684–7.

Index

Note: Page numbers of article titles are in **boldface** type.

A

Abdominal pain, in mastocytosis, 186–187
Acute spontaneous urticaria, 54, 57
Acute urticaria, **11–21**
    angioedema with, 26
    clinical features of, 14
    differential diagnosis of, 14–15
    epidemiology of, 11–12
    etiology of, 12–14
    in pregnancy, 150
    investigation of, 15–16
    mechanisms of, 14
    prognosis for, 17
    treatment of, 16–17, 151–153
Adrenergic urticaria, 59, 63–64
Agoraphobia, in chronic urticaria, 98
Alexthymia, in chronic urticaria, 97
Allergy tests, for urticaria, 59, 65–66, 130
Ammonium persulfate, contact urticaria due to, 161
Anakinra, for Schnitzler syndrome, 146
Anaphylaxis, in acute urticaria, 16–17
Angioedema, **23–31**
    classification of, 55
    clinical features of, 43–44
    diagnosis of, 59, 66
    in pregnancy, 153–154
    pathophysiology of, 2, 23–25
    quality of life impact of, **89–104**
    types of, 27–29
    urticaria combined with, 26–27, 126
    versus urticaria, 23–31
    without urticaria, 27–29
Angiotensin-converting enzyme inhibitors, angioedema due to, 28–29
Animal handlers, contact urticaria in, 162
Antibiotics
    contact urticaria due to, 161–164
    pediatric urticaria due to, 128
Anticoagulants, for chronic urticaria, 109
Antihistamines, 151–153
    for acute urticaria, 16
    for chronic spontaneous urticaria, 36–37
    for chronic urticaria, 106–107

Immunol Allergy Clin N Am 34 (2014) 197–206
http://dx.doi.org/10.1016/S0889-8561(13)00100-8
0889-8561/14/$ – see front matter © 2014 Elsevier Inc. All rights reserved.

Moving?

Make sure your subscription moves with you!

To notify us of your new address, find your **Clinics Account Number** (located on your mailing label above your name), and contact customer service at:

Email: journalscustomerservice-usa@elsevier.com

800-654-2452 (subscribers in the U.S. & Canada)
314-447-8871 (subscribers outside of the U.S. & Canada)

Fax number: 314-447-8029

Elsevier Health Sciences Division
Subscription Customer Service
3251 Riverport Lane
Maryland Heights, MO 63043

*To ensure uninterrupted delivery of your subscription, please notify us at least 4 weeks in advance of move.

Printed and bound by CPI Group (UK) Ltd, Croydon, CR0 4YY

03/10/2024

01040493-0004